ASPERGER SYNDROME IN ADULTHOOD

ASPERGER SYNDROME IN ADULTHOOD

A COMPREHENSIVE GUIDE FOR CLINICIANS

KEVIN P. STODDART
LILLIAN BURKE
ROBERT KING

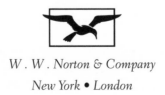

W . W . Norton & Company
New York • London

The text of this book is composed in Meridien
with the display set in Goudy.

Composition by MidAtlantic Publishing Services
Manufacturing by Quad Graphics, Fairfield
Production Manager: Leeann Graham

Library of Congress Cataloging-in-Publication Data

Stoddart, Kevin P., 1962-
 Asperger syndrome in adulthood : a comprehensive guide for clinicians / Kevin P. Stod-
dart, Lillian Burke, Robert King. -- 1st ed.
      p. cm.
 "A Norton professional book"--T.p. verso.
 Includes bibliographical references and index.
 ISBN 978-0-393-70550-8 (hardcover)
 1. Asperger's syndrome. 2. Asperger's syndrome--Diagnosis. 3. Asperger's syndrome-
-Treatment. I. Burke, Lillian. II. King, Robert. III. Title.
 RC553.A88S846 2012
 616.85'8832--dc23
                                    2012012246
 ISBN 13: 978-0-393-70550-8

W. W. Norton & Company, Inc., 500 Fifth Avenue, New York, N.Y. 10110-0017
www.wwnorton.com

W. W. Norton & Company Ltd., Castle House, 75/76 Wells Street, London W1T 3QT
1 2 3 4 5 6 7 8 9 0

To the families and individuals living with Asperger syndrome, with whom we have been so privileged to work.

CONTENTS

PREFACE

The past 15 years of our clinical lives have been an interesting journey. Among our discoveries is the number of adults—more than we could have previously imagined—seeking a diagnosis of Asperger Syndrome (AS) in their 20s and beyond. Undiagnosed individuals seeking help in their 40s, 50s and 60s is now common. They have been "missed" by pre-*DSM-IV* diagnostic systems, and because of lack of public awareness, clinical knowledge, and expertise. Sometimes, they have suffered tremendously because of their AS, and their quality life has been poor; others, although appearing successful in their vocation or relationships, still have had to contend with the effects of the core features of the syndrome. Both groups demonstrate that AS in adults can present as a disorder of extremes.

Adults living at the "higher functioning" end of the autism spectrum are who this book is about. At the place that has been called "the borderlands of autism," we need to be cautious to carefully apply diagnostic criteria, utilizing the best available assessment procedures, so as not to make a diagnosis of less value. We are faced with the difficult task of distinguishing when variation in ability to engage with others socially is within the typical range of functioning, versus when it is not and results in significant day-to-day problems. Some would argue that "Asperger Syndrome" as a diagnosis is now over-applied. We have not seen that to be the case. Instead, we have met many adults who have struggled to understand their social and behavioral differences without such a label.

I often wonder how our clinical work would be different in a world of services and supports which was knowledgeable about, and responsive to, the struggles of adults living with AS. Currently, we would argue, it is not as it should be. The greatest challenge facing people with AS is not necessarily their primary symptoms related to AS, or even the comorbid symptoms, but rather finding knowledgeable supports and services in their communities. Our reason for writing this book is to introduce clinicians to this clinical population and to promote effective clinical assessment and intervention. Misdiagnosis of AS, or inability to recognize AS is common in the mental health, medical, and social service fields, despite the bold attempts of those affected by AS to advocate for services. Adults with AS commonly have doors closed to them as many service providers feel unprepared to address their needs.

The rewards that come from working with adults with AS are many. We have been inspired as we see strengths and admirable resilience to the challenges that adults with AS experience: social, organizational, mental health, relationships, medical—often combined. Not only their own resilience and persistence, but also that of their family members and partners is remarkable. Rarely are we just treating AS in its pure form; more often than not we support adults with features that are comorbid to the syndrome along with the psychosocial "fallout" of living with a condition for years with poor or inadequate treatment. We can't forget the necessity of supporting and educating systems which surround the individual by helping them revise their assessment of adults who have not had the benefit of early and accurate diagnosis and treatment. This is challenging work.

When I was approached by Norton Publishers to author this book, I felt that it was both a daunting but necessary endeavor. Throughout the process, we have come to a greater knowledge of what we have learned over the past 15 years, but that also that we still know so little about this group of adults.

I would like to thank Lillian and Bob for helping me with this task. Their encouragement, hard work, and persistence over these past years of writing have been a blessing. Thanks also to our colleagues at The Redpath Centre for their support and comments on various drafts of the manuscript. Deborah Malmud, my editor at Norton has been helpful and incredibly patient; her vision for this book was our first inspiration. Thanks also go to her colleagues at Norton and to Vani Kannan, Associate Managing Editor. I have had the help of several graduate students including Kathleen White, Stephanie Moeser, Sarah Duhaime, Leila Abbaszadeh and Claudia Accardi—all have reviewed chapter drafts and retrieved relevant research. The children, adolescents, and adults with AS and their families that we have had the privilege to meet have been patient teachers. Finally, our gratitude goes to family and friends who have coped with numerous rough drafts of chapters, and many weekends and evenings that have been devoted to "the book."

Kevin P. Stoddart
Toronto, Canada

ASPERGER SYNDROME IN ADULTHOOD

Chapter 1

INTRODUCTION TO ASPERGER SYNDROME AND AUTISM SPECTRUM DISORDERS IN ADULTS

Despite the dramatic proliferation of research, clinical perspectives, and first-person accounts of Asperger syndrome (AS) in the last 15 years, much of this discourse has focused on the application of the diagnosis to children. The purpose of this chapter is to provide the reader with an introduction to the concept of AS and to issues that are germane to adults. Given the wealth of professional literature that is child-focused, it is also vital to explore the AS presentation in adulthood, considering Hans Asperger's (1944) observation that AS displays "persistence over time" in individuals. We have previously argued that a developmental lifespan perspective facilitates "greater understanding of the challenges of AS at transitional periods, and greater recognition of symptoms of AS at all ages, including wider discourse about the commonalities and differences between specific developmental periods" (Stoddart, 2005b, p. 27).

This volume will integrate our clinical experiences over the past 15 years and the published research, in an effort to improve understanding of, and the support provided to adults living with AS. The group of adults on the "mild end of the autism spectrum" is the focus of this book. Although there is research and practice literature that applies to all those on the autism spectrum, demand is increasing for practices that are specific to this higher-functioning cohort of adults (Barnard et al., 2001; Powell, 2002; Stoddart, 2005b; 2007a; Tantum, 2003). Without elucidation of effective clinical practices, adults with AS will continue to suffer from the current widespread lack of knowledge and expertise in the clinical community when they seek supports and services.

Pervasive developmental disorder is the term used to describe a cluster of five disorders in the *Diagnostic and Statistical Manual of Mental Disorders, Fourth Edition* (DSM-IV; American Psychiatric Association, 1994). These disorders include autistic disorder, Rett's disorder, childhood disintegrative disorder, Asperger's disorder, and pervasive developmental disorder (not otherwise specified). According to the DSM-IV, "Pervasive Developmental Disorders are characterized by severe and pervasive impairment in several areas of development: reciprocal social interaction skills, communication skills, and the presence of stereotyped behavior, interests, and activities. The qualitative impairments that define these conditions are distinctively deviant relative to the individual's developmental level or mental age" (American Psychiatric Association, 1994, p. 65). In this book we use the more popular terms autism spectrum disorders (ASDs) and Asperger syndrome (AS; as opposed to Asperger's disorder). We have provided DSM-IV-TR (American Psychiatric Association, 2000) diagnostic criteria for Asperger's disorder and autism in Figures 1.1 and 1.2.

HETEROGENEITY IN ASDS

CASE 1.

Lina is a 35-year-old woman diagnosed with autism. She lives in an ensuite apartment attached to a group home for persons with intellectual disabilities. Lina prefers time alone and becomes agitated when she is with peers for an extended period. Since childhood, she has engaged in many obsessive behaviors and always insisted on having things in specific places. She works part-time in a ladies wear store, where she unpacks clothing. When she arrives home, she goes through the refrigerator, the bookshelves, and other areas of the house to ensure

DIAGNOSTIC CRITERIA FOR ASPERGER'S DISORDER (299.80)

A. Qualitative impairment in social interaction, as manifested by at least two of the following:

   1. marked impairment in the use of multiple nonverbal behaviors such as eye-to-eye gaze, facial expression, body postures, and gestures to regulate social interaction

   2. failure to develop peer relationships appropriate to developmental level

   3. a lack of spontaneous seeking to share enjoyment, interests, or achievements with other people (e.g., by a lack of showing, bringing, or pointing out objects of interest to other people)

   4. lack of social or emotional reciprocity

B. Restricted repetitive and stereotyped patterns of behavior, interests, and activities, as manifested by at least one of the following:

   1. encompassing preoccupation with one or more stereotyped and restricted patterns of interest that is abnormal either in intensity or focus

   2. apparently inflexible adherence to specific, nonfunctional routines or rituals

   3. stereotyped and repetitive motor mannerisms (e.g., hand or finger flapping or twisting, or complex whole-body movements)

   4. persistent preoccupation with parts of objects

C. The disturbance causes clinically significant impairment in social, occupational, or other important areas of functioning.

FIGURE 1.1. DSM-IV-TR diagnostic criteria for Asperger's disorder. Diagnostic and Statistical Manual of Mental Disorders, Fourth Edition, Text Revision, p. 84. Copyright 2000 by the American Psychiatric Association. Reprinted with permission.

D. There is no clinically significant general delay in language (e.g., single words used by age 2 years, communicative phrases used by age 3 years).

E. There is no clinically significant delay in cognitive development or in the development of age-appropriate self-help skills, adaptive behavior (other than in social interaction), and curiosity about the environment in childhood.

F. Criteria are not met for another specific Pervasive Developmental Disorder or Schizophrenia

FIGURE 1.1. CONTINUED

that nothing was moved while she was gone. She likes creating menus, reading about and making drawings of wildlife, and has volumes of medical books that she reads and rereads. She is obsessed with germs and illness and exerts considerable effort to ensure that her ensuite is spotless at all times.

CASE 2.

Robert, a university professor in philosophy, was experiencing increasing problems in social interaction at work. He had been productive in his academic work, despite his struggle of many years with anxiety and depression. Increasing departmental administrative responsibilities and meetings exacerbated his problems with social and organizational tasks. His ex-wife suggested to him that he be assessed for AS, and he agreed. A positive diagnosis of AS and social anxiety disorder resulted in social and organizational accommodations being suggested and used at his workplace. He has sought individual therapy with someone knowledgeable about AS, and his daughter is now being assessed for an ASD.

CASE 3.

Thomas, now 40 years old, recently moved to a group home from a facility for those with developmental disabilities, where he had lived since age 6. Three other men live at Thomas's new home, which has 24-hour supervision. His meals are prepared and he receives assistance with his

DIAGNOSTIC CRITERIA FOR AUTISTIC DISORDER (299.00)

A. A total of six (or more) items from (1), (2), and (3), with at least two from (1), and one each from (2) and (3):

1. qualitative impairment in social interaction, as manifested by at least two of the following:

   a. marked impairment in the use of multiple nonverbal behaviors such as eye-to-eye gaze, facial expression, body postures, and gestures to regulate social interaction

   b. failure to develop peer relationships appropriate to developmental level

   c. a lack of spontaneous seeking to share enjoyment, interests, or achievements with other people (e.g., by a lack of showing, bringing, or pointing out objects of interest)

   d. lack of social or emotional reciprocity

2. qualitative impairments in communication as manifested by at least one of the following:

   a. delay in, or total lack of, the development of spoken language (not accompanied by an attempt to compensate through alternative modes of communication such as gesture or mime)

   b. in individuals with adequate speech, marked impairment in the ability to initiate or sustain a conversation with others

   c. stereotyped and repetitive use of language or idiosyncratic language

FIGURE 1.2. DSM-IV-TR DIAGNOSTIC CRITERIA FOR AUTISTIC DISORDER. DIAGNOSTIC AND STATISTICAL MANUAL OF MENTAL DISORDERS, FOURTH EDITION, TEXT REVISION, P. 75. COPYRIGHT 2000 BY THE AMERICAN PSYCHIATRIC ASSOCIATION. REPRINTED WITH PERMISSION.

d. lack of varied, spontaneous make-believe play or social imitative play appropriate to developmental level

3. restricted repetitive and stereotyped patterns of behavior, interests, and activities, as manifested by at least one of the following:

a. encompassing preoccupation with one or more stereotyped and restricted patterns of interest that is abnormal either in intensity or focus

b. apparently inflexible adherence to specific, nonfunctional routines or rituals

c. stereotyped and repetitive motor mannerisms (e.g., hand or finger flapping or twisting, or complex whole-body movements)

d. persistent preoccupation with parts of objects

B. Delays or abnormal functioning in at least one of the following areas, with onset prior to age 3 years: (1) social interaction, (2) language as used in social communication, or (3) symbolic or imaginative play.

C. The disturbance is not better accounted for by Rett's Disorder or Childhood Disintegrative Disorder.

FIGURE 1.2. CONTINUED.

activities of daily living. Thomas has a history of severe self-injury, and there is a behavioral program in place to manage these episodes. Thomas does not use speech, but he does communicate with some sign language and pictures. He is aware of his housemates when they intrude on his space, but otherwise he appears uninterested in them. He enjoys the attention of staff members, however, and will let then know when he wants something by poking their arms or pulling their shirts. His preferred activities are rocking back and forth to music, drinking Coke, and assembling Legos and puzzles. He also enjoys flushing toilets, running water from taps, and flicking lights off and on. He has been diagnosed with a severe intellectual disability and autism.

CASE 4.

Ellen, a young woman who reads fantasy novels voraciously, was struggling with the demands of university life in another city, and came for a psychological assessment. Her academic adviser had questioned if she had attention-deficit/hyperactivity disorder (ADHD). She still had a few close friends from early childhood and had managed to cope with the demands of both grade school and high school. As a child, she had been diagnosed with an unspecified learning disability and received numerous accommodations throughout her school years. With the support and advocacy efforts of her parents (both teachers), she was offered admission to a university. However, without academic supports and the assistance of her family, she failed her first year and was not offered admission for her second year. At our center, she was diagnosed with a learning disability and AS and now receives specialized academic counseling at her new college program.

At initial glance, it might appear that Lina, Robert, Thomas, and Ellen have little in common; however, they all have an ASD. One of the complications that has plagued this field is that ASDs are highly heterogeneous conditions (Willemsen-Swinkels & Buitelaar, 2002); there has also been a significant temporal effect in the widening of this variation.

At the beginning of our careers in ASDs (in the late 1970s and early 1980s), it was common for us to characterize individuals on the autism spectrum as having moderate to severe language impairment and intellectual disability. In the late 1980s and early 1990s in Canada, we were beginning to see some clients who we thought were "higher-functioning" individuals; at that time "Asperger syndrome" was little discussed in North America. Even after AS became a diagnosis in 1994, we see in retrospect that clinicians tended to apply the diagnosis to those who were functioning in the borderline to low average ranges of cognitive ability, and who had reasonable language skills, similar to individuals we now refer to as having "high functioning autism."

For the last five years, we have been seeing individuals for later-life diagnoses who have average intelligence and good verbal skills and who two decades earlier would not even have been considered as having an ASD. Supportive of our recent experience, Baron-Cohen (2009) argues: "Autism not only comes in degrees, but . . . it blends seamlessly into the general population. . . . Today the notion of an autistic spectrum is no longer defined by any sharp separation from 'normality'" (p. 71). Although some individuals with AS are high-achieving in their various fields of work, others struggle in relationships and in work well into adulthood.

DISCOVERY OF A MILD FORM OF AUTISM

Reflecting our belief that individuals with social differences have always existed, it is acknowledged by most professionals that recognition of individuals who have problems interacting socially existed before the identification of the syndrome by Dr. Hans Asperger. Despite differing names, very early papers by Schneider (1923), who discussed "affectionless psychopaths," and by Ssucherewa (1926; Wolff, 1996), who described "schizoid personality in childhood," provide evidence of this.

In the 1940s, papers published by two clinicians, both unaware of the other's work, would mark the commonly recognized beginning of early research and writings on ASDs. Leo Kanner, who practiced at Johns Hopkins in Baltimore, identified 11 children who had "autistic psychopathy" (Kanner, 1943). Coincidentally, only a year later, in 1944, Hans Asperger provided a description of what he termed "autistic pathology" and four cases which he saw in his clinic in Vienna (Asperger, 1944). His description of these boys, in German, remained obscure until Frith (1991) provided a translation (Asperger, 1944/1991). This publication served to raise awareness of milder forms of autism in English-speaking countries.

In the 1970s, publication was occurring on the subject of milder forms of ASDs, although it was little known. This included papers by Bartak and Rutter (1976); Chick, Waterhouse, and Wolff (1979); Isaev and Kagan (1974); Mnukhin, Isaev, and O'Tuama (1975); van Krevelen (1971); and Wolff and Barlow (1979). Although the translation of Asperger's work didn't occur until 1991, professionals in the field of autism were aware of his work in the previous decade, and the 1980s witnessed the emergence of several publications that had a significant influence on the later proliferation of AS as a diagnostic concept (Burgoine & Wing, 1983; Gillberg, 1989; Nagy & Szatmari, 1986; Szatmari, Bartolucci, & Bremner, 1989; Szatmari, Bartolucci, Bremner, Bond, & Rich, 1989; Szatmari, Bartolucci, Finlayson, & Krames, 1986; Szatmari, Bremner, & Nagy, 1989; Tantum, 1988; Wing, 1981; Wolff & Chick, 1980).

Most notably, Lorna Wing (1981) discussed children seen during her research and clinical work. She observed that children might show symptoms even during the first year of life: "there is a lack of the intense urge to communicate in babble, gesture, movement, smiles, laughter and eventually speech that characterizes the normal baby and toddler" (p. 117). She felt that imaginative pretend play does not occur in some children or is limited to a few themes, is enacted repetitively, and does not involve other children, except when peers are willing to follow the routine prescribed by the child. Half of Wing's clinical children walked at the usual age and were slow to talk; the other half talked on time, but were slow to walk. Although speech was impressive because of grammatical skills and a high level vocabulary, the content of speech was often impoverished (Wing, 1981).

Peter Szatmari and his colleagues in Canada compared gender- and age-matched children and adolescents with traits of AS to children and youth who were "isolated and odd" (Szatmari, Bremner, et al., 1989). Their criteria for the diagnosis of AS, while not meeting criteria for autism, included solitariness, impaired social interaction and nonverbal communication, and odd speech.

Early Descriptions of Adults with Autism Spectrum Traits and Possible Asperger Syndrome

Many of the early accounts of relatively able individuals with either ASDs or ASD traits are found in case histories of parents of children diagnosed with ASDs. It is noteworthy that Asperger himself recognized that the parents—most often, the father—had personality traits in common with their children. Asperger recorded his clinical impressions of Harrow's father, for example. Although couched in the pejorative professional language of the time, his notes provide useful personality and behavioral descriptions:

> The father, who brought the child to us, was a strange man, and very similar to his son. He appeared to be something of an adventurer . . . By profession he was a painter and a sculptor, but out of financial necessity he was making brooms and brushes. While there was severe unemployment at the time

we saw the boy, the contrast of the two jobs was certainly striking. The father, who himself comes from peasant stock, is a typical intellectual. He professed to be completely and painfully self-taught. One could make out from what he said that he had nothing to do with anyone in the village where he lived and where he must have been considered highly eccentric. He said himself that he was nervous and highly strung but that "he controlled himself to such an extent that he appeared to be indifferent" (Asperger, 1944/1991, pp. 51–52)

Ernst's father had similar traits:

The father was said to be very highly strung and irritable. By profession he was a tailor's assistant. Although we had known the boy for many years, we had seen the father only once. He was clearly eccentric and a loner. The mother did not like to talk about her domestic circumstances. However, it was plain that her life could not have been very happy due to the husband's difficult character. (Asperger, 1944/1991, p. 60)

Asperger (1944/1991) concluded that the traits observed were polygenetic and that it was a "vain hope to think that there may be a clear and simple mode of inheritance" (p.84). He remarked that of the 200 children that he had seen over a decade, "we have been able to discern related incipient traits in parents or relatives in every single case where it was possible for us to make a closer acquaintance" (p. 84). Although our own experience is similar, we cannot echo Asperger's observation that traits are apparent in every situation; however, this clinical issue has become a constant in our work with families. The implications of late diagnosis, diagnosis of a parent subsequent to the diagnosis of his or her child, and parenting with AS are addressed in Chapters 2, 5, and 7, respectively.

There are also references to the fathers of the children that Leo Kanner saw at Johns Hopkins Hospital and the Child Study Center of Maryland in his classic paper "Autistic Disturbances of Affective Contact," generally considered to be the first publication to describe the occurrence of autism in 11 children (Kanner, 1943). Although his descriptions are less detailed than Asperger's, the similarities of the fathers parallel the descriptions of their children. For example, Donald's father was described as "a successful, meticulous, hard-working lawyer who has had two breakdowns under strain of work.

When he walks down the street he is so absorbed in thinking that he sees nothing and nobody and cannot remember anything about the walk" (pp. 218–219). Similarly, Herbert's father, a psychiatrist, is described as "a man of unusual intelligence, sensitive, restless, introspective, taking himself very seriously, not interested in people, mostly living with himself, at times alcoholic" (p. 232). Alfred's father "does not get along well with people, is suspicious, easily hurt, easily roused to anger, has to be dragged out to visit friends, spends his spare time reading, gardening, and fishing. He is a chemist and a law school graduate" (p. 233).

In summary, Kanner (1943) noted: "In the whole group, there are very few really warm hearted fathers and mothers. For the most part, the parents, grandparents and collaterals are persons strongly preoccupied with abstractions of a scientific, literary or artistic nature, and limited in genuine interest in people. Even some of the happiest marriages are rather cold and formal affairs" (p. 250). Kanner agreed with his psychoanalytically-trained colleagues that factors in the family environment, such as the "emotional frigidity" in the families of children with autism, was a contributor to their autism (Eisenberg & Kanner, 1956), although he later retracted this view. Sadly, his early perspective set the stage for decades of blaming, during which professionals held parents responsible for their children's autistic traits (Bettelheim, 1967; Despert, 1951; Rank, 1949).

Others since Kanner have noted the tendency for autism to run in families. For example, Eveloff (1960), after a discussion of his work with 3½-year-old Mary and her presentation of autism, formulated the case using the widely accepted psychogenic paradigm of the era:

> The typical mother is cold, impersonal, and ritualistic. She may be sophisticated and charming on the surface, but this is a thin crust for profound narcissism. As Mrs X. has said: "I can get along with people quite well if I want to, but I don't want to." The fathers tend to be detached, perfectionistic, and intellectual. . . . These parents are in a sense successfully autistic adults. (pp. 101–102)

An early paper by Leon Eisenberg, a colleague of Kanner at Johns Hopkins, discussed the fathers of children with autism based on his review of 100 cases (Eisenberg, 1957). He wrote about "those personality characteristics which involve the ability to form meaningful relationships with other people and which influence marital and parent–child configurations" (p. 715). Eisenberg illustrated the "remarkable pattern of behavior among fathers of autistic children" with three detailed case studies. In summary, he writes:

> The characteristics exemplified in these illustrative vignettes recur with monotonous regularity in 85 of the fathers in this series of 100. They tend to be obsessive, detached and humorless individuals. An unusually large number have college degrees, as do their wives. . . . Perfectionistic to an extreme, they are preoccupied with detailed minutiae to the exclusion of concern for over-all meanings. . . . They have a capacity for concentration on their own pursuits amidst veritable chaos about them. One father, in describing this feature in himself, cited as an example the prototypical behavior of his own father who, in the midst of a train wreck, was discovered by a rescue squad working away at a manuscript while seated in a railroad car tilted 20 degrees from the vertical! (Eisenberg, 1957, p. 721)

These historical quotes are presented as illustrative of early descriptions of adults with AS traits, and although lacking in warmth or sensitivity, they do reinforce what we now know: that ASDs comprise a highly genetic disorder, and that this etiology holds important implications for all clinicians in this field. Because of the parent-blaming tendencies of the past, clinicians may have been reluctant to address this issue, as we are compelled to do, sensitively and proactively. The fathers (and mothers) of children with ASD have benefited from, and appreciated, the opportunity that they have had to discuss this issue, when it is significant.

Lorna Wing, from the Institute of Psychiatry in London (Wing, 1981), was one of the first to describe case accounts of higher-functioning *young* adults with ASDs who were seen for their own symptoms, and not those of offspring. Noteworthy was the psychiatric comorbidity she reported in these individuals. If they were not referred for these other disorders, they were referred because of "their problems in coping with the demands of adult life" (p. 118). For example, Mr. KN "presented as a psychiatric outpatient when he was aged 28, complaining of nervousness and shyness" (p. 125). He had been employed in clerical work for many years. Mr. LP "was admitted to a psychiatric hospital at age 24 because of a suicidal attempt"

(p. 126). He had, in fact, made several unsuccessful suicide attempts and had begun to have contact with psychiatrists in adolescence. Wing theorized that both depression and anxiety appeared late in adolescence or in early adult years because of a "painful awareness of handicap and difference from other people" (p. 118). Further, she noted that growing sexual awareness and the oddities that are tolerated in children become more obvious and less acceptable in a young adult. Perhaps the most significant contribution by Wing, for the purposes of this book, is her discussion of differential diagnosis and her perspective of AS as a normal variant of personality:

> As with any condition identifiable only from a pattern of abnormal behaviour, each element of which can occur in varying degrees of severity, it is possible to find people on the borderlines of Asperger's syndrome in whom diagnosis is particularly difficult. Whereas the typical case can be recognized by those with experience in the field, in practice it is found that the syndrome shades into eccentric normality, and into certain other clinical pictures. Until more is known of the underlying pathology, it must be accepted that no precise cut-off points can be defined. The diagnosis has to be based on the full developmental history and presenting clinical picture, and not on the presence or absence of any individual item. (p. 120)

Wing proposed that all the features that characterize AS can be seen, to some degree, in the normal population. The differentiating factor between those with features and those with a diagnosable case of AS is the effect of those features on daily functioning. This point is discussed further in Chapter 2.

EPIDEMIOLOGY OF AUTISM SPECTRUM DISORDERS

One needs to have only minimal contact with the field of ASDs to know that epidemiology has been a critical area of research in the last decade (Bertrand et al., 2001; Charman, 2002; Fombonne, 2001, 2003; Fombonne, Simmons, Ford, Meltzer, & Goodman, 2001; Fombonne & Tidmarsh, 2003; Lauritsen, Pedersen, & Mortensen, 2004; Prior, 2003; Webb et al., 2003; Wing & Potter, 2002; Yeargin-Allsopp et al., 2003). Many influences have brought concern of a potential increase in ASD prevalence to the forefront of autism research, such as the overwhelming increase of children with ASDs seeking services in parts of the United States (Croen, Grether, Hoogstrate, & Selvin, 2002), more awareness of ASDs in the media, and greater advocacy efforts for early intervention by parents of affected children and adults. Our experience shows us that a diagnosis of ASD, including AS, is now more frequently given in childhood and adulthood. Social service, medical, and educational systems involved with children and adults with ASDs are burdened with overwhelming numbers of requests for support.

Epidemiology, the study of the disease occurrence in a population and the reasons for the occurrence, is influenced by many variables that are also relevant to the epidemiological study of ASDs. These include changes in diagnostic classification, diagnostic precision, differing types of screening, the size of the population screened, and the relative rarity of some diseases. There has been improved case finding in recent studies of ASDs (Fombonne, 2003). For example, Fombonne (2003) reviewed 32 epidemiological studies published between 1966 and 2001. He suggested that the prevalence rate could be as high as 60 per 10,000. Despite this apparent increase, some researchers at the beginning of the new millennium argued that we should not conclude that the incidence of autism and other ASDs has risen (Fombonne, 2003; Fombonne & Tidmarsh, 2003; Tidmarsh & Volkmar, 2003; Wing & Potter, 2002).

More recently, Rice et al. (2010) stated that "ASD prevalence estimates using the current diagnostic criteria are approximately 6 to 7 per 1,000 and are about 10 times higher than earlier estimates" (p. 187). Population-based studies in Japan (Honda, Shimizu, Imai, & Nitto, 2005), Sweden (Kadesjo, Gillberg, & Hagberg, 1999), and the United Kingdom (Baird et al., 2006) have shown an ASD prevalence of more than 1% and as high as 2.7% in Norway (Posserud, Lundervold, & Gillberg, 2006). Rice also notes that less than half of children in these studies have cognitive impairment, as compared with the 75% figure often used in the past.

One of the most recent and large-scale American studies demonstrated that the range of ASD prevalence was 5.0 to 9.8 per 1,000 (Rice et al., 2010) and that there were significant increases in ASD identification between 2000 and 2004 in three of the four study sites. Rice and colleagues argue that an increase in ASD symptoms *cannot* be ruled out, and may not be entirely explained by improved case ascertainment. They found a prevalence rate of 9.8 (95% confidence interval [CI], 8.3–11.6) for Arizona, 9.0 (95% CI, 8.1–9.9) for Georgia, 8.6 (95% CI, 7.1–10.6) for Maryland, and 5.3 (95% CI, 4.4–6.3) for South Carolina. In Table 1.1 we include a summary of other U.S. epidemiological studies that show a trend for increased prevalence rates based on time period studied.

GENETIC THEORIES

The current research on the genetics of ASDs is likely one of the most exiting and well-funded areas of ASD research. We now know that the mode of genetic transmission is complex and that all ASDs share common genetic mechanisms. Both twin and family studies have implicated a significant genetic component and have included characteristics that comprise the broader autism phenotype (BAP) in family members. This phenotype may include social, cognitive, and communication characteristics that occur, but at a subclinical level. Bailey and colleagues (1995) found that the concordance for monozygotic twins was 60% for autism, but this rate rose to 92% when social and/or cognitive problems of the twins were included. Recurrence rates in siblings are thought to be between 2 and 7% (Smalley, Asarnow, & Spence, 1988), and between 10 and 20% of siblings may exhibit the BAP (Bolton et al., 1994; Piven, Palmer, Jacobi, Childress, & Arndt, 1997).

ASD traits across generations may be more significant in higher-functioning forms of ASDs, and, indeed, we have observed this to be the case in our practices based on detailed family history taking and clinical interview. In his comparison of the family history of 23 children with autism and 23 children with AS, Gillberg (1989) emphasized this point in his assertion that a significantly higher number of parents of the AS individuals had problems with social interaction and a restricted range of interests as opposed to those probands who were more severely affected. DeLong and Dwyer (1988) suspect that high-functioning autistic individuals have a positive family history of AS. They further argue that "high-functioning autism is generally a familial condition (or at least has a strong familial factor) related to Asperger's Syndrome and low-functioning autism has a much larger

15

TABLE 1.1. ASD Epidemiological Research in the United States

Study author(s) and publication date	Time period studied	Age range studied (years)	Prevalence and confidence intervals	% IQ < 70
Burd, Fisher, & Kerbeshian (1987)	1985	2–18	0.12 (0.00–0.20)	NR
Ritvo et al. (1989)	1984–1988	8–12	0.40 (0.31–0.50)	NR
Croen, Grether, Hoogstrate, & Selvin (2002)	1987–1999	0–21	1.1 (1.06–1.14)	NR
Yeargin-Allsopp et al. (2003)	1996	3–10	3.4 (3.2–3.6)	62
Bertrand et al. (2001)	1998	3–10	4.0 (2.8–5.5)	49
CDC ADDM (2007)	2000	8	6.7 (6.3–7.0)	36–61
Gurney et al. (2003)	2001–2002	6–17	4.4 (4.3–4.5)	NR
CDC ADDM (2007)	2002	8	6.6 (6.3–6.8)	45

NOTE: Adapted from the Centers for Disease Control (2010). NR = not reported.

factor of neurological damage, without strong familial factors relating to Asperger's Syndrome" (p. 598). They reported a 1% incidence of AS in first-degree relatives of autistic probands. The diverse presentation of ASDs combined with other disorders reminds us that although there are genetic factors at play, the expression of those factors may be determined by multiple variables.

Over the past decade researchers have shown interest in candidate genes on several chromosomes, including 7, 15, and 17 (Holden & Liu, 2005). Recent studies on chromosome 11 have found abnormalities and the deletion of part of a gene known as neurexin 1, a potential early clue to understanding the 50–100% increase in recurrence risk in a sibling's proband (a 5–8% rate of recurrence in affected families). Other chromosomes have been long identified for their contribution to ASDs. The most well-known is the fragile X (FraX) chromosome, which is thought to account for about 5% of cases of ASD. FraX is carried by females and exhibited in males; there have been case reports of identical triplets with FraX (Gillberg, 1983), as well as of identical triplets with AS who do not show FraX (Burgoine & Wing, 1983). We discuss FraX further in Chapter 4.

With the advancement of microarray technologies, recent publications have noted interest in, and the relevance of, copy number variations (CNVs) in the search for the genetics underlying autism (Cook & Scherer, 2008; Glessner et al., 2009; Pinto et al., 2010). CNVs are duplications, rearrangements, or deletions of sections of DNA. "Evidence is accumulating that multiple and rare de novo (and some inherited) CNVs contribute to the genetic component of vulnerability to ASD. . . karotypic and sub-microscopic CNV abnormalities have been known for some time, including the maternal 15q11-q13 duplications found in 1–3% of individuals with ASD" (Cook & Scherer, 2008, p. 920).

With respect to specific genetic mechanisms that may be responsible for the phenotype of higher-functioning individuals with ASDs, the oxytocin receptor gene (OXTR) has been of interest. Oxytocin is responsible for human attachment and social interaction and behavior (Bartz & Hollander, 2008; Hollander et al., 2003, 2007; Wermter et al., 2010; Yrigollen et al., 2008). Initial genetic studies have found some evidence for the association of oxytocin and ASDs (Wermter et al., 2010; Yrigollen et al., 2008). This finding has led to the exploration of the use of the hormone as a potential exploratory treatment (Bartz & Hollander, 2008; Opar, 2008).

ENVIRONMENTAL THEORIES

A genetic etiology in ASDs does not exclude the possible role of biological and environmental variables, including *in utero* influences (Szatmari, 2003; Herbert, 2010; Landrigan, 2010). If there has, in fact, been a true increase in the prevalence of ASDs, a possible explanation is the presence of a new or increased environmental or biological issue that is influential; it is therefore not possible to rule out gene–environment interactions. This dynamic appears to be getting more attention in the last decade. An example of a possible toxicity problem was the impact of the measles, mumps, and rubella (MMR) vaccine and the effect of the preservative thimerosal on developing brains, but this theory has been repeatedly disproven (Fombonne & Cook, 2003; Honda, Shimizu, & Rutter, 2005; B. Taylor et al., 1999), and thimerosal has been removed from vaccines.

Regional epidemiological studies have also been performed because of seemingly higher incidence in some of these locations due to the possibility of environmental factors, although higher incidence was not necessarily found in Brick Township, New Jersey, for example (Bertrand et al., 2001). During a recent symposium on the environment and autism, Landrigan (2008) proposed that two of the central questions facing environmental research are how we can accelerate the discovery of new knowledge about the preventable environmental causes of autism, and how to effectively translate these discoveries into clinical and community terms to improve treatments. He proposes that a large national prospective birth cohort study of children will help answer some of the questions being asked in environmental research on ASDs.

COGNITIVE THEORIES

Theory of mind (ToM) can be understood as an individual's ability to empathize and to identify and attribute thinking and feeling states to oneself and others (Baron-Cohen, 1991, 1995). This construct has led a growing body of literature on individuals with ASDs and their relatives (Baron-Cohen & Hammer, 1997; Baron-Cohen, Jolliffe, Mortimore, & Robertson, 1997). However, there are several arguments against a core deficit in ToM in autism, which include the fact that social problems predate the development of ToM, ToM does not explain issues such as repetitive behavior and executive function problems, is not consistently impaired, and is not specific to ASDs (van Engeland & Buitelaar, 2008).

The *extreme male brain* explanation has promoted increased interest in the empathizing–systemizing (E-S) theory of ASDs and in the parallel differences in typical male and female brains (Baron-Cohen, 2003, 2008, 2009; Baron-Cohen, Knickmeyer, & Belmonte, 2005; Baron-Cohen, Richler, Bisarya, Gurunathan, & Wheelwright, 2003; Baron-Cohen & Wheelwright, 2004; Nettle, 2007). Asperger himself was the first to make this observation in the context of ASDs: "The autistic personality is an extreme variant of male intelligence. . . . Boys . . . tend to have a gift for logical ability, abstraction, precise thinking and formulating, and for independent scientific investigation. . . . In the autistic individual the male pattern is exaggerated to the extreme" (Asperger, 1944/1991, pp. 84–85). Baron-Cohen (2009) proposes that males are better at understanding systems and systematizing, whereas females are better at empathizing:

> According to the empathizing–systemizing (E-S) theory, autism and Asperger syndrome are best explained not just with reference to empathy (below average) but also with reference to a second psychological factor (systemizing), which is either average or even above average. So it is the discrepancy between E and S that determines if you are likely to develop an autism spectrum condition. . . . Systemizing is the drive to analyze or construct systems. These might be any kind of system. What defines a system is that it follows rules, and when we systemize we are trying to identify the rules that govern the system, in order to predict how that system will behave. (p. 71)

Baron-Cohen (2009) notes that his theory has several strengths: (1) It is a two-factor theory that can explain both the social and nonsocial issues related to ASDs; (2) it can lead to new interventions; (3) it explains the difficulty with generalizing in ASDs; (4) it removes the stigma about the cognitive differences found in ASDs; and (5) it relates these differences to male and female differences found in the general population. The drawback of the theory is that there continues to be little evidence for it, and it may only apply to individuals at the mild end of the spectrum.

Weak central coherence was first recognized in Kanner's now classic article when he described the children he assessed, and it was later labeled by Frith (1989):

> A situation, a performance, a sentence is not regarded as complete if it is not made up of exactly the same elements that were present at the time the child was first confronted with it. If the slightest ingredient is altered or removed the total situation is no longer the same. . . . The inability to experience wholes without attention to the constituent parts is somewhat reminiscent of the plight of children with specific reading disability. (Kanner, 1943, p. 246)

Central coherence is the ability to draw together information to construct higher meaning and to understand situations according to context. Weak central coherence explains many traits of individuals on the spectrum, such as their attention to detail and the tendency to "miss the bigger picture." Weak central coherence produces a preference for local detail over global processing. Attention to this preference has implications for education (e.g., for learning and generalizing skills), for processing interpersonal situations, and for social skill development in this population. Although there has been considerable interest in the concept of weak central coherence in individuals with autism and their relatives, there has been inconsistent evidence from research for its relevance (Beaumont & Newcombe, 2006; Burnette et al., 2005; Happe, Briskman, & Frith, 2001; Jolliffe & Baron-Cohen, 1997, 2001). Nazeer (2006) offers his perspective, as an adult with ASD, on the concept of weak central coherence. He describes observing a peer, André, in a bar:

> André's solution, playing with ice in his glass, making a pattern on the bar with his fingertips, are not high tech, but they affect a narrow, uncomplicated purpose and he is in control. He can't pull the entire bar-going experience together into a coherent ball of dough, but he can do these other, less ambitious things and when he does, everything else becomes background. (p. 38)

NEUROLOGICAL RESEARCH

Research is rapid and ongoing into the neurological basis o\
and a comprehensive review is beyond the scope of this c\
(For recent reviews, see DiCicco-Bloom et al., 2006, and M
Rubenstein, & Hyman, 2006). Early increased brain growth in \
hood has been a consistent finding and appears to affect both
and white matter; however, the role of this early growth in
pathogenesis of autism is unclear (van Engeland & Buitelaar, 20\
Morphometric studies have also demonstrated complex pattern\
growth abnormalities in the cerebellum, cerebrum, medulla, a\
hippocampus. Postmortem brain weights, head circumference, sta\
ing, and volumetric calculations using MRI (magnetic resonanc\
imaging) have supported these findings. Furthermore, magneti\
resonance spectroscopy has illustrated regional decreases in concentration of neuron-related molecules such as N-acetylaspartate and
creatine. Neuropathological studies have demonstrated increases
and decreases in various types of cell density and multiple brain
ranges (Bauman & Kemper, 1985).

A deficient mirror neuron system (MNS) has proven to be an
interesting line of investigation in the neurology of ASDs (Wan,
Demaine, Zipse, Norton, & Schlaug, 2010; Williams et al., 2006).
"Mirror neurons are those brain cells that are active not only while
one is reacting but also when one is observing others in the outside
world. As autism is characterized by domination of one's 'inside
world,' these neurons are viewed as deficient in children with autism" (Hughes, 2009, p. 571). Despite its ability to correspond with
a deficit ToM hypothesis of autism, MNS theory has not won universal agreement (Leighton, Bird, Charman, & Heyes, 2008; Southgate
& Hamilton, 2008).

CONTROVERSY IN DIAGNOSIS AND NOSOLOGY

Should autism and Asperger syndrome be seen as distinct and
mutually exclusive diagnostic categories, or should Asperger
syndrome be seen as a subcategory of autism? This question
cannot be answered definitively from existing scientific data
(Frith, 1991, p. 2)

There remains considerable debate about the set of characteristics that defines AS. Central to this debate is the question of whether AS is qualitatively different from high-functioning autism (HFA; Mayes, Calhoun, & Crites, 2001). In their review of studies published by 2002 comparing AS to HFA, Macintosh and Dissanayake (2004) note that there is insufficient evidence to suggest that AS is different from HFA. However, a meta-analysis of 10 studies examining cognitive and adaptive behavior reported significant differences in these groups (McLaughlin-Cheng, 1998). In order to differentiate HFA from AS, studies have focused on variables such as clumsiness/motor performance (Ghaziuddin, Butler, Tsai, & Ghazuiddin, 1994; Manjiviona & Prior, 1995), neuropsychological traits (Miller & Ozonoff, 2000), and speaking style (Ghaziuddin & Gerstein, 1996). Mayes and colleagues (Mayes et al., 2001) note little agreement in favor of the "separation" of AS and autism:

> Differing relationships between Asperger's syndrome and autism were also postulated, including that Asperger's syndrome was: (1) "on a continuum with autism" (Klin, 1994) (p. 139), (2) not a separate diagnostic entity but on the autism spectrum (Wing, 1991), (3) "a mild variant of autism" (Gillberg, 1989), (4) equivalent to "high-functioning autism" (Schopler, 1985), (5) "a mild form of high-functioning autism" (Szatmari, Bartolucci, & Bremner, 1989) (p. 717), and (6) equivalent "to the DSM-III-R category of pervasive developmental disorder not otherwise specified (PDD-NOS), albeit in those with normal IQ" (Szatmari, Bremner, et al., 1989) (p. 558). (p. 264)

Historically, the ASDs have received a range of treatments in the DSM. In DSM-I (American Psychiatric Association, 1952) and DSM-II (American Psychiatric Association, 1968), autism was categorized as a type of childhood schizophrenia. Not until 1980 did the American Psychiatric Association publish separate criteria for autism in the third edition of the DSM (American Psychiatric Association, 1980, 1987). Here, the term *pervasive developmental disorder* (PDD) was used to describe a spectrum of impairments. Criteria for Asperger's disorder were first included in the fourth editions of the DSM (American Psychiatric Association, 1994, 2000) under the category of pervasive

developmental disorders (PDDs). The current text revision of the DSM-IV criteria for AS is seen in Figure 1.1, and for autistic disorder in Figure 1.2. According to the current DSM, two characteristics distinguish autism and AS: (1) delayed language development in autism but not in AS, and (2) at least average/near-average intellectual abilities necessary in AS but not in autism.

As with other psychological conditions (Clark, 2005; Pierre, 2008) the spectrum of ASDs has suffered from the tensions between "lumping" versus "splitting" of symptoms and disorders. Reflecting these tensions, "Asperger syndrome," as a distinct diagnostic entity, has a precarious future in the DSM-V, to be published in 2013 (American Psychiatric Association, 2010). It has been proposed that because there has not been any clear evidence to distinguish AS from other ASDs, it should be subsumed under the broader term *autism spectrum disorder*. Although there is a rational empirical argument to remove Asperger disorder from the DSM-V, its inclusion has also meant that we now have a much broader understanding of the range of social–communication impairments than previously. This broader understanding is especially helpful for adults with AS who have struggled for years without answers to their difficulties in relating to others socially. Many individuals with AS do not want the label *autism* applied to them because of the stigma and misconceptions associated with it. We believe that the clinical value of the term *Asperger syndrome*—its effect in promoting research and furthering understanding of the adults we describe in this book—has been immeasurable.

AUTISM SPECTRUM DISORDERS: DISABILITY OR DIFFERENCE?

Over the last few decades, ways of thinking about *disability* have evolved and the disability literature has grown exponentially. Out of this environment has arisen a movement to identify and acknowledge an autistic culture, considering ASD as a way of being, impossible to separate from the person. Relating the experiences of these individuals to those in the disability rights movement, many individuals with ASDs argue that they should not be thought of as disabled and that a "cure" is not needed for their autism. Youth and adults with ASDs are embracing those characteristics that define them. Similarly, parents have begun to admire their children's ASD qualities, although the search for a "cure" by others remains ever-present. Sinclair (1993) writes:

> . . . when parents say I wish my child did not have autism, what they're really saying is I wish the autistic child would have died and not existed and I had a different (non-autistic) child instead. Read that again, as this is what we hear when you mourn our existence. This is what we hear when you pray for a cure. This is what we know when you tell us that your fondest hopes and dreams, perhaps your greatest wish is that one day we will cease to be and a stranger you can love will move in behind our faces. (p. 2)

Donna Williams, an adult with ASD and author of the books *Nobody Nowhere* (1992) and *Somebody Somewhere* (1994), suggests that interventions can instead be effectively focused on comorbid mental health and medical symptoms:

> In my case, I have addressed the visual perceptual condition of scotopic sensitivity, gut and immune disorders, atypical epilepsy (all diagnosed in my 20's) affecting information processing ability and sensory perceptual problems, and finally serotonin-related impulse control issues affecting involuntary behaviours such as OCD, TS (Tourette's syndrome), exposure anxiety and rapid-cycling bipolar disorder, which previously had been a big impact on behaviour, communication and a fear of sensory and emotional overstimulation. (Williams, 2005).

We believe that it is important for affected individuals to discuss their perception of themselves and AS and whether or not they feel they have a "disability." Conversations such as these during the clinical encounter often lead to an exploration of the ways in which environments, prejudice, and lack of understanding of AS can be disabling, possibly more so than the "disorder" itself. Professionals vary widely in their perspectives on this point, but this philosophical issue, although difficult to grapple with, has significant implications for one's work with this clinical group.

CHARACTERIZING "ADULT OUTCOME"

When parents hear that their child has a diagnosis on the autism spectrum, one of the first questions they ask relates to prognosis: "Will my child be able to attend college, get a job, get married, and have children?" As clinicians, we want to provide families with hope and to encourage interventions that will maximize their child's potential to be successful. When we look to the research literature, we seek optimistic evaluations of outcome in adolescence and adulthood that we can share with these families. More often, however, studies do not reinforce our optimism.

ASDs, as we understand the spectrum today, are a relatively new diagnostic category compared to clinical disorders such as depression, anxiety, or schizophrenia, and outcome studies are available, but not prevalent. Those that exist may not be discrete in terms of the type of ASD being studied. As well, they typically summarize the outcome of those diagnosed as children and youth, versus those individuals diagnosed later in life. The former group tends to exhibit more severe forms of autism than the latter. Although existing studies do indicate which factors predict the degree and direction of outcome, they do not offer a high degree of optimism. Engström, Ekström, and Emilsson (2003) remind us that studies of adults with autism show a poor outcome, and although Howlin's (2000b) report indicates that those at the milder end of the spectrum achieve better outcome, it is not without struggles.

It is inherently problematic to assume that we can arrive at a uniform description of the presentation of AS in adulthood, just as this problem exists for other disorders identified in the DSM. Over the last 15 years of clinical practice, we have observed that variability in the presentation of the syndrome is broad in children and even broader in adults. This range has been noted in early descriptions (e.g., Frith, 1991). The variability in adult presentation is increasing beyond that which we would have predicted even a decade ago. In part, this increase is due to factors such as early intervention, the presence of knowledgeable and effective services, the acknowledgment of comorbid disorders, and awareness that symptom expression can be present in many individuals despite high achievement. Regardless of the problems inherent in a static, well-characterized adult presentation of AS, we believe that just such a description is important to further the process of effective identification and treatment.

Frith (1991) noted that individuals with AS can be "well-adapted and some are exceptionally successful." With respect to their social difficulties, she stated: "They do not seem to possess the knack of entering and maintaining intimate two-way social relationships, whereas routine social interactions are well within their grasp" (Frith, 1991, p. 4). This early characterization is certainly true in some cases, in our experience, but the increasing numbers of individuals with AS who are in committed and satisfying long-term relationships belies this statement. Frith also points out that variation can be due in part to comorbid issues such as behavior difficulties and learning disabilities and the ability of these individuals to find a niche in society. With respect to work, Asperger felt that adults could be capable and original in their field of work. Wing felt that this capacity for originality reflected their unique thought process and chain of reasoning.

So far, characterization of the adult presentation of AS has been undertaken through a number of pathways of inquiry. Studies of outcome often examine the eventual living circumstances of the person, including his or her educational achievement, housing, relationships, level of support required, employment, psychiatric functioning, as well as variables specific to the disorder (Engstrom et al., 2003; Renty & Roeyers, 2007). There appears to be three main groupings in the outcome literature: those emphasizing symptoms of ASDs, those examining the ability of the individual to take on a "typical" social role, and those considering quality of life (QofL).

In a review of longitudinal, retrospective, and cross-sectional studies of adolescents and adults with autism, Seltzer and associates (Seltzer, Shattuck, Abbeduto, & Greenberg, 2004) searched for outcomes that appeared with some consistency across the studies. They indicate that very few studies have looked at the "developmental course" of autism, and those that have studied changes in severity have investigated whether symptoms were altered in a positive or negative manner, and whether the individual continued to meet criteria for the diagnosis of autism. The variables of IQ, communication, and restrictive/repetitive behaviors and interests were often examined. Improvements in cognitive function and communication were not sufficient to substantially alter the impact of the diagnosis. Fewer improvements in the behavioral aspects of the disorder were noted than in IQ or communication. Their review suggests that "the core symptoms of autism abate to some degree during adolescence and young adulthood" (p. 236), although the improvement is not necessarily smooth and may not affect all presenting features of the disorder.

A comparative study examined the development of adolescents with AS and HFA, looking at the relationship between speech development and other characteristics of autistic disorders (Gilchrist et al., 2001). Those with AS had no developmental speech delay, whereas those in the group with HFA had experienced a speech delay. A third group experienced social impairments (conduct disorder; CD) but had no speech delays. IQ and behavioral profiles were also reviewed. The CD group was noted to have less severe social and communicative impairments than the AS or HFA groups, as well as a different IQ profile. Cognitive functioning of the AS and HFA groups showed significant differences on verbal tasks, but were not significantly different on perceptual reasoning tasks. The speech of those with AS was more mature than that of those in the HFA group. Also, early behavioral concerns experienced by the AS and HFA groups were similar, but with the AS group showing less severity. By adolescence, the difference in presentation of the AS and HFA had decreased, although the AS group continued to be better able to converse. The authors proposed that "individuals with autistic disorders may show similar communicative and social abnormalities despite differences in speech or other aspects of development" (Gilchrist et al., 2001, p. 236).

IQ was presented as the variable of interest in another study examining children with autism and those with AS (Szatmari, Bryson, Boyle, Streiner, & Duku, 2003). None of the children in the study had an intellectual disability. They were assessed at ages 4–6 and again at 10–13. Outcome was examined in terms of socialization, communication, and autistic symptomatology. The authors reported that "the children with AS had higher predictor and outcome scores in socialization and communication and lower scores on autistic symptoms" (p. 523). They also noted, however, that at different points in time, the predictive influence of the variables differed. The authors concluded that "determinants of outcome in children with autism are different than in the children with AS" (Szatmari et al., 2003, p. 526).

Seltzer and associates (Seltzer et al., 2004) noted that few of the studies looked at "contextual variables" as predictors of outcome. Comorbidity of psychiatric disorders and medical conditions in those on the spectrum are documented in the literature, but not adequately examined in relation to outcome in adulthood. As well, the authors remind us that parents of children and adolescents with autism face more demands than many other parents. They are noted to experience high levels of stress, psychiatric difficulties, and troubled relationships. Once again, the impact of these reciprocal factors of the living situation for individuals with autism during their developmental years has not been well addressed.

Berney (2004) reminds us that in autism, "overt" symptoms are intense in early childhood, whereas with AS, symptoms may not be recognized until adolescence. This is the time when the young person encounters the demands of social engagement and the expectations of increasing independence. Berney suggests that, because the disorder has gone unrecognized, the egocentric behavior of these individuals may have caused relationship strains. Furthermore, they may have not achieved their potential but have no way to explain their failure to do so, and they may be more dependent on family or others than in the case of their peers. In adulthood, the symptoms that presented in adolescence persist, particularly in the areas of communication, relationships, and areas of interest.

The psychosocial functioning of a group of adults (both men and women) on the milder end of the autism spectrum was examined by Engstrom et al. (2003). Of interest was their living situation, employment, financial and family support, and social adjustment. None of the individuals studied was married, although some reported a "partner" relationship. Of the 16 individuals interviewed, only one person lived with "minimal" support in terms of home living; others received varying degrees of family or system supports. When the levels of support were examined, 11 of the individuals were reported to require a high level of support from the public sector. Only one individual had competitive employment, one worked for a relative, one had a state-supplied position, and one was on a pension. The remaining individuals were employed through sheltered workshops, or they attended day programs. When the social adjustment of the individuals was rated, two received ratings of good and two of poor; the remainder was rated as fair. The authors note that when comparing their results with similar studies in the literature, they found "fewer cases with an overall good outcome," but as well, they identified "fewer cases with a poor outcome" (Eng-strom et al., 2003, p. 106).

Plimley (2007) considered adults with ASDs from a QofL perspective, drawing on the QofL literature related to those with intellectual disabilities. She used Shalock's model (1996) to identify the various aspects reflected in the QofL research, including physical and material well-being, relationships with others and social inclusion, personal growth and development, emotional health, self-determination, and rights. Plimley proposed that considering Shalock's domains and the QofL variables within each, and then adding an ASD focus for each, would provide a strong measure of outcome for adults with ASDs, and further, would provide information of value in the process of individual planning.

Renty and Roeyers (2007) suggest that QofL may offer a "more comprehensive, multi-dimensional outcome measure" for adults who have an ASD (p. 512). This type of research also allows input from the individual related to his or her sense of satisfaction and well-being. Those who participated in this study represented individuals from across the spectrum, but none had an intellectual disability. One quarter of participants had a college or university education, and a comparable number had competitive employment. Almost 70% were single, and the remaining were in or had been in an intimate relationship. Lastly, 75% were in a living situation where they received home support either by parents or by a service agency.

Bolte and Bosch (2004) use three cases that depict the differences between those on the opposite ends of the spectrum. The individuals described are probably very similar to those all of us working in the field of ASDs have met. Because our clinical work focuses on individuals who have AS, the case of "Richard L." was very familiar to us: an intelligent person with a university degree who had been employed, and had been assisted in his daily life (outside of work), by his wife. At age 69, his presentation was still that of a "socially awkward or inappropriate" person. He had few social contacts and engaged in his own special interests. "In direct social interaction he revealed a monologue flood of words, hard to disrupt and accompanied by exaggerated gestures. He repeatedly revolved around certain topics" (p. 12).

ASPERGER SYNDROME: A "SPECTRUM WITHIN A SPECTRUM"?

In our work with those who have AS, we have identified three points along the "spectrum" where individuals tend to cluster. All of the authors have worked in settings that support individuals with intellectual disabilities and mental health problems. In these settings, we have encountered individuals who have AS, and although they don't fall within the mandate of the developmental disability sector, they sometimes present "as if" they have an intellectual disability due to the extreme impairment of either their symptoms of AS, or of AS in association with other disorders. This first group of individuals are most like those described in the outcome studies above: unable to develop or sustain relationships, hold competitive employment, or perform activities of daily living without external supports.

At the other end of this AS spectrum are individuals who are educated, successful in their chosen profession, and have either current or past intimate relationships. These individuals are more akin to Richard L. (Bolte & Bosch, 2004). They engage intensely in their areas of interest, and in social situations, may lecture others on their interests without being aware of cues that their interests aren't shared. Although they have achieved some degree of success in employment, they continue to be socially awkward or naïve, and often come to our practice for relationship counseling, to inquire about appropriate accommodations to support them in their place of employment (often related to sensory or social issues), to address high anxiety or depression, or to assist them in working through specific problems that have presented in their lives (e.g., parenting or relationship issues).

We believe that we may be more aware of this group because they would not qualify or be appropriate for services in the developmental services sector, and because they are financially able to pay for private support or have insurance through their employer that will cover this treatment. Also, we have not identified ourselves as a service provider for individuals with *autism*, but *Asperger syndrome* and co-morbid conditions instead. Although many of our clients may not receive systemic support in their activities of living, many do rely on spouses, parents, paid financial planners, and others, who offer support in a natural manner, decreasing the appearance of disability. As well, common themes emerge in our first interactions with them: They were bullied in school; they never felt that they fit in; they recalled observing others and practiced taking on the appearance of those who were successful; in social and employment situations, they "perform." An evaluation of outcome has not been completed within our center, but our estimate, based on about 450 cases over the past 2 years, would suggest that these individuals represent 30% of those we see.

Between the two ends of the "*AS spectrum*" are those who, again, are not "disabled enough" or "ill enough" to access services within the developmental or mental health sectors. Berney (2004) refers to this state of affairs as "therapeutic limbo." These individuals have not, however, achieved the success of the group we see in private practice (described above). We access this middle group only when someone brings them to our attention, often following some critical event. They may have gone for long periods without appropriate supports because they don't meet the criteria of the two main support systems that could assist them (i.e., developmental or psychiatric), and without ability to pay and awareness of where to look, they may end up in a crisis psychiatric bed, incarcerated, in a hostel, living with an elderly family member, or receiving financial support from a sibling. Unfortunately, many of these individuals have gone to college, have attempted to engage in relationships and to gain employment, but have encountered repeated failures in schooling, employment, or relationships. Some of their difficulties may be related to executive functioning, such as problems in planning and organizing, managing time, regulating their emotions, and transitioning between tasks. Other struggles may reflect concurrent disorders such as general anxiety, social anxiety, extreme sensory responses, or obsessive–compulsive disorder. Some of these individuals have been able to engage in volunteer activities a few hours a week or obtain part-time employment with support.

A study of those diagnosed in childhood compared to those diagnosed as adults identified, as predicted, that those with a concurrent intellectual disability would have a poorer outcome (Marriage, Wolverton, & Marriage, 2009). However, of those with average functioning who fell at the milder end of the spectrum, there was a range of outcomes from "an isolated individual living on a disability pension to a married university professor" (p. 326). The authors indicated that regardless of when the diagnosis occurred, participants tended to function substantially below their potential (based on IQ). They suggested this sub-par performance might be due to social and sensory issues that "made negotiating educational, vocational and community settings difficult" (p. 326). As well, the authors noted impairments in executive functions, which, as we discussed earlier, may affect employment or relationships. They also indicated that family was often "protective" of those who had been diagnosed as children, reflecting Berney's (2004) reference to dependency in adults with ASDs. Marriage and associates (2009) propose that when the adult with ASD is successful, this is often achieved at a later point in life than would occur with other adults.

Barnhill (2007) explored the difficulties in research on adult outcomes. She refers to reports by individuals with AS and their families that indicate an appearance of normality, but without an experience of fitting in. In her review of outcome studies, she noted that problems with employment; comorbid health, neurological and mental health disorders; sensory and motor issues; and social impairments were all impediments to positive outcomes. Barnhill further noted that current treatments address the symptoms, but not the "underlying impairments" of the disorder. She urged that, "to improve outcomes of adults with AS, it is imperative to increase public awareness of the condition so that diagnoses can be rendered earlier and appropriate supports can be provided" (Barnhill, 2007, p. 122).

A phenomena that has occurred with the increased attention to AS is the identification of famous historical figures who have contributed to art, science, math, literature, or other fields, and who may have had AS (Abrahamson, 2007; Arshad & Fitzgerald, 2004; Fitzgerald, 2000, 2002; Gillberg, 2002a; Ledgin, 2002; Sacks, 2001). Although this is an interesting and possibly useful line of academic inquiry and reinforces the fact that individuals with social difficulties have always existed (although it is impossible to know for certain whether these historical figures had AS), there may also be some dangers to this association. The main concern is that affected individuals and family members may expect that this level of achievement is common in individuals with AS. There is, however, no evidence to support this expectation. The benefit that we have seen is that the diagnostic label is seen as positive for some individuals when they proudly realize the *genetic lineage* that they are now a part of, and their potential to accomplish great things, despite (or possibly because of) their social difficulties.

In summary, we would suggest that the concept of a well-defined "adult outcome" in AS may be a misnomer. Because individuals with AS and ASDs are highly heterogeneous, especially in adulthood, it is naïve to think that "adult outcome" would be easily captured by empirical study. Clearly, the outcome literature is not studying the individuals with AS who are "well-functioning" and (possibly because of this) who have received diagnoses in the later adolescent years and adulthood. Because these "well-functioning" individuals are, from a nosological perspective, on a spectrum of disorders, it is important to identify and value both risk and protective factors (found from studies of those at different points on the spectrum) that may have influenced their developmental trajectory. However, it is also important to consider what additional risk and protective factors may exist for this newly rediscovered "well-functioning" group of adults with AS. It is likely that we have not yet found the *end* of the autism spectrum in adulthood.

We conclude with a quote from Tantum (2000) which echoes our experience:

> Asperger's (1944) statement that 'autistic psychopathy' has a good prognosis now seems to be more accurate than it has ever been. To some degree earlier detection and the provision of specific education have improved prognosis, as Asperger himself thought they did. The recognition of a much larger group of people with Asperger syndrome, but with sufficiently good social functioning to have missed diagnosis previously, has also changed our understanding of what a person with Asperger syndrome can achieve. (p. 61)

SUMMARY

The field of ASDs has had a complex history, marred by confusion and controversy. It has also produced exciting discoveries and developments that continue to the present. Embedded in this clinical history are the stories of adults with AS and AS traits, significant for their role in providing credibility to our current experiences in the field. Presently, compelling but alarming studies are emerging in the areas of cognition, genetics, neurology, and epidemiology. Clinicians and researchers are recognizing the immense influx of individuals who are less characterized by traits of autism, communication impairments, and cognitive delays, but who are nevertheless struggling. Consequently, the empirical research on adult outcome, although informative, has yet to fully capture the *well-functioning* individuals with AS with whom we have had experience in recent years. Although the research and clinical lenses of the past 15 years have focused on children and youth, in North America we are moving forward with a greater commitment to adults with AS. It is hoped that this volume plays some small role in the evolution of research and practice with respect to this fascinating and underserved group of adults.

Chapter 2

ASSESSMENT OF ASPERGER SYNDROME IN ADULTS

CASE EXAMPLE: FIRST ASD DIAGNOSIS IN ADULTHOOD

As I walked down the hallway to the waiting room to meet my new client, I mentally reviewed what I knew about him. Paul's wife Janice referred him to me for an assessment. Paul was trained in drafting, but was unable to keep employment, despite his educational background and skills. His family heard about AS on television and after following up with Internet research, they decided Paul might be affected by AS. I greeted Paul, his parents, and his wife in the waiting room. He appeared older than someone in his 30s. Paul responded to my greeting awkwardly, seeming reluctant to disengage from the Newsweek *he was reading.*

In my office, his parents provided a developmental and social history and were relieved to be able to talk to somebody about their observations. Paul met his developmental milestones early. As a preschooler, he was able to read, spoke like an adult, and appeared advanced relative to other children. He liked to draw and build with blocks and Legos®. He did not play with other children, preferring instead to lecture adults about dinosaurs, and later about bridges. Although his fine motor skills were good, his gross motor skills were not. He did poorly when his parents attempted to involve him in sports, and he did not engage in outdoor games. Paul had no friends, despite being enrolled in activities such as Scouts. His parents spoke of his social withdrawal, inability to converse and initiate social contact with others, and odd routines and obsessions. They discussed the constant need to provide him with instrumental supports until he married, something they had not needed to do with their other children. They detailed the social and emotional difficulties Paul faced during college and throughout the various jobs he had held.

Appearing frustrated, his wife revealed her observations of Paul in social situations and her need to support him in day-to-day life. She noted his withdrawal from social gatherings and discomfort with small talk. If he engaged in conversation, he dominated the group, talking "at" them about one of his obsessive interests. He had gotten them into considerable debt by impulse buying, requiring her to take on the responsibility of finances as well as the general upkeep of the house. When they had relaxation time, he went off on his own, building model bridges or researching new ones on the Internet. He largely ignored her interests and was rarely affectionate. She was surprised after their marriage to discover he did not enjoy any of the activities in which they had engaged while dating. Once married, he spoke more openly about disliking her suggestions of what they could do together. On the few occasions they traveled, his wife did all the planning, and Paul spent his time photographing local bridges.

Paul was quiet for much of the interview with his wife and parents. When he did speak, he replied with brief, concrete responses. He showed little affective response and at times appeared disconnected from the people in the room. He seemed comfortable with family members completing or adding to his answers.

I then met with Paul alone. When asked about his interest in bridges, the photographs that he had taken, and the drawings and models he made, he became surprisingly animated. I found it difficult to interrupt and redirect him to other topics. When he talked of bridges he did so fluently, but when asked questions about his behaviors or the reactions of others, he had difficulty providing answers. He eventually did, but sometimes voiced a few possible responses until he came up with the right one, as if he had trouble matching his answers with some mental template. When asked to define words on cognitive testing, his responses seemed verbatim from a dictionary. He was aware he had social difficulties but did not understand what they were. He admitted he had problems talking about feelings.

Despite the increased awareness of ASDs in both professional and public arenas, affected individuals continue to enter adulthood without having received an accurate diagnosis and suitable supports and services. The purpose of this chapter is to provide a clinical rationale for a diagnosis in adulthood and the multidisciplinary diagnostic process that should ideally occur. Although previously noted in Chapter 1, it is helpful if clinicians are aware of the ongoing debate by researchers about diagnostic nosology; we therefore highlight this concern here. A discussion of the pathways to adult diagnosis is followed by a description of the process used to collect relevant information in the assessment process. Twelve diagnostic areas for assessment are summarized, along with our understanding of differential diagnosis and the outcome of the assessment.

PATHWAYS TO ADULT DIAGNOSIS

The purpose of the diagnostic assessment is not only to provide a diagnostic label, but also to help individuals understand what is contributing to their own or others' discomfort or lack of success with developmentally appropriate tasks (Stoddart, 2005b) and to help them find ways to improve their quality of life (Burke, 2005). Specifically, a diagnosis may provide access to funds or programs (e.g., disability benefits), promote a more positive self-understanding, provide opportunities to overcome or compensate for comorbid concerns (e.g., sensory or organizational), and facilitate better relationships (e.g., spousal and work relationships). It may also improve health (e.g., awareness of food sensitivities), provide opportunities to affiliate with those who are similarly affected, enable individuals to receive specialist treatment, and alert them to the presence or potential development of mental health concerns.

Individuals may be referred for assessment and diagnosis in adulthood for many reasons, coming to us through various diagnostic and service pathways. For some, symptoms of AS may not have been recognized in childhood. Some undiagnosed adults may have

problems finding or keeping employment or maintaining relationships (Stoddart, 2005b). Others may have been treated for another
disorder (e.g., depressive, obsessive, or compulsive symptoms) in
the mental health system, and a clinician recognized the features of
AS (Attwood, 2007). Still other adults seen in our practice have
been assessed or treated in the developmental services sector (as
they were perceived to have had an intellectual disability), and the
features of ASD were not recognized. Some may have received a
diagnosis as a child, but they have experienced new difficulties getting supports or services (Stoddart, Burke, & Temple, 2002a). Still
others are parents or relatives of diagnosed children or youth who
come to be assessed themselves, following the ASD diagnosis of a
family member.

The major cluster of referrals we receive is from parents of young
adults. The following e-mail was sent by the parent of a woman
suspected of having AS. It poignantly illustrates the desperation that
many parents feel in their desire to help their adult child receive a
suitable assessment and accompanying services and supports:

> My daughter is now 34 years old, unemployed, alone, friend-
> less, and desperately unhappy—a "square peg" who, with
> courage and persistence, tries futilely to fit herself into the
> "round holes" offered by the world. I firmly believe she has
> either Asperger Syndrome or Non-Verbal Learning Disorder
> [NVLD], though in a brief and unsatisfactory visit to the local
> mental health hospital several years ago, I was told she did not
> exhibit the signs of Asperger Syndrome. As she was angry and
> crying throughout the half-hour we were given, and no tests
> were administered or relevant questions asked, I am not sure
> how they reached that conclusion.
>
> Her behavior is inexplicable and frustrating to her family:
> distant, uncommunicative, intelligent but lacking in "common
> sense," resistant even to positive change, persistent in efforts
> proven to be unproductive or counterproductive. Though
> there are no overt signs to indicate she is different from most
> of the world, she does not "get it" socially at all, and is inca-
> pable of reading or responding to the emotional needs of oth-
> ers. I am the only family member who has not, for all practical
> purposes, walked away from her because of her seeming indif-

ference to us and our lives. She has only recently acknowledged that literature on NVLD and Aspergers, which I gave to
her and begged her to read, accurately describes how she experiences the world. Though no longer resistant, she remains
passive about doing anything to see how she might improve
the quality of her life.

If the information and resources available today had been
available when my daughter was younger, I would have
known what to do and, as the parent, would have been able to
be sure she got the help. But what do you do with an adult,
especially one who is alternately passive or actively resistant?
Who continues to rely on you for all kinds of support? When
you believe that individual has a disability that makes it difficult or impossible for her to see how she can help herself? How
can I determine what I can reasonably expect from her? How
can I stop trying to find ways to improve her quality of life
when she is my child? How can I salvage my own life while
not abandoning her? She is not sufficiently "overtly disabled"
to access any social assistance, but who can live on that any-
way? At the same time, how can I, at 58 years old, contem-
plate supporting her forever?

This e-mail is important for two reasons: It highlights the distress
a parent may feel on behalf of her child, and it introduces the importance of the diagnoses of AS in women. The literature tells us that
while diagnoses of ASDs in males continue to increase, the referrals
and diagnoses for women have not followed this pattern (Wilkinson,
2008). As well, for women, when a diagnosis is made, it tends to be
at a later age. Wilkinson notes that there appear to be many reasons
for the "gender gap," including socialization to one's gender role,
greater abilities to cope with stressful situations, and the appearance
of better social skills (or less visible poor social skills). Our clinical
experience supports the idea of a "gender gap."

Self-referrals are another major source of clients in our practices.
Many individuals who have AS have reached adulthood with the
awareness that others see them as "different." They frequently have
the sense that something about them is lacking, but have been unable to identify what that is. Many people who self-refer for a diagnostic assessment have found information on the Internet or have

seen programs on television that describe their difficulties. Often, they seek self-assessment measures, and many come to their first appointment with lists of symptoms or printouts from tests they have found on the Internet suggesting that they have AS. Although some clients who self-diagnose are mistaken and their symptoms suggest some other problem, we have found that usually they are correct. This being said, we do not wish to promote self-diagnosis. However, with this client group, many would not receive a diagnosis if they had not been self-informed and referred, and their concerns should be taken seriously. Below is an e-mail from a woman who self-assessed and concluded that she had AS.

> I am 51 years old and just figured out this year why I have been having such awful difficulties all my life. Last year I found out I have Tourette's syndrome. But it still did not explain why I am so different. I stumbled upon Asperger Syndrome, and the list of characteristics could have been written about me! After my family had me check off quite a few more items than I thought I should check, I am exhibiting at least 90% of those characteristics. I have also done all the tests by reputable Asperger specialists I found on the Internet and my scores are, without fail, well above the average for people with AS.
>
> I need my self-diagnosis validated by a specialist, because many people (including my husband) still don't believe me. I am not just making up excuses for being "weird and unacceptable" by saying I can't help being this way. This is me! They claim with a little more "willpower" and trying harder, I could be more "normal" (meaning more like them, but why do I have to be like them?). They don't know that I have all my life used up all my energy, trying so hard to be like others, without success. I am sick of pretending to be somebody I am not. I want to be "allowed" to be me, without everybody trying to change me constantly!

Individuals who have received a diagnosis of AS in adulthood may respond in various ways. Those who self-refer often show relief, indicating that the diagnosis confirms what they knew. If the person has been referred by others, and has been aware that he or she has difficulties, then they may react in the same manner as the person who self-refers.

However, if the assessment has been requested by someone other than the individual, and the affected person is either unaware of the difficulties others see, or content, regardless of the difficulties, then this diagnosis may create discomfort. In this case, the person may need support to deal with the repercussions of the assessment. A "label" may be difficult for some individuals to accept. An expectation may be held by family, friends, or employers that now that they know what the problem is, the person should do something. For the person diagnosed, this will not be easy; he or she will need to seek support, and this may not be something he or she wishes to do.

If a spouse or partner who has found the relationship difficult is the referring person, the diagnosis may help him or her be more understanding or supportive of the person. Alternatively, it may confirm for the spouse that it is time to terminate a relationship with which it has been difficult to cope, and which they can find no way to improve.

MULTIDISCIPLINARY ASSESSMENT

To give an individual the best opportunity to address all aspects of AS, he or she should be seen by professionals who can assess the impact of AS within their scope of practice and make suitable recommendations. Whereas the option of an integrated multidisciplinary assessment is often available for children, it is rarely available for adults. For example, a psychiatrist may make a diagnosis of AS and prescribe medications to reduce anxiety or obsessive–compulsive behaviors, but may not assess the person's cognitive profile, which affects his or her vocational or other areas of functioning. The psychologist, who assesses cognitive discrepancies, may be unable to address the sensory and motor needs of the individual to the extent that an occupational therapist would. Other professionals may include a medical specialist who addresses digestion or other medical problems, and an audiologist who would test for central auditory processing issues. Occupational therapy, speech and language pathology, social work, and behavior therapy are some of the disciplines to which the diagnosing clinician may refer. Therefore, the ideal assessment that leads to optimal intervention is one that includes professionals who can address all the needs of the person in an integrated manner (Stoddart, Muskat, & Mishna, 2005; Burke, 2005).

It is often left to the adult being assessed, or the lead professional to organize a multidisciplinary assessment by colleagues who are familiar with mild presentations of ASDs. The clinician should be aware of the possible need to refer the individual to another professional and attempt to network with other professionals in his or her community to gain knowledge of potentially useful resources. In order to avoid overwhelming the adult being assessed, or his or her family, the lead clinician or clinicians should assist in prioritizing the assessments and interventions that need to occur. We have seen cases in which the individual with AS becomes obsessed by, and overwhelmed with, an assessment process that attempts to address all of their concerns. Although this is understandable when an individual is seeking answers for difficulties after a long period of having no answers or help, there is a danger that a prolonged assessment process can overshadow the efforts needed to make progress on intervention priorities.

Although we feel that the "assessment process" cannot artificially be separated from the "intervention process," an explicit and goal-directed intervention approach is eventually required. The clinical issues presenting in adults with AS often overlap. Although it may be difficult to ascertain the relative influence of various factors on a client's overall clinical presentation, it is nonetheless important that each be assessed and addressed by the most appropriate member of the multidisciplinary team.

DIAGNOSTIC CRITERIA AND DEBATE

The specific criteria for diagnosis of disorders on the autism spectrum are found in the DSM-IV-TR, subsumed under the category of pervasive developmental disorders (American Psychiatric Association, 2000). The criteria for diagnosis can also be found in the *International Statistical Classification of Diseases and Related Health Problems–10* (ICD-10; World Health Organization, 2007). Clinicians should adhere to the current diagnostic criteria when considering the diagnosis. Symptoms of pervasive developmental disorders in these manuals include those that are communicative, social, and behavioral. In addition, age of onset and developmental delays in speech, language, and cognition are addressed. It is important to remember that not every individual presents with all the characteristics of the disorder as articulated in the diagnostic criteria. Please refer to Figure 1.1 in Chapter 1 for the DSM-IV-TR (American Psychiatric Association, 2000) criteria for AS.

Many clinicians and professionals in the field of ASDs have concerns with the current DSM-IV-TR (American Psychiatric Association, 2000) diagnostic criteria for AS, or express confusion about the differentiation between AS and "high-functioning" autism (Klin, Volkmar, Sparrow, Cicchetti, & Rourke, 1995). Most experienced clinicians follow the diagnostic criteria and voice their concerns through proper channels, such as in the literature. Klin, Pauls, Schultz, and Volkmar (2005) reviewed three diagnostic approaches. Although there is a substantive body of research, so far the "absence of a validated definition prevents the development of standardized instrumentation that could enhance reliability of diagnostic assignment and make possible cross-site collaborations that are essential to both behavioral and biological research" (p. 222). In addition, they state that some clinicians ignore the DSM-IV-TR (American Psychiatric Association, 2000) criteria for diagnosis, which may cause confusion to families, clinicians, and researchers. Others have also addressed the potential impact of this inconsistency for those who are engaged in research on AS and related disorders (Ghaziuddin, Tsai, & Ghaziuddin, 1992a). Reading the current professional literature and attending seminars help clinicians stay informed about new findings, as well as about debates within their field. Although it is important to be informed, it is also essential that clinicians refrain from incorporating opinions or findings into the diagnostic process that are discrepant with DSM-IV-TR (American Psychiatric Association, 2000) criteria.

Our concerns about the idiosyncratic utilization of diagnostic labels stems from situations where individuals come to us after seeing an inexperienced clinician. In these cases, a diagnosis on the autism spectrum has been made based on some loosely defined criteria. This type of poorly informed diagnosis may have caused difficulties for the individual with understanding his or her disorder or receiving suitable funding and services. For example, a young man presented to us with a diagnosis of AS. He had an IQ at the boundary of mild intellectual disability and borderline functioning, with classic features of autism. He had a well-developed vocabulary and had been seeing a clinician who had estimated, but not tested, his cognitive ability. His diagnosis of AS led to much higher expectations being placed on him than he could achieve, leading him to experience high levels of anxiety. He was unable to work without the support from a local agency for those with intellectual disabilities. However, the diagnosis of AS precluded him from receiving services in the developmental services sector.

We also need to caution against clinicians overemphasizing commonly discussed symptoms. Every person presents with his or her own constellation of symptoms. For those who are more competent, they have likely attempted to modify issues they're aware are problematic. For example, we have seen individuals who have previously been assessed and a diagnosis of AS has been dismissed based on a symptom that has been overemphasized by the clinician, such as ability to make eye contact. Although many individuals with ASDs do not make good eye contact, there are those who fixate on others' eyes. There are also individuals who have practiced tolerating eye contact, or who use methods such as looking at a person's nose or at a spot behind their head to make it appear that they are engaging in eye contact.

Some individuals meet the criteria for the diagnosis of autism and are intellectually high-functioning. These individuals may have experienced a delay in language development, but in all other ways, reflect a person with AS. Some children with autism who developed fluent language skills have been found to present as similar to those with AS (Szatmari, Bryson, Streiner, et al., 2000). Szatmari (2005) has proposed that the criteria for the distinction between autism and AS would more logically be evidence of a specific language disorder, rather than a delay in developing speech. He suggests that under these circumstances, those who are now classified with high-functioning autism (because of speech delay) would instead be considered as having AS. Countering this perspective, other research comparing those with AS and high-functioning autism found differences between the two groups. For example, one study found differences in the areas of ToM and verbal memory (Ozonoff, Rogers, & Pennington, 1991).

Many clinicians would prefer to avoid a diagnosis of pervasive developmental disorder not otherwise specified (PDD-NOS) because it is "general and lacks clinical specificity" (Bonfardin, Zimmerman, & Gaus, 2007, p. 118). Countering this, Scahill (2005) points out that this diagnosis is fitting when the person shows social impairment, but does not meet the criteria for other disorders on the autism spectrum. According to DSM-IV-TR, PDD-NOS is to be used when there is a severe impairment in social interaction and difficulties in communication and/or behavior. Currently, if a clinician is to stay within the DSM-IV-TR criteria, there are times when the only correct diagnostic choice may be PDD-NOS.

Given the current diagnostic controversy, we suggest that it would be most suitable to provide the diagnosis that best fits the DSM-IV-TR criteria and also to make a statement of explanation (e.g., the individual presented as someone with AS but did not meet the criteria of "no language delay"). This qualification allows for a change in diagnosis later if the DSM criteria change and if the person wishes the diagnosis to be revisited. This situation would be comparable to the situation of those diagnosed with autism before 1994, who requested reassessment once the diagnosis of AS was included in the DSM-IV (American Psychiatric Association, 2000).

INFORMANTS IN THE INTERVIEW

When a child is assessed, the examiner may observe the child in the home and school settings, and parents and teachers act as informants about the child's development, skills, and behaviors (Schnurr, 2005). However, when an adult is assessed, some of these options are not possible or desirable. For example, it would not typically be advisable for the assessor to attend the individual's place of employment or observe his or her skills in a postsecondary setting, because doing so would stigmatize the individual and possibly create social and employment difficulties. There are alternative opportunities for observation, however. Because individuals may respond differently to structured versus unstructured situations, or to familiar versus unfamiliar persons (Burke, 2005), altering the conditions in which assessment occurs can help to gain a better understanding of the person's range of responses. This approach might involve, for example, observation while sharing a coffee with the individual in the clinic's cafeteria and engaging him or her in casual conversation. The individual's response in this unstructured environment can then be contrasted with his or her behaviors and social–communication abilities when assessment measures are administered in a quiet and highly structured environment.

The adult who attends an appointment for a diagnostic assessment is the primary informant, as he or she is providing information about his or her perceptions, emotions, and experiences. However, individuals with AS are not always reliable informants, as they may be unaware of how they present to others and may not always feel connected to their emotions or to the social environment. It is preferable, therefore, that another person who knows the individual attends the appointment to provide a more rounded or accurate picture. If that is not possible, the clinician may schedule a separate session or a telephone interview with someone who can provide another perspective.

We have seen many cases where the absence of additional informants led to false diagnoses or a false negative diagnosis of AS. Usually, a family member is the best additional informant, because that person can also provide historical information about early milestones, social development, and school experiences. This person may offer opinions in response to direct questions by the assessor or by completing standardized measures (discussed shortly). Many, such as spouses of affected partners, offer information through e-mails or a telephone conversation at referral.

Throughout the information collection process, care should be given not to undermine the adult; the purpose for involvement of the family member therefore needs to be carefully explained. This is especially salient in situations where an older parent is reporting on an adult child in his or her late 20s or 30s. We have found that in adult psychiatry, the use of family members as informants is sometimes not valued and may be perceived by the clinical setting as lacking respect for the patient. If the adult is older, the parent may no longer be alive, or may be aging and have difficulty recalling information accurately. A sibling, spouse, or friend can then serve as a possible informant. Sometimes photo albums, if available, can help the informant remember important information. Documents may also be available, such as old report cards, other school records, or previous reports and assessments by physicians, psychologists, or other health care providers (Attwood, 2007). It is currently our practice to send the individual or a family member with whom we are in contact a questionnaire about early development as well as current functioning. The questionnaire format allows time for historical information to be gathered prior to the appointment, and then the returned questionnaire becomes a guide for the clinical interview, allowing the individual and family to review and expand on relevant information.

CLINICAL OBSERVATIONS

Clinical observations begin at the first contact with an individual. If it is by telephone or e-mail, is the person concise or very detail-oriented in describing concerns? Is he or she able to provide relevant information, appropriately schedule an appointment, and end a conversation? Does the person provide too much information or present as extremely mechanical? At first meeting, does the person make eye contact, shake your hand, and use appropriate greetings? How does he or she respond to the receptionist in the office or to other clients in the waiting room? What is the presentation of voice volume, pitch, and prosody?

When interviewing the adult, the clinician attends not only to the overt responses given; observation of communication, social, and behavioral characteristics is also important. For example, if a person describes items or events in sophisticated terms, the clinician may ask for clarification and sometimes find that the person has only a superficial understanding of what he has said. If an individual identifies problems in social situations, it is useful to investigate in more detail to obtain that person's understanding of what would be fitting in such situations. Sometimes, a person tells us that he is better able to communicate with others on the Internet and that it is more difficult talking face-to-face. If an individual does engage in conversation, does she "lecture" rather than discuss? Does he jump into a topic, leaving out the beginning and significant details, and expect you to know what he is talking about? Does she have difficulty if you change the topic, or does she join in a conversational topic after others have moved on to a new subject? One individual equated conversation to watching the puck during a hockey game: Just when it lands somewhere sufficiently for him to focus on it, it moves quickly in another direction.

Box 2.1 lists the issues that should be addressed throughout the interview and assessment that will guide the clinician to a diagnostic decision. Some individuals will display only a few of these features, and others will present with many.

As well as noting behavior, one should also note the appearance of the individual. This focus may provide clues to other factors that need to be considered. How is the person dressed—sloppy, too casual, provocatively, or overdressed? An individual who comes to an appointment in a sweat suit may have an aversion to heavy materials such as denim or corduroy, or may be unable to tolerate tight or "scratchy" clothing. A person who is dressed in an old-fashioned or excessively professional style may not be aware of the current fashion or of fashion's importance in the social world, or the clothes may be bought by a parent. Well-styled clothes from another fashion era may indicate an obsessive interest. Tinted glasses or use of sunglasses indoors may cue the clinician to vision sensitivities or to difficulties in establishing eye contact. Hygiene is also important. Is his hair clean and brushed? Does he have body odor? Is he unshaven? Observation may also cue to forms of obsessive or compulsive behavior, anxiety, or self-injury. Does she have cuts or scars? Does she have unusual patches of hair loss (suggesting trichotillomania)? Are her hands, arms, or legs scarred from repeated picking of sores? Is she excessively thin? Are nails bitten? Are hands or skin rough, red or chapped?

Not only is observation of the individual important: observation of the behavioral interactions between family members can provide useful information. For example, a mother whose adult son was being assessed left work in the middle of the day to bring him a snack during the assessment, reflecting a high level of parental involvement. Other family members may respond to questions in the assessment that are meant for the identified client, or treat the individual in other idiosyncratic or infantilizing ways. We would expect these responses from parents of children or those with intellectual disabilities, but not for an adult child with average intellectual functioning. From this, we conclude that there is something about the client that makes the family believe that he or she is less capable or needs to be cared for. Often, we meet with parents of young adults who are attending university or just beginning independent life. The parents have had to become excessively involved in the young per-

---

BOX 2.1. FEATURES TO ATTEND TO DURING THE ASSESSMENT
INTERVIEW

COMMUNICATION/SOCIAL INTERACTION:

- Odd or flat inflection during speech
- Use of sophisticated words/terms; outdated terms
- Use of idiosyncratic words (e.g., says heavy when sad)
- Poor comprehension
- Word-finding problems
- Concrete statements
- Does not initiate conversation
- Speaks without adequately introducing the topic
- Talks at rather than with you
- Talks obsessively or intensely about a specific interest
- Appears disinterested when others speak
- Difficulty with change in topic
- Joins a conversation when it has moved on to a new issue
- Looks to others for confirmation or assistance
- Delayed responding
- One-word answers
- Problems relating to social or emotional events
- Difficulty making/maintaining eye contact
- Uses speech from learned sources to communicate (e.g., lines
  from movies)

MANNERISMS, ACTION PATTERNS, AND BEHAVIORS:

- Apparent problems related to time, space, planning, prediction, organization
- Obsessive or compulsive patterns (e.g., patterns of face/body
  touching; needs to repeat certain words/phrases; pulls at
  clothing or other objects)
- Unusual mannerisms or anxiety-related behaviors (e.g., rocking, picking at clothes or skin)
- Discusses emotional issues in terms of actions
- Acts out past events when talking about them (e.g., using
  alternate voices and body movements)
- Normalizes things that others would find unusual

---

son's life because the individual is not paying bills, attending classes, eating, or attending to personal hygiene. The parents are confused, comparing the needs of this adult child with their other (sometimes younger) children or with their son or daughter's peers who appear more competent in daily functional skills.

Although we would like to test for all possible issues, often there are no tools available to assess a potential clinical problem that are appropriate for use with adults. Informal methods of assessment are useful to explore findings that either have been identified through standard test measures, or for which there is no measure available. Therefore, we believe it is helpful for the clinician to have informal methods available for use to gain a better understanding of the person. One example is ColorCards (Harrison, 1996), which depict pictures of people expressing emotions in a variety of situations. These cards can be used to examine an individual's understanding of emotions or social interactions. As well, the clinician may engage a person in a simple game or task to further observe executive function, browse through a magazine to discuss current events, involve the client in a discussion of a favorite topic, or ask him or her to bring in written work (e.g., if in college, a written project).

Although we have emphasized the importance of careful clinical observation in this chapter, we also strongly caution against overvaluing clinical observation to the exclusion of other methods of assessment. For example, the professional, well-dressed, articulate woman who presents with excellent eye contact and with ability for insight and self-reflection may, to the naïve clinician, "present" as if she does not have AS. We know that the symptoms that women present may be more subtle in nature. Novice clinicians may report "It is impossible that this woman has AS!" with the template in their mind of the highly socially awkward male who avoids any eye contact and is not successful in employment or relationships. To rely exclusively on observation and a cursory evaluation of their psychosocial functioning is to do a disservice to individuals coming to us for diagnosis, especially well-functioning individuals with AS. Just as we cannot necessarily observe depression in individuals who come to us for a diagnosis of depression, so too, we may not necessarily observe AS. In part, these false negative diagnoses also result from overvaluing certain AS characteristics over others (such as lack of eye contact) in order to inform a diagnostic impression.

AUTISM SPECTRUM MEASURES

Instruments developed for use in the assessment and diagnoses of ASDs vary in format and type of respondent; they include observation protocols, interview protocols, self- and other-report questionnaires. Some have been developed to distinguish between disorders on the autism spectrum, but more often, they provide confirmation of symptoms for a specific disorder. Many have been developed and normed for children, but because the upper end of the age range is 18 or 22 years, they are often used for adults in the absence of adult-specific measures. At the onset of the assessment, the clinician does not know if, in fact, the individual has an ASD or for which ASD the person may meet diagnostic criteria. Therefore, one or more of these instruments can be used.

Both Howlin (2000a) and Campbell (2005) have reviewed several measures and identified difficulties with sensitivity, reliability, and validity. Campbell (2005) stated that of the tools he reviewed, all presented with inadequate psychometric data, but he did indicate they "hold promise as clinical instruments" (p. 25). These tools, in themselves, are not adequate for diagnosis, but they do help identify symptoms to supplement clinical impressions. We do not recommend any specific instrument, but we do provide information on some of the tools available.

A concern in assessing adults with ASDs, including AS, is that it has been necessary for clinicians to use instruments intended for other purposes and abstract the information necessary for the current purpose. For example, we often use instruments developed for children, find individual or informal methods to identify symptoms of the disorder, and supplement findings with checklists, interview, and observational information (Burke, 2007). For assessment specific to adults with AS, there are no protocols that are seen as superior instruments comparable to those used to identify autism, particularly in children, such as the Autism Diagnostic Observation Schedule (ADOS; Lord et al., 2001) or the Autism Diagnostic Interview—Revised (ADI-R; LeCouteur, Lord, & Rutter, 2003). Although the two measures cited are sometimes used by clinicians in assessing adults believed to have an ASD, we have found these most useful when the person has an intellectual disability or borderline functioning, and they are used to determine if the person also has an ASD.

For individuals who are very high-functioning and very competent in their studies or their field of employment, these measures may not be appropriate. As well, there are some questionnaires listed below that have been recently developed specifically for adults. However, at this point, reviews do not identify any one measure as exceptional. Most identify symptoms of a named ASD (e.g., autism or AS), but do not distinguish between different forms of ASDs. Regardless of the specific tools a clinician prefers to use in a diagnostic assessment, it is also necessary to rely on the observational and interpretive skills of clinical experience.

Interview Protocols

• The Asperger Syndrome Diagnostic Interview (ASDI; Gillberg, Gillberg, Rastam, & Wentz, 2001) is a brief interview, comprised of 20 questions over six symptoms areas. It does not distinguish between those who have AS and those with autism who are higher-functioning.

• The Autism Diagnostic Interview—Revised (ADI-R; LeCouteur et al., 2003) does assist in identifying a good early history in terms of symptoms of an ASD. However, there are problems when using it with adults. First, it presumes that there is someone available who has a detailed history of the person who can respond to questions. Second, it does not allow one to adequately offer a profile of the person at the current time. It takes approximately 1½ hours to complete. Experienced clinicians will have developed their own interview to integrate this information. Therefore, this measure may be most useful for a less experienced clinician to acquire the necessary historical information. In our practice, this is a good measure for assessment of children when there is a query of an ASD.

Observation Protocols

• The Autism Diagnostic Observation Schedule (ADOS; Lord et al., 2001) was originally developed for use with children. It does not distinguish between disorders on the autism spectrum. The current schedule has an assessment protocol for adolescents and adults who are fluent speakers (Module 4), and includes questions about emotions and relationships that are appropriate to individuals with AS. For an experienced clinician, the questions and activities offered by the ADOS that are appropriate for the adult with AS are likely already incorporated into the clinician's typical method of assessment. For a clinician working with both children and adults, and both autism and AS, this measure would be important. However, for clinicians who work primarily with adults and with those who do not have intellectual disabilities, we have found it is neither cost-effective nor efficient.

Questionnaires and Scales

• Adult Asperger Assessment (AAA; Baron-Cohen, Wheelwright, Robinson, & Woodbury-Smith, 2005) is comprised of two separate screening tools: the Autism Spectrum Quotient (ASQ) and the Empathy Quotient (EQ). The ASQ was developed to examine characteristics of autism in adults who have average cognitive abilities (Woodbury-Smith, Robinson, Wheelwright, & Baron-Cohen, 2005). The EQ was developed as a 60-item self-report questionnaire, and it demonstrated that individuals with high-functioning autism and AS have an "empathy deficit" (Baron-Cohen & Wheelwright, 2004). The combined assessment identifies symptoms present in AS, and the authors of the scale suggest that their criteria are more stringent than those in DSM-IV, so that that if criteria are met in this assessment, they are also met for DSM-IV.

• The Asperger Screening Questionnaire for Adults (ASQ-A; Stoddart & Burke, 2011) has been in clinical use in our practice for several years and was developed because of our need to have our clients report and rate their own symptoms of AS. On the ASQ-A, the individual rates his or her experiences on a 5-point scale across symptom areas. The ASQ-A typically takes between 20 and 30 minutes to complete and does not distinguish between AS and other ASDs.

• Asperger Syndrome Diagnostic Scale (ASDS; Myles, Bock, & Simpson, 2001) contains 50 statements that are rated as Observed or Not Observed across five subscales: Language, Social, Maladaptive, Cognitive, and Sensorimotor. Results are reported as the probability of AS, ranging from Very Likely to Very Unlikely. An informant responds to the questions, and the measure can be completed in 10–15 minutes.

• Australian Scale for Asperger's Syndrome (ASAS; Garnett & Attwood, 1998) was developed to help parents and teachers identify symptoms of AS in children. At the time it was written, most available measures addressed symptoms of autism and not AS. The scale was published in Attwood's book (1998) and intended for children. However, it is mentioned here because Attwood stated in his more recent publication (2007) that an adult version would be published. At the time this chapter is being written, an adult version by the original authors is not yet available.

• The Autism Spectrum Disorders in Adults Screening Questionnaire (ASDASQ; Gillberg, 2002b; Nylander & Gillberg, 2001) was developed for use with outpatients in a clinical setting. This 10-question screening taps basic symptom areas through yes/no responses. It does not distinguish among ASDs.

• The Gilliam Asperger's Disorder Scale (GADS; Gilliam, 2002) is a 32-item measure that was developed for children and adolescents. Although it is often used with adults, some questions reflect behavior more typical of children. It requires rating of the individual on characteristics of the disorder based on four subscales: Social Interaction, Restricted Patterns of Behavior, Cognitive Patterns, and Pragmatic Skills. It also provides questions on developmental issues as well as current behaviors. These are not included in scoring but do provide useful information to the clinician. Scores are reported regarding the probability that the individual has AS, and the scale can be completed in 10–15 minutes.

• The Gilliam Autism Rating Scale—Second Edition (GARS-2; Gilliam, 2006) is, as the GADS, a scale developed for children and therefore carries the same constraints in its use with adults. It is similar in format to the GADS, requiring someone who knows the individual to rate him or her on the characteristics of autism. Areas rated are Stereotyped Behaviors, Communication, and Social Interaction. Ratings for the diagnosis of autism range from "very likely" to "unlikely" and the scale can be completed in 10–15 minutes.

• The Krug Asperger's Disorder Index (KADI; Krug & Arick, 2003) is reported to be useful to distinguish AS from high-functioning individuals with autism. It is recommended for individuals 6–22 years, takes about 20 minutes to administer, and is composed of 32 items. Campbell's review of five measures assessing AS (2005) suggested that all had substantive weaknesses, but the KADI appeared to have the strongest psychometric properties.

- Ritvo Autism and Asperger's Diagnostic Scale (RAADS; Ritvo et al., 2008) has been developed to identify the presence of autism or AS in adults, but it does not distinguish between the disorders. The person being assessed rates characteristics of autism and AS in him- or herself, both in the past and at present. Scores suggest the presence or the likelihood of AS or autism.

TWELVE ASSESSMENT THEMES

The diagnostic assessment is completed by a psychologist, psychiatrist, or other medical doctor, optimally with other members of an assessment team. It should first address the clinical criterion for the diagnosis according to DSM-IV-TR (American Psychiatric Association, 2000). Scahill suggests that the steps to diagnosis should include a "categorical diagnosis, dimensional assessment, and evaluation of the individual patient's symptoms" (Scahill, 2005, p. 21). *Categorical diagnosis* refers to the results generated by questionnaires and observational measures related specifically to the characteristics of an ASD. *Dimensional assessment* refers to evaluation of other dimensions of functioning, such as intelligence, behavior, and adaptive functioning. *Patient symptoms* refer to the specific difficulties of the individual being assessed, or which the referring person is reporting.

Below, we detail 12 themes that should be a part of a comprehensive diagnostic assessment: (1) developmental and service history, (2) cognitive profile, (3) communication skills, (4) social functioning, (5) interests and repetitive behavior, (6) adaptive and life skills, (7) executive functioning, (8) sensory functioning, (9) motor functioning, (10) theory of mind, (11) mental health, and (12) emotional understanding. The first five areas are critical to ensure that the individual does, or does not, meet diagnostic criteria. If in the interpretation of these it is identified that another disorder may be present, such as a learning disability, other measures will be introduced such as tests of achievement or of learning and memory. Areas 6–12 are also significant but not essential to include if they do not potentially address the clinical question(s) being posed, or if they have been explored in an assessment previously. Difficulties in these areas are not exclusive to people who have an ASD. Nevertheless, some of these have been reported repeatedly in the research literature, and can provide support for a diagnosis of an ASD. As well, they may be causing the person difficulties in their daily life and require attention (Burke, 2005).

We should note that there are occasions when a comprehensive assessment may not be required. We often omit a full cognitive assessment measure or utilize an abbreviated scale of cognitive ability if we are diagnosing an older or retired person, when an individual is functioning successfully in his or her area of employment or interest, or when previous cognitive assessments have been completed. In these situations, we still gather a detailed history, conduct a clinical interview, engage in observation, and ensure that relevant questionnaires and screening measures are completed.

Developmental and Service History

It is our preference to begin the assessment by gathering a biopsychosocial history. This detailed history of developmental and personal events in the individual's life should be done prior to administering tests and questionnaires (Burke, 2005). The ability to distinguish AS from another ASD may lie in the historical and current cognitive functioning, language development, behavioral presentation, and adaptive living skills. As well, there are disorders with similar presentations to ASDs, such as personality disorders (e.g., avoidant, schizoid, or schizotypal) and OCD (Fitzgerald & Corvin, 2001; Szatmari, 1998). The early presence or pattern of symptoms may therefore be an important contribution to a differential diagnosis.

The clinician should have a list of relevant questions related to early development and current behavior to ask during the interview, or request that a history questionnaire be completed by family members. Schnurr (2005) suggests that anything unusual in developmental milestones should be noted, particularly with language and communication development and social behavior. Questions should also identify difficulty with transitions, changes, coping behaviors, and repetitive or stereotypic movements, intense levels of interests or repetitive conversation about those interests. Many of the developmental concerns that we address when taking a developmental history are presented in Box 2.2.

Many adults who come to us for a diagnostic assessment have had an extensive but unproductive service history with mental health,

---

BOX 2.2. KEY AREAS TO CONSIDER IN DEVELOPMENTAL/PERSONAL
HISTORY

- Prenatal difficulties and birth history
- Age of acquiring milestones (sitting, standing, walking, crawling, toileting, feeding self)
- Eating or sleeping difficulties
- Age of babbling, acquiring speech (single words, phrases, functional speech)
- Use of gestures
- Social behavior (e.g., showing fear of strangers during infancy, making eye contact, initiating social contact with peers)
- Accepting or displaying affection
- Excessive anxiety/anger/tantrums
- Repetitive or stereotypic behavior
- Health (e.g., childhood diseases, ear infections, seizures)
- Health or mental health concerns of other family members
- Early observations by family or related reports of medical practitioners or educators
- Play behavior at various ages
- Overreaction to small issues or to change
- Early fascinations, fears, or obsessive behaviors
- Extreme sensory responses
- Involvement in group activities (e.g., play groups, organized sports, cubs/scouts)
- Friendships—quality, number, activities
- School performance
- Problem behaviors
- Areas of intelligence, resilience, and strength

---

social service, education, or medical providers. Inquiring as to their experience with past service providers is not only a useful approach for joining therapeutically with many adults, but also for understanding past diagnoses and response to various treatments or services. For example, an unsuccessful trial of stimulant medication from a community psychiatrist may be helpful diagnostically and narrow future treatment options. Presence of an extensive history with developmental service providers may highlight that functional skills were a problem in the past, and that intellectual capacity was questioned. Standard marital counseling without acknowledging the contribution of AS traits may have been futile. As well as inquiring about past interventions from the adult being assessed, historical reports are helpful in bringing detail to the developmental, service, and diagnostic pathways. Having had little or no history with service providers may also contribute to the current clinical picture and diagnostic formulation.

Cognitive Profile

Early research on cognition in those with AS suggested that there might be patterns of intellectual ability that could aid in distinguishing those with AS from those with autism. As early as 1994, preliminary studies suggested stronger verbal skills compared to visuospatial skills in those with AS (Ellis, Ellis, Fraser & Deb, 1994). In those with autism, variability between skills has been a frequent finding, and nonverbal (i.e., visuospatial) skills have been reported as stronger in those with autism (Tager-Flusberg & Joseph, 2003). There is logic to this, as communication difficulties are one of the diagnostic features of autism. However, other research has shown that some individuals who are high-functioning and have autism also have stronger verbal skills (Ozonoff, South, & Miller, 2000), presenting with an overall cognitive profile similar to those with AS. The cited research did indicate there were subtest differences, however, with comprehension in those with AS being stronger than that in high-functioning individuals with autism. Although these trends have been observed and researched, the results have not been found consistently, and therefore differential diagnosis should not depend on the presence of these patterns.

By definition, those with AS have no significant delays in cognitive development. When individuals present for assessment and diagnosis, their level of intellectual ability should be confirmed, as many people have never had psychometric testing. We do sometimes see those who present with a "cloak of competence" (Egerton, Bollinger & Herr, 1984), a term reflecting the tendency in those with developmental disabilities to appear more competent than is actually the case. If the individual has completed an academic program at secondary school, and particularly if he or she has gone to college, we would assume the presence of at least average intelligence. However, we often find comorbid learning disorders or other neurological impairments that affect the person's functioning, and so recommend comprehensive assessment in most cases. When it is not necessary to do a comprehensive intellectual assessment, we have found it is still useful to do a cognitive screen, because such a measure confirms the individual's abilities, identifies areas of strength and weakness, and provides an opportunity to observe the individual's responses and actions in a structured setting (Burke, 2005). If the person either has experienced learning difficulties or has been considered as being gifted, he or she may have been assessed through the school system, and that information should be accessed and reviewed when possible.

In most clinical settings, the Wechsler scales are the primary tools for intellectual assessment. Therefore, if the person has never been assessed, or if there are concerns that there may be a learning disability in addition to, or instead of an ASD, a full assessment should be undertaken. Currently, the Wechsler Adult Intelligence Scale—Fourth Edition (Wechsler, 2008) would be used. This scale provides not only an overall estimate of intellectual functioning, but also index scores for "Verbal Comprehension," "Perceptual Reasoning," "Working Memory," and "Processing Speed." As well as aiding in the identification of a learning disability, this scale can give useful information about appropriate vocational planning. If it is believed that a full assessment is not needed, a brief assessment tool such as the Wechsler Abbreviated Scale of Intelligence (WASI; Wechsler, 1999) should offer the clinician a rapid way to screen the person's cognitive skills. Two verbal and two performance (nonverbal) tasks provide a Verbal, Performance, and a Full-Scale IQ. This measure meets the "general validity and reliability requirements for a brief test of intellectual functioning" (Garland, 2005, p. 134).

During assessment, specific areas of concern may be identified and a more in-depth testing of one or more skills is desirable. Most clinicians who do assessment have several preferred tools to supplement initial cognitive testing, if needed. We frequently do further testing on memory, visual–motor integration, and academic skills. If a diagnosis of learning disorder is being entertained, a measure of academic achievement will be essential.

Communication Skills

According to the DSM-IV-TR (American Psychiatric Association, 2000), a person who meets diagnostic criteria for AS cannot have significant delays in language development. This area of substantial debate and confusion is addressed elsewhere in this chapter. The adult with AS may be very competent and articulate in his or her speech. However, historical information may identify early delays in developing speech and language.

Because an adult did not experience a significant delay in language development, it does not mean that he or she will not have other difficulties or peculiarities in speech and language processing and communication (Lindblad, 2005; Attwood, 2007). If a speech and language pathologist (SLP) is available at the time of assessment, it is helpful to have this professional's participation. If it is not possible to have an SLP at the assessment and if the individual has not been seen previously by an SLP, then the clinician must assess for features noted below.

The person who has AS may have trouble in the use and interpretation of nonverbal communication skills. As children, most of us learn through interaction and experience to use and understand the communicative gestures within our culture. Those with AS will have more difficulty in understanding or interpreting eye gaze, emotional voice tone, body language, facial expressions, and other nonverbal forms of communication (Lindblad, 2005). In regard to receptive language skills, the person with AS may have a superficial understanding of what others say and have difficulty with irony or sarcasm, colloquial use of words, and other indistinct forms of communication. The individual will also experience expressive difficulties. He or she may have a well-developed vocabulary, but may not have a true understanding of what words mean. As well, he or she may have word-finding problems or take longer to synthesize information, and so responses may be delayed.

It is sometimes desirable to assess the receptive and expressive oral vocabulary of the individual. The need for this type of assessment would be indicated if the person's vocabulary skills were unclear or if there appeared to be a discrepancy between oral receptive and expressive vocabulary skills. The Comprehensive Receptive and Expressive Vocabulary Test—Second Edition (CREVT2; Wallace &

Hammill, 2002) can be used for individuals ages 4–89 years. It takes little time to administer and is easily scored.

Difficulties in oral discourse can cause considerable problems in social conversation because the person may become lost as the conversation shifts. The presence of (social) anxiety may contribute to these difficulties. During an interview, practiced phrases or unique voice characteristics may be observed, such as problems with pitch and volume regulation or unusual accents. These may be described by the person or by others. Although a person who has AS is typically a good reader, written output may be difficult, possibly because of the receptive and expressive difficulties, noted above, as well as working memory and other executive functioning deficits, or fine motor or sensory problems that affect the physical task of writing.

Pragmatics, or speech in the social context, is an important issue to address in an assessment (Burke, 2005). The individual with an ASD, including AS, may misinterpret what is occurring in a social communication or may not use speech properly in an interaction. For example, the person may get into difficulties for being blunt or rude (e.g., referring to someone by his or her ethnic origin; calling them fat). The person may also misunderstand the intent of others and become intensely angry about something he or she has not interpreted correctly.

Several tests of pragmatics are available, and each may address different aspects of social communication. Examples are the Awareness of Social Inference Test (McDonald, Flanagan, Rollins, & Kinch, 2003) and the Test of Pragmatic Language—Second Edition (TOPL-2; Phelps-Terasaki, & Phelps-Gunn, 2007). We have found the Test of Pragmatic Language to be useful for assessing adults with ASDs, including AS. Originally a test for children under 13, the current revision provides normative information up to age 18 years, 11 months. Both verbal information and drawings are used to represent social contexts and interactions. Individuals must analyze the situations and identify fitting communicative responses. Although, once again, there are difficulties in using assessment tools designed for children when assessing adults, there are few available alternatives at this time. We have found that even adults with AS who are very intellectually capable have trouble on this test, and it therefore does provide us with information relevant to the individual's challenges. Although it does not assess all aspects of pragmatics, it does assess six components of social communication. If extensive testing is needed, the person should be referred to an SLP.

Social Functioning

Difficulty in social understanding and functioning is one of the primary characteristics of AS (Engstrom et al., 2003). The individual's early social history is important to assess when gathering information on early childhood development. The clinician should then address the same issues in adolescence and adulthood. Does the person initiate social contact with others, such as invite them to shop or go to the movies? Can the person tolerate small talk at the workplace? Does the person focus on a specific interest during his or her social interaction with others, while excluding other people without those interests or preoccupations?

Social functioning is measured by some of the instruments (previously described) that assess symptoms of ASDs. As well, when a comprehensive assessment is being done which utilizes the WAIS-IV, the examiner may wish to use the Advanced Clinical Solutions (ACS: Psychological Corporation, 2009), which contains activities to address social cognition. Use of measures such as the Social Problem-Solving Inventory—Revised (D'Zurilla, Nezu, & Maydeu-Olivares, 2002) and the Social Functioning Questionnaire (Tyrer et al., 2005) has been reported in research with adults (Huband, McMurran, Evans, & Duggan, 2007), although not those with AS. The Social Problem-Solving Inventory—Revised (D'Zurilla et al., 2002) is a measure of positive and negative problem orientation, problem definition and solving, and decision-making. It also examines issues in resolution, such as carelessness and impulsivity, and is a self-report inventory that comes in a short version. At times, we will use the informal Test of Social Know-How (Dewey, 1991), which presents individuals with social dilemmas and situations and asks them to rate the appropriateness of various responses to them.

Sometimes, individuals take on prescribed roles that assist them in social contexts. For example, we have seen people involved in teaching, sales, law, and the ministry, all of whom describe the social aspects of their work as a "performance." The script they develop and the stereotypic persona of their profession gives them confidence in social settings. One teacher identified that she did well with lectures, but could not spontaneously respond to her students' questions. She had them write questions down and provided answers later. The wife of a marketing executive who had AS stated that when she saw him "perform" at work, he was a different person as compared to the person she saw at home, where he withdrew socially.

Occasionally, people take on an extreme persona that seems delusional in nature. Attwood (2007) notes this situation when the individual takes on the appearance and behaviors of superheroes or fantasy characters. If the person cannot "separate" from the identity he or she has assumed, clinical intervention may be required. A final concern is involvement with "fringe" groups, as that is where individuals with AS often find acceptance. Some individuals with whom we have worked have been involved in illegal enterprises or have joined cult-like religious groups where their social role is clear, but where they have been taken advantage of.

Interests and Repetitive Behavior

The second major area addressed in the DSM-IV-TR diagnostic criteria is an individual's tendency to exhibit "restricted, repetitive, and stereotyped patterns of behavior, interests, and activities" (p. 84, American Psychiatric Association, 2000). According to the DSM-IV-TR, this type of behavior might be seen in an "encompassing preoccupation with one or more stereotyped and restricted patterns of interest that is abnormal either in intensity or focus . . . inflexible adherence to specific, non-functional routines or rituals, stereotyped and repetitive motor mannerisms or twisting, complex whole-body movements, or persistent preoccupation with parts of objects" (p. 84).

As with an individual's social difficulties, the restricted, stereotyped, and repetitive patterns of behaviors or interests will have been evident since childhood. The adult, his or her parents, or other family members typically report intense interests with activities that might revolve around general themes; specific interests may vary over the years. For example, an individual who is interested in science may display a range of interests within the scientific field over time. Some adults report strong interests and abilities with technical and scientific subjects, others with philosophy and theories, and still others have exhibited superb skills in language and writing (e.g., Jansen, 2005). Such preoccupations may lead to functional use and productivity in employment (Grandin, 1992). At other times, they lead to problematic behaviors and failure to complete necessary tasks of daily living. An individual's social interaction may revolve around his or her special interests. We often ask if the individual talks incessantly about his or her interest, or is unaware of social cues by others that they are not as passionate about the subject. Interests may be unusual for the person's age or gender and involve repetitive thoughts and activities.

A hallmark of AS is difficulty with changes in routines, schedules, or patterns of behavior. Non-functional routines might include behaviors that are not appropriate given the situation. For example, a wife of a man with AS complained that he wore an old ripped shirt and boxer shorts to bed on his honeymoon because he had always dressed this way in bed.

Rarely do we see "persistent preoccupation with parts of objects" in adults with AS, as it is articulated in the DSM-IV-TR (American Psychiatric Association, 2000). More often, the assessor will discover, or will hear from informants, about the person's inability to "see the big picture" or to "see the forest for the trees," which is most likely reflective of a central coherence problem (Stoddart, 2007b). Repetitive behaviors might include behaviors that are symptomatic of anxiety or other mental health diagnoses, such as pacing, skin picking, rocking, spinning, frequent checking, or washing. It may also be helpful to determine the sensory function of some of these behaviors. Stoddart (2007b) has suggested that the proclivity to substance addictions, problem gambling, and excessive use of the Internet and video games might be perpetuated by the tendency to engage in repetitive cognitions and activities.

Adaptive and Life Skills

According to DSM-IV-TR (American Psychiatric Association, 2000), individuals with AS should not show a delay in adaptive behaviors, except in the area of social skills and understanding. Scales of adaptive behavior, which are always used in the diagnostic assessment of those with intellectual disabilities, are frequently used to assess those with AS. Despite the DSM-IV-TR (American Psychiatric Association, 2000) requirement that there should be no delay outside of social skills, in our practices we have found that individuals with AS tend to have lower adaptive skills relative to their intellectual ability. In discussion with family, this deficit seems to be related to an absence of interest in, or perceived need to do certain activities (e.g., domestic chores, budgeting). Alternatively, the difficulty is related to some other disorder, such as obsessive compulsive traits (e.g., not wanting to come into contact with any germs, not opening mail) or executive dysfunction (e.g., being unable to initiate or organize). Some individuals have difficulty understanding or predicting time or distance. For example, we were told of a person leaving the same amount of time to make a 200-mile trip as she would to drive across town. We have also met professionals who cannot plan beyond the month they see on the calendar.

Scales available for rating adaptive skills include the Vineland Adaptive Behavior Scales, Second Edition (VABS-II; Sparrow, Cicchetti, & Balla, 2005), and the Adaptive Behavior Assessment System, Second Edition (ABAS-II; Harrison & Oakland, 2003). The VABS-II has several formats, but none is self-report. The ABAS-II adult scales can be administered through interview, completion by informant, and completion by the patient. Scales are also available to assess adaptive skills that are administered directly by the clinician to the individual, such as the Independent Living Scales (ILS; Loeb, 1996). On the ILS, the person is asked to show his or her ability to use the telephone, write checks, use money, and respond to questions about maintaining home, finances, and other issues relevant to leading an independent adult life.

Executive Functioning

Executive functions are skills that direct and organize complex behaviors, such as inhibition, flexibility, set maintenance, planning, and organizing (Ozonoff & Griffith, 2000; Roth, Isquith, & Gioia, 2005). Although executive functioning difficulties are not diagnostic for AS, the literature has repeatedly identified executive functioning difficulties in affected individuals (Goldstein, Johnson, & Minshew, 2001; Szatmari, Tuff, Finlayson, & Bartolucci, 1990).

Several aspects of executive function can be tested through "hands-on" activities and instruments during neuropsychological testing. Ozonoff (1998) describes areas of testing, including flexibility, planning and organization, and inhibition. She discusses tests and notes areas to observe during testing, such as (1) the approach taken in solving tasks (e.g., trial and error or step-by-step); (2) whether the person gets stuck on one approach to problem solving; and (3) whether the person has difficulties with inhibition.

Those experienced in neuropsychological testing have preferred measures they use to test for executive functions. Some prefer to examine constructs individually, using tests such as the Wisconsin Card Sort Test (WCST; Grant & Berg, 1948; Heaton, Chelune, Tally, Kay, & Curtiss, 1993), which identifies difficulties in changing set, perseveration, and conceptual understanding. Ozonoff (1998) discusses the WCST and notes that it is now available via computer administration. The noted author cautions that children with autism who are high-functioning have been found to score better using the computer than the traditional card administration.

When a comprehensive assessment is required using the WAIS-IV, the Advanced Clinical Solutions (ACS; Psychological Corporation, 2009) may provide adequate assessment of Executive Functions. It contains measures of both perceptual and verbal aspects of EF. Other composite tests of EF are available, such as the Delis-Kaplan Executive Function System (D-KEFS; Delis, Kaplan & Kramer, 2001) and the Behavioural Assessment of Dysexecutive Syndrome (BADS; Wilson, Alderman, Burgess, Emslie, & Evans, 1996), each comprised of several tests that allow for various aspects of EF to be evaluated. The D-KEFS contains nine tests which can be administered and interpreted individually if desired. The BADS is comprised of six tests and two questionnaires. Chamberlain (2003) notes that tests of executive function have been criticized for assessing single abilities in artificial contexts. However, authors of the BADS state that they have developed tasks that are more closely related to real-life situations, which allows better prediction of challenges in executive functioning.

For identifying executive function deficits during a diagnostic assessment with adults, we have found that it is efficient to utilize a questionnaire format, observation, and specific testing on areas identified as difficult. The Behavior Rating Inventory of Executive

Function—Adults (BRIEF-A; Roth et al., 2005) is a 75-item questionnaire that is available in both informant and self-report formats. The person and/or someone who knows the person well completes the scale, rating behaviors as occurring "Never, "Sometimes," or "Often." Resulting scores can be viewed for individual aspects of executive function (e.g., self-monitoring, shifting sets, and emotional control) or as broader index scores (i.e., the Behavior Regulation Index and the Metacognitive Index). An overall Global Composite Index is also calculated.

It should be noted that there is some overlap between symptoms of EF difficulties and Attention-Deficit/Hyperactivity Disorder (ADHD), which is discussed in Chapter 4. If history and symptoms suggest a possible diagnosis of ADHD, this should also be pursued. Checklists are available to supplement information from history and interview including the Conners' Adult ADHD Rating Scales (CAARS; Conners, Erhardt & Sparrow, 1999), the Brown Attention Deficit Disorder Scales (Brown, 1996) or the Adult ADHD Self-Report Scale (ASRS-v1.1; Adler, Kessler & Spencer, 2003).

Sensory Functioning

People with ASDs, including AS, may have extreme responses to sensory input, at either the high or the low end (hyper- or hyposensitivity; Aquilla, Yack, & Sutton, 2005). Those who are hypersensitive to some sensory aspect of the environment may be distracted and unable to attend. They may become anxious or frightened and engage in problematic behaviors or display a panic reaction. Alternatively, they may find the response stimulating and become obsessed with accessing that sensation. People who are hyposensitive may be unaware of sensory features in their environment and miss information that is important for social or safety reasons. Individuals with extreme sensory responses that interfere with their daily functioning should be seen by an occupational therapist for assessment and consultation.

The Adolescent/Adult Sensory Profile (Brown & Dunn, 2002) is designed for an individual to rate his or her experience in several areas of processing, including taste/smell, movement, vision, touch, activity level and auditory processing. Results identify experiences in four quadrants: low registration, sensation seeking, sensory sensitivity, and sensation avoiding. The ratings within the quadrants range across five levels from "Much Less Than Most People" to "Much More Than Most People."

The Adolescent and Adult Sensory Processing Disorder Checklist (see www.Sensory-Processing-Disorder.com) is a measure available on the Internet that was brought to our attention by an occupational therapist. Although it does not provide a score, it does allow sensory issues to be identified in a number of categories and appears to be a practical method to identify concerns.

Motor Functioning

Early literature on those with ASDs identified motor functioning issues, and the literature on AS has included "clumsiness" as a primary feature. There has been some speculation that the specific motor difficulties experienced by those on the spectrum may help us differentiate the disorders (Szatmari, 1998; Smith, 2000). Ghaziuddin, Tsai, and Ghaziuddin (1992b) reported concern that "clumsiness" has not been well defined in the studies that have been carried out. Smith (2000) promotes the idea of studying "underlying perceptual and/or motor planning deficits" (p. 107) as a more pragmatic route to understanding the motor difficulties seen in individuals with AS. Although there are many tests for individual motor functions, at present we could not find an appropriate measure to screen for a range of possible motor issues in adults, and therefore address these concerns through clinical interview only.

We have seen individuals who have trouble in gross motor planning and have had difficulties climbing stairs or engaging in sports. We also frequently see individuals who have difficulties with fine motor functions and cannot write in cursive. An individual who is reported to have motor functioning issues should be referred to an occupational therapist.

Theory of Mind

To have a theory of mind (ToM) means that individuals are aware of their own thought processes and the emotional needs and responses of themselves and others. ToM is an important contributor to self-awareness and to social empathy (Attwood, 2007). The absence of ToM has been referred to as "mind blindness" (Baron-Cohen, 1995). Without ToM, one would not be self-aware in terms of emotions and behavior (e.g., after exploding in a rage, does not understand how he or she appears to others). As well, the person would not be able to take another's point of view, so would always appear self-centered and lacking empathy. In the clinical setting, ToM can be identified during conversation or by using questions, pictures, and vignettes. Deficits are suggested when an individual has difficulty in recognizing joking or sarcasm, lying, deceit, and the subjective nature of beliefs and desires. Problems in ToM make it difficult for a person to understand or predict his or her own or others' behavior.

It has been suggested that individuals with AS may experience less impairment in ToM than others on the autism spectrum (Ozonoff & Griffith, 2000). Some research has shown that individuals who have AS can pass tests examining ToM, reflecting the difference between individuals with autism and those with AS. However, it has also been argued that in such studies, the tasks used in testing require a relatively low mental age (Baron-Cohen et al., 1997). If higher-functioning individuals with autism or AS pass such tests, one cannot necessarily infer intact ToM. The noted authors have used a more advanced test of ToM with very high-functioning individuals and have found significant weakness.

Important retrospective information can be gathered about an individual's ToM *"in situ"* by gathering information from family members and partners and asking an individual about others' responses to particular social or relationship scenarios. This line of questioning is particularly helpful if the spouse or family member is present in the room so that he or she can confirm or dispute the information. Some individuals are not cognizant that they lack ToM, whereas others have a keen awareness that they have little or no understanding of what others are thinking or feeling. Still other individuals are not aware that others have thoughts or perspectives which are *different* from their own.

Mental Health

We discuss mental health issues related to AS at length in Chapter 3. However, for assessment purposes, it is important to acknowledge that there is a high incidence of mental health difficulties in individuals who have AS (Szatmari, 2007). In fact, almost all of the adults whom we see clinically have struggled with anxiety, depression, or both, at some time in their life, and this source of discomfort is often one of the major reasons for seeking assessment or therapy. The most common mental health issues that coexist with AS appear to be anxiety, depression (Konstantareas, 2005), OCD, and substance abuse (Stoddart, 2005a). In affected females, we see a significant occurrence of eating disorders, including anorexia nervosa, bingeing–purging, and excessive exercise, which may relate to obsessive or sensory issues (Attwood, 2007). Individuals may also present with concurrent bipolar disorder (Gutkovich, Carlson, Carlson, Coffey & Wieland, 2007; Raja & Azzoni, 2008), and there is a growing body of literature suggesting some individuals with AS may present with delusional symptoms (Abell & Hare, 2005) suggesting the presence of a psychotic disorder.

Tantum (2000) points out that some of the disorders that coexist with AS are unrelated to the fact that the individual has AS. However, other disorders such as dyslexia or bipolar disorder may occur more frequently because the person has AS. The author suggests this may be related to heritability. He further points out that anxiety, which is frequently present in those with AS, may be exacerbated by features of an ASD, such as failure in developing relationships, or social responses. We believe there is a need for the clinician to make this distinction and to engage in suitable treatment.

Sometimes a person reports that he or she feels depressed or anxious whereas at other times the person is unaware. One man told us that he did not know he had anxiety because it had always been his constant state. After suffering panic attacks, he was given antianxiety medication. It was only after experiencing reduced anxiety that he realized he had always been anxious. We attempt to evaluate a person's psychological and emotional status during assessment. Sometimes this is through available standardized instruments, and sometimes this is accomplished more informally through observation and clinical interview.

The ideal is not only to elicit the individual's report on his or her experience of anxiety and depression, but also to have someone who knows the person well rate the patient's emotional experience based on observed behavior. For self-report, measures such as the Beck Depression Inventory–II (Beck, Steer & Brown, 1996), the Beck Anxiety Inventory (Beck & Steer, 1990) and the Clark-Beck Obsessive-

Compulsive Inventory (Clark & Beck, 2002) may be utilized. Although no appropriate instruments are readily available for mental health rating by others, we sometimes use the Emotional Problems Scales (Prout & Strohmer, 1991). Although developed for individuals with a mild intellectual disability, we have found this instrument is adequate for use with those suspected of having an ASD. It is available in both "Self-Report" and "Behavior Rating" (by others) formats; we use both formats for comparison.

Emotional Understanding

Individuals who have an ASD, including AS, are believed to have difficulty reading the facial expressions of others, showing empathy, and interpreting their own or others' emotions within a context. However, research in this area has not provided consistent results (Frith, 2004). Frith suggests that this difficulty is most obvious for complex emotions. In our practice, we see some individuals who do appear to be able to read basic emotions of others and recognize emotional cues. More often, however, both individuals and their families report that they struggle with emotional understanding, and unless this is pointed out to them, they remain naïve about others' feelings. As well, their awareness of their own feelings may appear superficial or tied to actions.

"Alexithymia refers to people who have trouble identifying and describing emotions and who tend to minimize emotional experience and focus attention externally" (Bagby, Parker, & Taylor, 1994, p. 23). The Toronto Alexithymia Scale–20 (TAS-20; Bagby, Parker, & Taylor, 1994) is a measure of one's ability to identify and describe feelings, including the focus and intensity of the feelings. It consists of 20 items within three subscales. Although we could not find evidence that it has been used extensively with individuals with ASDs, it has been utilized in empathy research of those with ASDs (Bird et al., 2010). As well, it has shown utility in identifying alexithymia in relatives of individuals with ASDs (Szatmari et al., 2008).

In addition to screening instruments, we have found that informal methods of assessing an individual's emotional understanding are often useful to supplement anecdotal information and clinical observations. An example is the use of "ColorCards" (Harrison,

1996) to determine if a person has trouble with interpreting emotional expression. Some pictures on these cards show close-ups of people displaying obvious facial expressions. Others show groups in which the facial expressions are subtler and the emotion needs to be derived from the context. Individuals being assessed have told us (correctly) that, for example, the person in a picture is happy. When asked, they may say they know this because the person is smiling or they can "see their teeth." When they see other pictures where a person is engaged in a family activity or some other event but not smiling, the person may say (incorrectly) that the pictured individual is mad or sad because he or she is not smiling.

This process is useful to ground further discussion of emotions with the person. We may ask an individual how she knows a specified friend or relative (e.g., brother) is happy, angry, or sad. She may describe the facial expression, but more often she provides a description of actions (e.g., he waves his hands and talks loudly). Often, we find the person either does not attend to, or is unaware of, the emotions of those close to him or her. A common misunderstanding for those who are married occurs when a spouse is not showing strong affect or emotional involvement. If their spouse is sad or withdrawn because of something that has happened and is not expressing it verbally, the individual with AS assumes that there is nothing wrong. The spouse feels rejected, believes that his or her partner does not care, and the affected person has no idea that this has occurred.

Family members typically report that the individual rarely labels his or her feelings, and usually the person with AS acknowledges this. Some tell us they know how they feel, but do not understand the need to talk about it. Others tell us that they have difficulty labeling their feelings. We frequently find that these individuals expect others to know how they feel without their having to talk about it. Because of the tendency to present with either less facial expression than others, or with affect that is not appropriate to the context, people with AS can be "hard to read" emotionally, except for instances of intense anger or rage. Regardless of the person's situation, emotional response and awareness provide important information for increasing social adaptation and providing treatment. Box 2.3 summarizes the assessment process described in this chapter.

BOX 2.3. SAMPLE ASSESSMENT PROTOCOL

1. Clinical interview

2. Developmental and service history

3. Tests administered:

   - Gilliam Asperger's Disorder Scale
   - Gilliam Autism Rating Scale
   - Asperger Screening Questionnaire for Adults
   - Wechsler scale (WAIS-IV OR WASI)
   - Advanced Clinical Solutions for the WAIS-IV and WMS-IV
   - Adaptive Behavior Assessment System
   - Comprehensive Receptive and Expressive Vocabulary Test
   - Test of Pragmatic Language
   - Social Problem-Solving Inventory
   - Behavior Rating Inventory of Executive Function
   - Adolescent/Adult Sensory Profile
   - Beck Anxiety Inventory
   - Beck Depression Inventory
   - Clark-Beck Obsessive-Compulsive Inventory
   - Brown ADD Scales
   - Emotional Problem Scales
   - Toronto Alexithymia Scale
   - Test of Social-Know-How

4. Informal testing and observation of communication and behavior patterns, executive functioning and theory of mind, social interaction and understanding

---

DIFFERENTIAL DIAGNOSIS AND THE BROADER AUTISM PHENOTYPE

There is a risk of misdiagnosis if a complete investigation is not conducted or if a clinician is not experienced in certain disorders. Sometimes an individual who has been given a different diagnosis presents for assessment. The person is looking for clarification of the diagnosis or for an alternative diagnosis. As well, an individual may present with a query of possible AS, bringing substantial evidence to support his or her belief. Initially, the assessing clinician needs to remain open to many alternatives. Although clinicians use tools to assess for the presence of symptoms of AS or other ASDs, there is a risk that if they consider the results too narrowly, they might not obtain an adequate history or conduct a broad enough interview, resulting in an diagnostic error (Stoddart et al., 2002a).

Often, the differential diagnosis will be between the three diagnoses on the spectrum: autism, AS, or pervasive developmental disorder, not otherwise specified (Fitzgerald & Corvin, 2001). However, there may be other disorders that present similarly to ASDs. Disorders that may sometimes be confused with AS include schizophrenia, schizoid personality disorder, attention-deficit/hyperactivity disorder, obsessive–compulsive disorder, affective disorders, semantic pragmatic disorder, and nonverbal learning disability (Szatmari, 1998; Fitzgerald & Corvin, 2001).

Often when a diagnosis is given to a child with an ASD, a parent may comment that he or she is much like this child. Other times, the clinician may see characteristics of the child in the parent, although the parent does not meet the criteria for a diagnosis. Increasingly there is evidence that suggests a genetic causation for ASDs (Nicholson & Szatmari, 2003).

Research by Piven and colleagues (1997) examined family history in terms of communication and social deficits and the presence of stereotypic behaviors, common features of ASDs. In families where there were multiple cases of ASDs, they found individuals without a diagnosis of an ASD who nevertheless presented with some features of an autistic disorder. The authors reviewed several studies that had appraised features of autism in family members who did not have an ASD, including language and reading ability, executive function, cognitive performance, and personality traits (Dawson et al., 2002). The authors further reported on research in cognitive neuroscience and genetics that has advanced the concept that many genes may contribute to the susceptibility of developing an ASD. They suggest that more research is needed to help us understand the symptoms of ASDs and the systems that lead to variability in presentation.

ASSESSMENT OUTCOME

When individuals meet with a professional for an assessment and diagnosis, they are expecting an outcome that will make some positive or helpful effect on their lives. The clinician should be sensitive to the direction of the impact of the diagnosis (positive or negative for the person and his or her family). Feedback should include information about the diagnosis, given in a clear manner. Realistic recommendations should be made based on the issues raised in the assessment. The clinician should offer referrals to other professionals, when appropriate, and provide a written report for the individual and offer further discussion later if the person requires additional explanation about what has been identified. It is often useful to have the person who has been assessed invite a family member or close friend to be present at the feedback session in case he or she does not remember or understand all the information given (Burke, 2005).

In our practices, we have seen individuals who have learned to compensate for difficulties and do not see a need for any change or support. Often, they agree to come to the assessment to appease a parent or spouse. Discussion with this person is important to determine what difference a diagnosis might make in his or her life. Sometimes the client decides to continue with the assessment and take advantage of recommendations and supports. Occasionally, a person may state that a diagnosis would not change his or her life in any way and that he or she does not wish to be labeled. To pursue the diagnostic assessment with this individual would not be advisable. Instead, counseling with the referring person to help him or her develop strategies for coping and for talking through their concerns would be more fitting, leaving the door open for future involvement. At times, the individual suspected of having AS may be reluctant to be labeled, but will want to continue contact with a professional to address some of the problems in his or her life. In such cases, pursuit of a diagnostic label may be off-putting, and if the clinician continues to pursue such a focus, the individual may cease all professional involvement. A formal diagnostic label may be pursued after establishing a good therapeutic alliance or professional relationship with the person.

SUMMARY

Individuals with AS who have reached adulthood without receiving a diagnosis likely have experienced isolation, rejection, confusion, and possibly extreme distress due to the obvious disconnect between their cognitive ability, perceived motivation, and their lack of social awareness and skills. Assessment and diagnosis may provide a better understanding of why this disconnect has happened for the person and for those around him or her. The assessment should be completed by a clinician experienced in ASDs, and should examine not only the possibility of AS, but also of alternate or coexisting disorders. Standard measures should be utilized when they are available, supplemented with a solid history, informal assessment, observation, and anecdotal information. Results should offer the person realistic recommendations that address access to information and resources, help him or her learn cope with, compensate for, or overcome the difficulties experienced, and that improve his or her quality of life.

The undertaking of adult diagnosis requires continued and focused research into the specific characteristics of AS relative to other ASDs in order to develop a universal diagnostic profile. We require further research about the presentation and prevalence of comorbid issues and traits to assist in determining whether these reflect specific diagnostic subgroups on the autism spectrum. Comprehensive, sensitive, and age-specific assessment tools require development, and existing measures demand further psychometric evaluation and refinement. The social and emotional costs of late diagnosis, in addition to the positive impact of diagnosis, may be uncovered in much-needed longitudinal studies. Such research will undoubtedly reinforce the importance of early and accurate diagnostic procedures for this group.

The following e-mail from an individual we diagnosed illustrates the relief and hope that can result from an accurate diagnosis, even received later in life:

I just got home, and I burst into tears. Thank you both so much. When you are on your rocking chairs, look up and remember me amongst others I am certain that you've helped so much. I "knew," however, objective naming is paramount to actualization. So much of my life makes SENSE now, where before,

I was hemming and hawing and rowing my little boat over that mountain right behind the Little Engine . . . that can. I can.

Your work is important. It has, in no small feat, changed my life, my perspective newly enabled, I go onwards. Although, I guess I have to accept now that regular humans were indeed my parents, and no one is coming to pick me up. Ah well. One fantasy let go, a new dream realized. I'm allowed. Thank you.

Chapter 3

MENTAL HEALTH SYMPTOMS IN ADULT ASPERGER SYNDROME

CASE EXAMPLE: MENTAL HEALTH SYMPTOMS IN ASPERGER SYNDROME

As Tom hesitantly approached the clinic reception desk, his gaze was noticeably downcast, his posture stooped, his arms swinging out of tandem with his legs. He was dressed in a full-length black coat, inappropriate for the mild spring weather. After answering the receptionist's request for his name, he sought refuge in a chair in the far corner of the waiting room.

During the assessment interview, Tom explained that panic attacks were interfering with his ability to complete his job as a pizza delivery person. Despite achieving good marks in high school, he had recently quit college after attending a concert there. He explained that while waiting outside the concert, his peers had engaged in "a secret social code to which he had not been given privy." Unfamiliar colloquialisms, the exchange of "high fives" and other foreign hand signals left him feeling bewildered and precipitated a panic attack, leading to his immediate departure from campus and resulting in withdrawal from school the next day.

Over time, Tom spoke of his fascination with cityscapes. He brought to my office large-scale, detailed drawings of plans for the urban expansion of a city he had once driven through, having detailed per capita needs for police enforcement, schools, water, electricity, recreation, and strategic locations for ambulances and fire services. He disclosed a distressing sense of loneliness and the perception that a peer's invitation at work to buy him drinks and dances from exotic dancers was an ultimate act of friendship. He was recently warned by police that his unannounced visits to a female acquaintance's home, bearing gifts and flowers, were unwelcome, and he was at risk of being charged with trespassing.

Retreating further to solitude, with much courage Tom disclosed that he watched pornographic movies in his bedroom, aware that this would engender strong family disapproval given the religious beliefs of his parents. He expressed a compassionate, humanitarian concern for children he felt might be conceived on the production sets of these movies, and ultimately felt that his continued involvement in this activity would be punished by "the sperm police." He expressed the belief without any other delusions, hallucinations, or disorganized behavior, that semen shot through the television screen would infect his body with cancer cells. This guilt was compounded by a series of ego-dystonic intrusive thoughts that great harm would come to his family if he did not tap his fingers on the lane change indicator in his car in a specific sequence, to temporarily quell his overwhelming anxiety.

Tom's diagnosis of AS at age 23 was accepted as a mixed blessing: an answer to the sense of alienation that he had experienced most of his life, but also a challenge to incorporate into his identity and reconcile with the possibility that some of his life dreams may not come to fruition. I was faced with deciding if his perception of reality was arising in the context of a psychotic disorder or attributable to a strong social conscience and an idiosyncratic style of perceiving the world.

The intent of this chapter is to review common mental health conditions and symptoms that the clinician will encounter when working with individuals on the autism spectrum. Specifically, we describe anxiety disorders (including social anxiety disorder, panic disorder, obsessive–compulsive disorder, and post-traumatic stress disorder), mood disorders (including depression, suicide and suicidal ideation, and bipolar disorder), psychotic disorders (including schizo-phrenia, paranoia, and delusional disorder), personality disorders (including schizoid and borderline personality disorders), eating disorders, and gender identity disorder. In conclusion, we provide a detailed discussion of methods with which to assess mental health and behavioral disorders, including self- and other-report measures, interview, and observation measures. We begin this summary with a reflection about the importance of first-hand accounts in providing a subjective perspective on mental health concerns in the context of AS and a summary of prevalence studies.

UNDERSTANDING EMOTIONAL EXPERIENCE THROUGH PERSONAL ACCOUNTS

Considering the relative scarcity of scientifically based evidence, our understanding of the emotional lives of adults with AS has been heightened by individuals with ASDs and their families. A host of books, Internet sites, and blogs have allowed professionals insights into the emotional lives and mental health of these individuals, at-titudes toward prescribed psychotropic medication, and the signifi-cant diversity of response to these.

Daniel Tammet (2006) describes the sensory experience of an adult with AS, providing a vivid account of the phenomenon of synesthesia, a neurological mixing of senses. He notes: "Mine is an unusual and complex type through which I see numbers as shapes, columns, tex-tures and emotions" (p. 2). This sensory experience has allowed him the ability to calculate large numbers in his head without any undue effort, eventually allowing him to set a world record by memorizing and recalling pi to 22,514 digits. On the impact on his emotional state, he comments: "Numbers are my friends and they're always around me. Each one is unique and has its own personality. The number 11 is friendly and number 5 is loud, whereas number 4 is both shy and quiet. It's my favourite number, perhaps because it reminds me of myself" (p. 2). It would be easy to understand that this description could be viewed by clinicians as symptomatic of a psychotic disorder.

Dr. Temple Grandin and Shawn Barron (2005) describe their unique journeys in developing social skills and finding purpose in their lives. They emphasize differences in their journeys, but acknowledge the pervasiveness of anxiety in the lives of individuals with ASDs. Both describe adolescence as a socially isolating and anxiety-provoking transitional period. Grandin stresses the need to address sensory issues, in the context of a structured, positive, behavioral-oriented, sensory-friendly program with extended opportunities for practice.

Unfortunately, current diagnostic standards fail to recognize the spectrum of diversity among individuals, causing parents such as Paradiz (2002) to despair:

> The professional literature on autism, which I rely on for information about Elijah's [her son] way of life, is impossible to embrace wholeheartedly. Elijah fits the diagnostic picture and yet he is being framed by a language that cannot shake its negativities and technicalities, a language so cautiously self-involved with clinical precision that it overlooks the problem of its own ephemeral standards and presumptuous conventions. (p. 60)

PREVALENCE OF MENTAL HEALTH CONCERNS

Although there is a range of opinions about what should be considered a psychiatric disorder, we support the definition offered by Ghaziuddin (2005): "Any behavioral or emotional disorder which causes a significant degree of distress or impairment to the individual, the family, or to the community" (p. 7).

When considering mental health disorders in those who have AS, the literature lacks clarity. Many studies combine those with AS and with other ASDs and often do not discriminate between those who have an ASD and those who have a comorbid intellectual disability. The literature has also focused on children or combined research subjects across age ranges. Further, there is some question about the appropriateness of some measures and methodologies used to identify mental health problems in those with ASDs.

In the developmental disabilities field, individuals with both an intellectual disability *and* a psychiatric disorder are said to have a "dual diagnosis." This term should not to be confused with the meaning in the broader psychiatric community (i.e., diagnosis of a psychiatric and a substance abuse disorder). There is some evidence to suggest that those with comorbid intellectual disability (ID) and an ASD may be more prone to developing secondary mental health disorders than those with ID alone. A Canadian study found the prevalence of psychiatric disorders to be 44% in a group of adolescents and young adults with autism and ID, compared with only 17% for those with ID alone (Bradley & Bryson, 1998).

However, more recent studies, reviewed by Underwood, McCarthy, and Tsakanikos (2010), indicate that results are not this clear. Although many individuals with ASD and ID do experience mental health difficulties, the more problematic issues may relate to behavioral difficulties and social and adaptive skills deficits. The noted authors indicate that larger sample sizes and better established clinical tools are needed to clarify this issue. Matson and Boisjoli (2008) state that "Adults diagnosed with ASD and comorbid Axis I diagnoses have been neglected . . . in the area of scale development and diagnosis" (p. 284). Their study attempted to establish the psychometric properties of the Autism Spectrum Disorder—Comorbidity for Adults (ASD-CA), for use with those who have an ASD and concurrent ID. A later study by LoVullo and Matson (2009) using this measure did show significant differences between those with ID, those with ID and ASD, and those with ID, ASD, and psychopathology. Their findings indicated that "the ID + ASD group scored significantly higher than the ID group on most subscales except for Conduct Problems" (p. 1293).

In a study of psychiatric disorders and AS in children and youth, Ghaziuddin, Weidmer-Mikhail, and Ghaziuddin (1998) discovered in a small sample of 35 patients with AS ($M = 15$ years of age) that 23 (65%) presented with psychiatric disorders. These included attention-deficit/hyperactivity disorder (ADHD), oppositional defiant disorder, Tourette syndrome, depression, obsessive–compulsive disorder, generalized and separation anxiety, and learning disabilities. A survey of hospitalized children with psychiatric diagnoses found that 3.2% of subjects qualified for a diagnosis of ASD as well (Sverd, Sheth, Fuss, & Levine, 1995).

In our own study of 100 comprehensively assessed adults (21 years and over) with ASDs seen in an agency for individuals with developmental delays, 13 subjects had one mental health diagnosis, 3 subjects had two mental health diagnoses, and 1 subject had three diagnoses. Of these 18 mental health diagnoses, 50% included OCD, OCD traits, and anxiety; 15% were tics or Tourette disorder; 10% were psychosis, depression, and "other disorders"; and 5%, schizophrenia (Stoddart et al., 2002a). Complementing our findings, the published clinical literature has provided clinical case descriptions of mental health problems in young adults with AS (Hare, 1997; Simblett & Wilson, 1993; Wing, 1981).

In a study of psychiatric outpatients, Nylander and Gillberg (2001) discovered that out of 1,323 adults, at least 1.4% met diagnostic criteria for AS, again suggesting a significant overlap between mental health problems and ASDs. In another screening of adults admitted to a psychiatric unit, five were found to have previously undiagnosed AS out of 2,500 cases (0.2%; Raja & Azzoni, 2001). In this group, two patients had depressive symptoms and four presented with obsessive–compulsive symptoms. In a study of adults with ASDs who were psychiatric patients, those with ASDs were compared to a non-ASD group (Ryden & Bejerot, 2008). Before referral to the program, the authors reported that most common psychiatric diagnoses received by the ASD individuals were depression and OCD.

In a European study of individuals referred for clinical services, 122 persons with ASDs were identified, all with normal levels of intelligence (Hofvander et al., 2009). Of these, 5 had autistic disorder, 67 had AS, and 50 had a diagnosis of pervasive developmental disorder not otherwise specified (PDD-NOS). The authors noted that those with PDD-NOS had a higher prevalence of ADHD than did those with AS. Of the total group, 12% were found to have a psychotic disorder, and 16% experienced substance abuse issues. Many in the group were diagnosed with an anxiety disorder, including 15% with generalized anxiety disorder, 13% with social phobia, 11% with panic disorder or agoraphobia, and 6% with a specific phobic disorder. Other diagnoses given included personality disorders and impulse control disorders.

Through examination of various clinical samples, clinicians and researchers have increasingly begun to explore the risk of individuals with ASDs developing comorbid psychiatric illness in adulthood. The implications of not proactively addressing the comorbid mental health issues in ASDs concern clinicians working in the field of autism, as well as the individuals themselves and their families. Berney (2004) reminds us that a diagnosis of a psychiatric comorbidity in an individual with AS "on its own is of limited value, but it is the gateway to a great deal of information, specialist groups and resources, including financial support" (p. 343).

Almost one-third of the parents surveyed in the United Kingdom (Barnard, Harvey, Potter, & Prior, 2001) indicated that their offspring with an ASD had already suffered with a mental illness, and late diagnosis of AS was associated with developing mental illness. "Where diagnosis was late [mental health problems] rose to 45% of those diagnosed in their 20's and 50% of those diagnosed after the age of 30" (Barnard et al., 2001, p. 22). Symptoms of illness included depression (56%), nervous breakdown or "near breakdown" (11%), and suicidal ideation or attempted suicide (8%). An adult (eventually diagnosed with ASD) described the ramifications of the previous and inaccurate diagnoses in this report:

> I suffered severe depressions resulting in self-injury, thoughts of suicide, hopelessness, failure and self-hatred. I couldn't do anything for myself. I had to be told to wash and be taken to the bathroom and I didn't eat and became very underweight. I was given various types of drugs and anti-depressants. I was diagnosed as a result of the depression. The first diagnosis was schizophrenia and then severe clinical depression with suicidal tendencies. (Barnard et al., 2001, p. 13)

Fifty-nine percent of parents surveyed in this study felt that the responsibility for their child was not adequately addressed by either the mental health sector or the developmental disability sector. This sentiment was even more pronounced in the parents of people with AS, 64% of whom expressed this view. Clinicians and consumers in North America would readily agree that the situation here for adults with ASDs reflects the picture described in the United Kingdom:

> Currently many people on the medium to higher part of the autism spectrum (and particularly those with Asperger syndrome) are assessed as being ineligible for Learning [i.e., developmental] Disability services on the basis of having an IQ over 70, with no reference to their social and communication difficulties. They are then commonly passed to the mental health team, but are ineligible for support services until they suffer an acute deterioration of their mental health. (Barnard et al., 2001, p. 14)

Ghaziuddin (2005) contends there may be several reasons why the prevalence of psychiatric comorbidities in ASDs is not understood.

These include the lack of trained and experienced professionals accustomed to assessing and diagnosing individuals with ASDs and psychiatric comorbidities, the stigma thought to be associated with receiving a psychiatric label, the "vagaries" of the current diagnostic system that discourage the giving of more than one diagnosis to individuals with ASDs, and the belief that psychiatric symptoms appearing in response to an environmental factor or event should not be considered "disordered" (pp. 8–9). Adding to these reasons is the issue of diagnostic overshadowing (discussed later in this chapter) and the lingering myth that individuals with autism do not experience emotions. The shortage of data about psychiatric illness in *adults* with ASDs is, in part, because of the lack of services for this group, the problems inherent in identifying large clinical and non-clinical samples, and the delayed interest in this older sample of individuals, given the historical focus on ASDs in childhood.

The challenges of settling on definitive psychiatric diagnoses in individuals with developmental disabilities and challenging behaviors have been well established (Reiss & Aman, 1998). Given the risk, however, that a single challenging behavior or mental health trait may have various antecedents (considered from a biopsychosocial perspective), some individuals have advanced a methodology that acknowledges that illnesses have periods of relapse, recurrence, remission, and natural histories, and typically affect multiple domains of an individual's life (i.e., behavioral, cognitive, and affective). Recognizing the limits of existing categorical approaches to diagnosis in individuals with idiosyncratic forms of communication, others have advanced the need to (1) establish operationalized definitions of anticipated signs or symptoms of formulated illness(es), (2) document their presence or absence over time with a suitable method of data collection, (3) regularly review the data to support or refute diagnostic hypotheses, and (4) help individuals and their care providers make well-informed decisions (King, 2006; Lowry, 1997; Pfadt, Korosh, & Sloane Wolfson, 2003).

ANXIETY DISORDERS

The inside home of an autistic can feel like a safe refuge. Autistics are extreme examples of people who just need to be more cloistered. Not all are shy, but all do need to feel the calm of their inner experiences. It centres and soothes some of the anxiety that comes from outside confusion. It's comforting to know that you have a portable sanctuary. (O'Neill, 1999, p. 18)

Anxiety disorders are likely the most common mental health concern the clinician faces in treating individuals with ASDs. The class of anxiety disorders includes general anxiety disorder, social anxiety disorder, panic disorder, obsessive–compulsive disorder (OCD), and posttraumatic stress disorder (PTSD; American Psychiatric Association, 2000); these are relevant for our discussion of anxiety disorders presenting in adults with ASDs.

White, Oswald, Ollendick, and Scahill, (2009) have provided a useful summary of the studies on anxiety disorders in children and youth with ASDs published between 1990 and 2008, totaling 40. Twelve of these papers focused on prevalence rates of anxiety in this population. The authors point out that although there have been no-large scale epidemiological studies of anxiety disorders, the existing research suggests a wide range of prevalence rates. From 11 to 84% of individuals with ASDs experience some form of anxiety, including simple phobias, generalized anxiety disorder, separation anxiety disorder, OCD, and social phobia. They also note: "There is some evidence that the prevalence of anxiety may differ across the specific diagnoses. Children with AS appear most likely to experience anxiety, followed by [those with] PDD-NOS, and then AD" (autistic disorder; Thede & Coolidge, 2006; Weisbrot, Gadow, DeVincent, & Pomeroy, 2005; p. 219). This finding parallels our clinical experience in that we see greater levels of anxiety in those with AS, compared to adults with other higher-functioning ASDs, although anxiety disorders are common across the autism spectrum. It is likely the range of measures and other methods of assessment used, variety of informant(s), samples studied (i.e., clinical versus community-based), and the psychiatric disorders included in these studies leads to much of the variance in the prevalence rates reported.

Russell and Sofronoff (2005) compared children with AS to peers who were clinically anxious. Their results indicate that children with AS who had not been given a diagnosis of anxiety were equally anxious to non-AS children who were considered to be clinically anxious. As well, the parents of the children with AS reported a higher degree of obsessive–compulsive behaviors and fears of physical injury than did the parents of the non-AS controls. Tonge, Brereton, Gray, and Einfeld (1999) reported that children with AS are more anxious and disruptive than children with autism or pervasive developmental disorder not otherwise specified (PDD-NOS). They speculated that this phenomenon may arise because children with AS are more likely to seek out interactions with their peers, creating more opportunities for social rejection, ridicule, and failure in response to core social and communicative deficits. Others would argue that anxiety is pervasive among all children with ASDs, to varying degrees, because of their need to for sameness and adverse reactions to unpredictable environmental changes.

White et al. (2009) and others point out the problem of differentiating between anxiety that can be subsumed under the diagnosis of ASDs versus anxiety that is beyond the scope and intensity of that seen in ASDs. It cannot be assumed that an individual has a "diagnosable" anxiety disorder because he or she has an ASD; however, there are situations when a separate diagnosis of anxiety disorder is warranted. If an individual's anxiety levels are significantly affecting daily functioning beyond that which is typically seen in conjunction with an ASD and require focused and specific treatment, then a diagnosis of a comorbid anxiety disorder is helpful.

Clinical experience suggests that individuals with ASDs and anxiety disorders may present differently than individuals with anxiety disorders but without ASDs. Although we rely on traditional means of assessing anxiety levels, such as standardized measures and clinical report, we have previously noted that individuals with ASDs may both under- and overreport symptoms because of their cognitive profile, the presence of alexithymia, their poor understanding of emotions, poor emotional recall, and poor understanding of "typical" levels of anxiety. We have also observed that individuals with ASDs tend not to report the presence of anxiety that is experienced bodily (e.g., faintness, weakness, tremors, headaches), with the possible exception of stomach and bowel upset, which seems to be common. The clinician should therefore also rely on behavioral indicators to identify the presence of anxiety, such as repetitive behaviors, insomnia, social isolation, and sensory-seeking or -avoiding behaviors (King, Fay, Turcotte, Weildon, & Preston, 2002; McBrides & Panksepp, 1995; Powell, Bodfish, Parker, Crawford, & Lewis, 1996).

Burke (2005) notes the impact of "empty time," referring to unstructured periods when the individual is unsure about what to do and engages in seemingly nonfunctional activity (pacing or other repetitive actions) to reduce anxiety and uncertainty. Similarly, repetitive behaviors such as seated rocking or pacing may function to reduce anxiety and distress or allow the individual to cope with sensory overload. A 65-year-old man with AS, whom we assessed several years ago, presented as quite calm, but we observed very subtle rocking in the interview with him. Another young man repeated certain segments of the clinical interview and could not stop talking at the end of the appointment due to his anxiety. Multiple authors and individuals with AS have provided both hypotheses and subjective explanations for seemingly nonfunctional routines and behaviors. These contributions have raised concern that attempts to treat intense areas of interest or insistence on sameness and ritualized behavior pharmacologically or behaviorally may diminish helpful and adaptive means developed by individuals in their attempt to cope with anxiety.

Displays of anger and aggression may also be indicators of anxiety. One young man with AS was aggressive toward his parents because he was anxious about any changes occurring in the house, about people in the house doing things differently (e.g., putting the milk on the top shelf of the fridge instead of on the door), of people breaking into the house, or "breaking the rules" in the neighborhood. Previous clinical investigations had suggested that he receive anger management training, but had overlooked the combined effect of his ASD and the comorbid contribution of an untreated anxiety disorder. Another individual became extremely anxious when his father wanted to buy a new car and his mother, a new washer and dryer. These fears can be understood as originating from some of the key precipitants in individuals with ASDs (see Chapter 2), but their intensity was even uncharacteristic of an individual with AS.

The etiologies of most psychiatric disorders are thought to be a combination of both environmental and genetic influences (Lesch, 2004). Similarly, there are both genetic and contextual rationales for the high prevalence of anxiety disorders in individuals with ASDs, and specifically in individuals with AS. As for environmental contributions, it is important to recall that some of the core features of ASDs are sensitivity to changes in routines, changes in the behaviors of people, the stress resulting from changes and transitions, difficulties with problem solving (Channon, Charman, Heap, Crawford, & Rios, 2001), and the sensory experience that is present in all environments. Therefore, individuals with ASD are predisposed to having heightened responses to these situations. On the potential contribution of sensory sensitivities, O'Neill (1999) writes:

> The autistic brain functions in a way that means autistics can focus attention like a laser beam, excluding most other stimuli. At the same time, this type of brain has a different way of orienting to various stimuli, so the individual may strongly react to a tiny sound that nobody else can hear. Or the individual may be unable to tune out background noise that is a mere hum to everyone else. (p. 20)

A genetic rationale for the high prevalence of anxiety disorders in this population is supported by the current research that is available on the psychiatric histories of family members of children and youth with ASDs. Although parents of children with other ASDs and AS are commonly examined together in this body of research, the findings are unequivocal: Parents of individuals with ASDs experience significantly elevated rates of anxiety disorders compared to the general population and when compared to parents of individuals with other developmental and medical disabilities. Some of these studies assert that the onset of anxiety disorders is an important feature to consider, given the considerable stress known to accompany raising a child with a disability. Research suggests that for this group of parents, there is a significant onset rate of anxiety disorders before the birth of the child with ASD (Stoddart, 2003, 2005a).

Yirmiya and Shaked (2005) completed a meta-analysis of 17 studies examining data relating to psychiatric problems in parents of children with ASDs. Inclusion criteria required that the autism parent sample be compared to a control group of parents, permitting the calculation of effect size (i.e., the influence of group membership) for each study. Two effect sizes were calculated; one included 37 effect sizes aggregated over all psychiatric difficulties, and the other included 70 effect sizes in which the specific psychiatric issues were represented separately. Although the effect sizes were small, parents of children with ASD showed significantly more psychiatric difficulties compared to parents of children with either Down syndrome or mental retardation. Mothers and fathers of children with autism showed higher levels of psychiatric disorders compared with mothers and fathers of all other children.

A disregard of family mental health history has also been identified as an example of diagnostic overshadowing—that is, attributing behaviors of concern to the disability rather than to a comorbid disorder (Reiss, Levitan, & Szyszko, 1982). It is important to obtain a comprehensive family history of mental health concerns during the assessment phase of treatment (Reiss et al., 1982), given the current state of knowledge about the genetics of DSM-IV-TR Axis I diagnoses (Buitelaar & Willemsen-Swinkels, 2000). Previously identified patterns of comorbidity are helpful in diagnostic formulations, given the higher likelihood that an individual with one Axis I diagnosis will have another. In addition, awareness of the history of treatment responsiveness to drugs in particular classes among family members guides the clinician in choosing medication for the current client.

Social Anxiety Disorder

Social anxiety disorder (or social phobia) involves a marked and persistent fear of not meeting expected social standards and may be associated with demanding social situations, such as giving a lecture. Social anxiety is the most common anxiety disorder in the general population and the third most common psychiatric disorder, trailing behind depression and alcoholism (Figueira & Jacques, 2002). In distinguishing typical social anxiety from that which may require treatment, two questions might be asked: "(1) 'Does the patient avoid the phobic situation, or endure it only with intense anxiety?' (2) 'To what extent has the shyness impaired the patient's job, family, or personal life?'" (Figueira & Jacques, 2002, p. 42).

It seems obvious that individuals with impaired social skills and ability to interact socially will have some degree of social anxiety. In fact, some of the individuals we see in practice, who later receive a diagnosis of AS, have a preexisting accurate diagnosis of social anxiety disorder. According to the DSM-IV-TR (American Psychiatric Association, 2000), the diagnosis of social anxiety disorder should not be made in individuals with AS, because the AS label takes precedence. However, we feel that awareness of symptoms that reflect social anxiety can be beneficial to individuals with ASD and aid them in their pursuit of focused and specific treatment for their social anxiety. The interventionist can target the specific area of distress and adapt treatments for social anxiety that have been empirically validated in the general population.

A clear distinction between core symptoms of AS and those of social anxiety disorder has been discussed by the Social Anxiety Institute (2007). Individuals with social anxiety disorder display extreme interpersonal hypersensitivity, often avoid crowded or busy social environments, and are vulnerable to developing comorbid major depressive disorder and/or panic disorder. Precipitants to, and perpetuators of, the pervasiveness of anxiety in individuals with AS have been identified as including feelings of social inadequacy arising from an acute awareness of being different and increased nervous system overarousal, leading to overreaction to low-level stimuli.

In Table 3.1 we list possible antecedents and perpetuators of social anxiety, based on the existing research in the fields of ASD and social anxiety, and on our clinical practices. We have found it useful to have our clients with social anxiety and AS rate the relative contribution of each factor during assessment so that we can better attempt to ameliorate the symptoms in ongoing treatment. We use the Redpath Social Anxiety Checklist (Stoddart, 2010) to serve as a guide for treatment and as a point of discussion in our cognitive–behavioral therapy (CBT) groups for adults with AS. We also advise, when using standardized scales to assess anxiety, that the clinician utilize a scale that addresses social anxiety specifically or has a social anxiety subscale embedded in it, such as in the Multidimensional Anxiety Questionnaire (MAQ; Reynolds, 1999).

Panic Disorder

Although we feel that panic attacks occur commonly in adults with AS, the literature is sparse on assessing and treating panic disorder in these individuals. Pardhe and Nandy (2006) reported on 10 cases of children, ages 8–12, suffering from panic attacks. The authors stated that the children's "obsession with time, place, person is so high that any change in such condition could make them upset or anxious" (p. 45). The children were treated over a 3-month period

TABLE 3.1. REDPATH SOCIAL ANXIETY CHECKLIST (STODDART, 2010)

Please rate the degree to which each of the following contributes to your social anxiety.

POSSIBLE FACTORS INFLUENCING SOCIAL ANXIETY	NOT AT ALL	A LITTLE	QUITE A BIT	A LOT
1. Poor social skills (e.g., standing close, talking too much)				
2. Lack of perspective-taking (i.e., seeing others' point of view)				
3. Missing important social cues (e.g., facial expressions)				
4. (Social) Anxiety runs in the family (e.g., genetic basis)				
5. Few opportunities for social interaction				
6. Lack of desire for social contact				
7. Lack of common interests for age or gender				
8. Sensory overload and unpredictability in social situations				
9. Lack of success when social interaction is attempted				
10. Past or present bullying and exclusion by peers				
11. Heightened awareness of your social differences				
12. Poor organizational skills (e.g. when making social plans				
13. Inflexible thinking (i.e., problems agreeing on activity)				
14. Heightened awareness of your own anxiety				
15. Misunderstanding social behaviors of others				
16. Unpredictable social behavior of others				
17. Repetitive negative thoughts about social situations				
18. Prosopagnosia (i.e., "face-blindness")				
19. Imposed eye contact with others				
20. Lack of structure/activity in social situations				
21. Problems paying attention to activity/ conversation				

by a combination of diverting activities, early preparation preceding events that precipitate the panic response, relaxation training, systemic desensitization, vicarious conditioning, and allowing for their thoughts to flow more freely. The treatment produced a reduction in both frequency of attacks and severity of symptoms.

It is important to understand that the catastrophic interpretations associated with the precipitation of a panic attack, in response to overarousal or physiological signs and symptoms of anxiety, are much more literal and concrete than those voiced by individuals without AS. We have seen individuals who have suffered panic attacks and severe anxiety reactions due to over-arousal from the environment, sensory reactions, concrete thinking, and confusion due to lack of logical thought processing. One young man's mother said that if her son thought he'd done something wrong, he believed his father would have a heart attack. Although in this case the young man didn't have an outright panic attack, he spent the day with extremely high anxiety that interfered with performance of any activity. One client responded to a fire alarm test by running from the building and pounding her head on a brick wall. Another person misplaced an item in the kitchen and when he could not find it, thought that he might have swallowed it—a thought that triggered a panic response.

Obsessive–Compulsive Disorder

Restricted, repetitive, and stereotyped patterns of behavior, interests, and activities are essential criteria for AS (American Psychiatric Association, 2000). These may include: "(1) encompassing preoccupation with one or more stereotypic and restricted patterns of interest that is abnormal either in intensity or focus, (2) apparently inflexible adherence to specific nonfunctional routines or rituals, (3) stereotyped and repetitive motor mannerisms (e.g., hand or finger flapping or twisting, or complex whole-body movements, (4) persistent preoccupation with parts of objects" (p. 84). The use of the words *stereotyped* and *nonfunctional*, as well as anecdotal references to "obsessive" interests held by adults with AS, has unfortunately led to semantic confusion among clinicians and nonclinicians in attempts to identify the presence of comorbid OCD in individuals with AS. Lorna Wing (1981) noted: "Repetitive interests and activities are part of Asperger's syndrome, but the awareness of their illogicality and the resistance to their performance characteristic of the classic case of obsessional neurosis are not found in the former" (p. 122). Original and novel interest in hobbies, mathematical talents, musical and artistic talents are often colloquially referred to as obsessions, but do not fulfill the DSM-IV-TR (American Psychiatric Association, 2000) definition of an obsession (Diagnostic Criteria for 300.3 Obsessive–Compulsive Disorder):

1. recurrent and persistent thoughts, impulses, or images that are experienced, at some time during the disturbance, as intrusive and inappropriate and that cause marked anxiety or distress
2. the thoughts, impulses, or images are not simply excessive worries about real-life problems
3. the person attempts to ignore or suppress such thoughts, impulses, or images, or to neutralize them with some other thought or action
4. the person recognizes that the obsessional thoughts, impulses, or images are a product of his or her mind (not imposed from without as in thought insertion (American Psychiatric Association, 2000, p. 462)

Similarly, stereotypies are highly consistent behaviors characterized by repeated, rhythmic, topographically invariant movements or movement sequences that may be functionally significant. Examples include hand flapping, body rocking, characteristic facial expressions, hand and arm movements, and repeated vocalizations that are not compatible with the DSM-IV- TR (American Psychiatric Association, 2000) definition of compulsions:

1. repetitive behavior (e.g., hand washing, ordering, checking) or mental acts (e.g., praying, counting, repeating words silently) that the person feels driven to perform in response to an obsession, or according to rules that must be applied rigidly
2. the behaviors or mental acts are aimed at preventing or reducing distress or preventing some dreaded event or situation; however, these behaviors or mental acts either

are not connected in a realistic way with what they are designed to neutralize or prevent or are clearly excessive (American Psychiatric Association, 2000, p. 462)

Several studies have tried to clarify the topography of compulsions in individuals with ASD to distinguish the symptoms of comorbid OCD from core features of ASD. Using the Yale–Brown Obsessive Compulsive Scale, McDougle and colleagues (1995) compared 50 patients with OCD to 50 age- and sex-matched individuals with ASDs. Overall, repetitive behaviors noted in the ASD group were observed to be less organized and complex than those displayed by individuals with OCD. Specific compulsions, including repetition, ordering, hoarding, telling or asking, touching, tapping, rubbing, and self-damaging or manipulating behaviors were more common in individuals with OCD. McDougle et al. (1995) noted that the individuals with ASD were otherwise less likely to show repetitive behaviors associated with cleaning, checking, or counting. With obsessions, individuals with ASDs were more likely to have obsessional themes of aggression, contamination, and a need for symmetry.

McBrides and Panksepp (1995) noted, in individuals with ASD, an absence of a clear anxiety response to an interruption of repetitive behaviors, a lack of correlation between completion of repetitive behaviors and anxiety reduction, and a frequent association between affects of excitement and happiness and the performance of repetitive behavior. They suggest alternative formulations to understand the etiology of repetitive behavior in individuals with ASDs. Others have developed a tabular guideline (see Table 3.2) to aid clinicians in distinguishing forms of repetitive behaviors potentially observable in individuals with developmental disabilities and ASDs (King, Fay, Prescott, Turcotte, & Preston, 2004).

Posttraumatic Stress Disorder

It is well known that individuals with developmental disabilities and ASDs often have suffered long histories of abuse and neglect (Mansell & Sobsey, 2001), although no known studies have specifically reported the prevalence of abuse and treatment responses in adults with ASDs. The Abuse and Disability Project at the University of Alberta surveyed 215 victims of sexual abuse or sexual assault and their advocates. Strikingly, in 46.6% of cases surveyed, abusers had

TABLE 3.2. Variables Distinguishing Repetitive Behaviors in Individuals with ASD from other Conditions.

	Voluntary or Involuntary (V/IV)	Onset	Rhythm	Observed Behavior	Response to Medication	Common Associated Conditions
Stereotypies	V Non-goal-directed	Slower, no obvious antecedents	Repetitive, rhythmic	Whole/partial body movement; object manipulation	Variable response to multiple medication classes; exacerbated by dopamine antagonists	DD, OCD, TS, anxiety disorder
Insistence on Sameness	V	Slower, intentional, goal-directed	Rigid, repetitive	Routines, repeated routes, resistant to change	No consistent response	Anxiety disorder
Obsessions	IV Irrational, intrusive	Abrupt	NA	Thoughts, impulses, images	Better with SSRIs, mixed results with atypical antipsychotics	OCD, anxiety disorder
Compulsions	V	Slower, intentional, following rules or goal-oriented	Repetitive	Ordering, touching, checking, hoarding, need for symmetry	Better with SSRIs, mixed results with atypical antipsychotics	OCD, anxiety disorder

(Continued)

TABLE 3.2. (CONTINUED)

	VOLUNTARY OR INVOLUNTARY (V/IV)	ONSET	RHYTHM	OBSERVED BEHAVIOR	RESPONSE TO MEDICATION	COMMON ASSOCIATED CONDITIONS
Self-Injury	V/IV	Variable	Variable	Simple or complex muscle movements	Variable response to multiple medication classes	DD, OCD, TS, BPD, anxiety disorder
Tics	IV	Abrupt, rapid non-goal-directed	Nonrhythmic	Simple or complex, motor or phonic	Better with traditional antipsychotics (e.g., haloperidol and pimozide) and atypical antipsychotics (particularly risperidone), clonidine; worse with stimulants (e.g., methylphenidate)	Medication-induced (e.g., stimulants), TS, metabolic disorders
Dyskinesia	IV	Variable, non-goal-directed	Chorea: jerky, non-rhythmic; athetosis: slow, whithering; dystonia: slow, sustained	Orofacial; extremities less common	Better with atypical antipsychotics and vitamin D (equivocal evidence); worse with traditional antipsychotics and antiparkinson agents	Spontaneous metabolic disorders, brain injury, degenerative disorders (e.g., Huntington's chorea)

(Continued)

TABLE 3.2. (CONTINUED)

	VOLUNTARY OR INVOLUNTARY (V/IV)	ONSET	RHYTHM	OBSERVED BEHAVIOR	RESPONSE TO MEDICATION	COMMON ASSOCIATED CONDITIONS
Akathesia	IV	Insidious, non-goal-directed	Nonrhythmic	Limbs	Better with anticholinergics (e.g., benztropine mesylate), benzodiazapines (e.g., clonazapam), beta-blockers (e.g., propranolol); worse with SSRIs, dopamine antagonists	NA
Echolalia/ Verbal Perseveration	V/IV	Immediate or delayed	Repetitive	Speech	No consistent response	TS

Note: BPD = borderline personality disorder; DD = developmental disability; OCD = obsessive–compulsive disorder; NA = not applicable; SSRIs = selective serotonin reuptake inhibitors; TS = Tourette syndrome. Adapted from King, Fay, Prescott, Turcotte, and Preston (2004).

a relationship with the victim specifically related to the victim's disability. Emotionally and behaviorally negative outcomes were experienced by 97.9% of victims (Mansell & Sobsey, 2001). Similarly, a large study by Sullivan and Knutson (1994) concluded that children with disabilities were over three times as likely to be abused as children without disabilities. They suggested a list of factors contributing to a heightened vulnerability to sexual abuse in individuals with developmental disabilities (DD). These include (1) placement in atypical social circumstances (living in isolated, segregated settings); (2) the use of behavioral suppressing, sedating and psychotropic medication in this population; (3) socialization as overly compliant and submissive to authority figures; (4) inadequate sociosexual knowledge and opportunity for age-appropriate sexual relationships; (5) social disempowerment; and (6) communication deficits creating obstacles to disclosure.

Jerry and Mary Newport (2002), a married couple who both have AS, describe several vulnerability factors arising from inherent deficits in communication and social skills in individuals with AS, placing them at risk of entering abusive relationships. These include misinterpreting the social intentions of others, an intense sense of loneliness and isolation, impaired self-esteem, failure to understand social codes and rules, and developing an overvalued interest in others without reciprocation, leading to stalking-like behaviors. We have seen a number of individuals in our practice who have been taken advantage of due to their naivety regarding the intent of others. Attempts to pursue these situations legally have not been successful because the person has "consented," although in fact, he or she was deceived. The consent was believed to be valid, however, because the individual was seen to be cognitively competent.

Tom, the individual introduced at the beginning of this chapter, was "befriended" by a peer in a pizza shop for which both he and this individual delivered pizzas. Unaware of social rules, Tom accepted an invitation by this individual to join him in an adult entertainment hotel. Tom subsequently believed the entertainers when, while intoxicated, he was told that they would like to marry him. He experienced significant shame when his therapist discussed the reality of this situation with him.

It is important to remember that PTSD does not arise only from sexual abuse or domestic or societal violence. Individuals who experience or witness any form of trauma may present with symptoms of PTSD. Such traumas include motor vehicle accidents, (perceived) mistreatment while in institutional care, catastrophic weather events, war or threat of war, and even serious illness or surgery with unexpected pain and physical restriction. We are aware that those with AS may be the subject of serious bullying in their early years and of other forms of social rejection later on (Konstantareas, 2005). Bradley and Burke (2002) discuss conditions which cause vulnerability and promote resilience in those with developmental disabilities. Negative social experiences may lead to the person responding with symptoms of PTSD. We propose that this also applies to those with ASDs.

Making the diagnosis of a comorbid PTSD is challenging in adults with AS, given the overlap between core symptoms of AS and criteria for PTSD. In addition, it may be difficult for adults with AS to verbalize the difference between sensory overload experiences and dissociative phenomena such as flashbacks, depersonalization, and derealization. Though important to diagnose, it is also important not to overdiagnose PTSD, acknowledging that most individuals (with and without AS) who are exposed to trauma that has the potential to produce PTSD, do not in fact develop this disorder (Kulka et al., 1990). This is an area in need of further research. Furthermore, it is important to explore protective factors in individuals with AS that allow them to respond with resilience to traumatic experiences.

MOOD DISORDERS

> There was no cataclysmic event that triggered her suicide. There was no portentous statement made in the days leading up to it. She left no note. The toxicology report showed a combination of drugs in her system. She had swallowed the contents of most of her bottles and jars, even the nutritional supplements. She had done it in the bathroom, which was where they were kept, in a large cabinet with a mirror door. She then went downstairs and peeled back a corner of the tarpaulin that was covering the swimming pool during the winter and climbed into the water and the rotting leaves and mulch. (Nazeer, 2006, p. 173)

Mood disorders include major depressive disorder, bipolar disorders and their variants, as well as mood disorders related to medical conditions or substance abuse. The clinical criteria for these disorders as well as descriptions of mood episodes can be found in DSM-IV-TR (American Psychiatric Association, 2000).

In describing the untimely death of his friend, Nazeer (2006) reminds us of the possible devastating effects of untreated mood disorders in adults with AS. We will never know the multiple variables contributing to Elizabeth's death. Her access to pills suggests that she may have had a comorbid mood disorder. The presence of supplements suggests that prescribed medication alone was inadequate to address her distress. Her failure to leave a note suggests that she felt alienated and alone in an anxiety-provoking, overwhelming world. Climbing into pool water amidst rotting leaves and mulch suggests that she had a severely impaired self-esteem, possibly arising from being teased as a child, experiencing significant challenges in establishing relationships, finding friends and love, despite the best efforts of her existing friends and family.

Depression

Ghaziuddin (2005) has reviewed potential causes of depression in individuals with AS. He notes that many individuals with AS "become aware of their limitations, especially in adolescence" (p. 141). In support of this, Butzer and Konstantareas (2003) investigated the correlations among depression, temperament, social skills, awareness of disability, and psychopathy in children with AS. Their findings indicated that children with severe symptoms of AS also presented with low mood. Those children who had stronger social skills experienced less depression. Parents who rated their children on depression gave higher ratings than the children rated themselves. As well, the more aware the children were of their disability, the greater depression they appeared to experience; this finding was also based on parental report.

Estimates of the prevalence of depression in those with autism and AS range from 4 to 38% (Stewart, Barnard, Pearson, Hasan, & O'Brien, 2006). These authors summarized 27 articles of comorbid ASDs and depressive disorders. Fifteen of the articles were based on case studies of individuals; some had their first episode of depression in childhood and others in adulthood. Of the cases studied, most relied on third-party accounts that were based on observed behavior or facial affect. Depressed mood was most often cited as the marker of depression; other symptoms included loss of interest, changes in eating or sleeping habits, psychomotor slowing, aggression, incontinence, and reduction in self-care.

Hellings (1999) cited three large prevalence studies of the rates of affective disorders in individuals with intellectual disability and ASD. Each of these studies found similar rates of affective disorders, ranging from 3.9 to 8.9% of individuals (Charlot, Doucette, & Mezzacappa, 1993; Meins, 1996; Reiss & Rojahn, 1993). She expressed concern, however, that these studies lacked uniformity and used different samples, ages, informants, methodology, and time frames. Ghaziuddin (2005) suggested that "reports from autistic clinics and psychiatric units suggest that depression is probably the most common psychiatric disorder across the lifespan of an autistic individual" (p. 130). He noted that "at least one child in Kanner's original series had a tendency to lapse into 'a momentary fit of depression'" (Kanner, 1943, p. 241) and that "many of the children described by Asperger had features suggestive of mild depression" (p. 130).

Characteristics such as sleep difficulties, altered eating patterns, and social withdrawal/avoidance are seen in both those with ASDs and those who are depressed (Stewart et al., 2006). The presence of communication difficulties may also interfere with the detection of depressive symptoms. Stewart et al. (2006) suggest that the measures used to identify depression in those with ASDs are inadequate, resulting in lost treatment opportunities for some individuals. Our experience suggests that many behavioral signs of depression seen in the general population are also significant in this clinical group, including loss of interest in usual activities, loss of energy, psychomotor retardation, and a lack of emotional responsiveness.

Suicide and Suicidal Ideation

There is little in the literature that is specific to suicide in those with AS. However, suicide or suicidal ideation is alluded to in a number of articles on ASDs, such as the reference by Stewart et al. (2006) indicating that in the case studies they reviewed, only one individual spoke of suicidal thoughts. Fitzgerald (2007) makes reference to discussion of suicide in those with AS by Gillberg (2002b), Ghazuid-din (2005), and others. They purport that suicidal thoughts and at-tempts are not uncommon in adolescents and adults with AS. Shtayermman (2007) recently examined suicidal ideation in adoles-cents and young adults with AS. The findings suggest that many ado-lescents and young adults with AS experience suicidal ideation.

In the introduction to this section on mood disorders, we were reminded that those with AS can succumb to the need to escape from the overwhelming events of life through suicide. In our prac-tices, we have seen a number of individuals who have presented with suicidal ideation and who have made attempts to end their lives. Methods have included jumping, cutting, hanging, and over-dose. One individual told us that it was a temptation that needed to be faced head on and overcome. Another told us that when life be-came difficult, it was always in the back of his mind as "a way out." We often reframe thoughts of suicide successfully as a "dysfunctional cognitive escape," and note that it is important to replace this "es-cape" with healthier ways of coping with a stressful or painful situ-ation. These healthier forms—for example, meditation, positive cognitive reappraisal, modifying the environment or situation, and help-seeking behaviors—can then be taught to the person.

Bipolar Disorder

According to the DSM-IV-TR (American Psychiatric Association, 2000), bipolar disorder (BD) has been subcategorized into bipolar 1, bipolar 2, and BD not otherwise specified. The term *bipolar affective disorder spectrum* has been introduced to include variations of these disorders. Bipolar 1 requires an episode of mania, but not necessarily depression. Bipolar 2 reflects at least one episode of both hypomania and of depression, but not necessarily mania. The terms *cyclothymia, substance-induced mood disorders, mood disorders secondary to a general medical condition,* and *schizoaffective disorder—bipolar subtype* reflect variations of mood as defined in DSM-IV-TR (American Psychiatric Association, 2000). The symptoms of the hypomanic, manic, and depressed phases of BD are typically described verbally as subjective experiences by the affected individuals. In mania, these symptoms include a self-perceived inflated self-esteem and grandiosity and the subjective experiences of racing thoughts or flight of ideas. In the depressed phase of the illness, these symptoms include a sense of worthlessness, hopelessness, a lack of future orientation, and thoughts of self-harm. Bipolar episodes are functionally impairing and are not due to direct physiological effects of a substance or general medical condition (American Psychiatric Association, 2000).

BD has been identified in first-degree relatives and probands with high-functioning variants of autism, especially AS, at higher rates than in the general population (DeLong & Dwyer, 1988; DeLong, 1994). Some authors have reported cases of adults with comorbid AS and BD (Raja & Azzoni, 2008). According to the authors, the rate of co-occurrence of these disorders has been difficult to determine due to the diagnostic issues in both AS and pediatric BD. Also confusing is the fact that the early presentation of BD in childhood may appear to be a unipolar depression or another disorder such as OCD or ADHD, with the manic features appearing only later. Other clinicians (Kerbeshian, Burd, & Fisher, 1987; Kerbeshian, Burd, Randall, Martsolf, & Jalal, 1990; Steingard & Biederman, 1987) presented early case reports describing BD in individuals with ASD. Each of these case reports documented responsiveness to lithium carbonate, a mood stabilizer identified as the maintenance drug of choice in practice guidelines for BD (Yatham, Kennedy, O'Donovan, Parikh, & MacQueen, 2005).

Considerable work has highlighted the need to focus on observable behavioral changes to identify the hypomanic, manic, and depressed phases of BD in adults with AS and other ASDs. In mania, these changes include alterations in sleep pattern (a decreased need), energy level (an increased amount), distractibility (decreased productivity in vocational and leisure activities), increased talkativeness, an increase in goal-directed activities, and an increase in excessive activities that have a high potential for painful consequences. In the depressed phase of the illness, observable and measurable changes in behavior include an alteration in sleep pattern (either increased or decreased hours of sleep per night), a decrease or increase in appetite and weight, impaired concentration (again, decreased productivity in leisure and vocational pursuits), and a decreased interest in previously enjoyed activities (anhedonia).

King and McCartney (1999) have presented a method with which to objectively support or refute hypotheses of BD in individuals with DD and ASD in response to treatment recommendations.

They describe a 6-point mood scale based on operationalized defini-tions of behavioral equivalents of the depressed, hypomanic, and manic phases of BD. This method uses a bipolar chart, which, when presented in graphic form, provides a longitudinal perspective on course of illness, allowing informed decision making regarding treat-ment recommendations to be made by individuals and their substi-tute decision makers. The authors initially utilized this method to report on an individual with ASD. Strikingly, when in the manic phase of his BD, the intensity of this individual's core symptoms of autism, specifically his ability and interest in interacting socially and communicating nonverbally, increased significantly. These changes suggested that the neurochemical alterations inherent in mania may have a positive effect on the core symptoms of ASD. King subse-quently refined this method, providing detailed instructions to assist in implementing this methodology. This work was based on Lowry's initial model of symptomatic behavior (Lowry & Sovner, 1992).

King (2000) has also described 26 outpatients with BD and DD, noting that 54% of the sample had the rapid-cycling variant of this disorder (i.e., four or more episodes of depression, hypomania, or mania in a given year). Rapid-cycling individuals noted to have a late onset of increased cycling included a high proportion of females who also had a higher rate of thyroid dysfunction. King (2000) re-viewed the pharmacological treatment of mood disturbances, ag-gression, and self-injurious behavior (SIB) in individuals with ASD. He notes that drugs acting on the brain neurotransmitters (dopa-mine, serotonin, norepinephrine, endogenous opioids, glutamate, and gamma-aminobutyric acid [GABA]) have all been explored in the treatment of aggression and SIB. While acknowledging the multi-determinate nature of these noncore features of ASD, King and others (Gordon, State, Nelson, Hamburger, & Rapoport, 1993; Lewis, Bodfish, Powell, Parker, & Golden, 1996) also note that these challenging behaviors are indicators of an underlying mood disor-der. He concludes with the opinion that no single drug or class of medication has emerged as consistently effective in the treatment of mood disorders in individuals with ASD. In tabular form, he pres-ents a "global picture of the pharmacological strategies that have been described with respect to persons with pervasive developmen-tal disorders (PDD) and aggression, self-injury or mood distur-bance" (p. 440).

We see many individuals who have experiences that may lead clinicians to misinterpret their behaviors as indicative of BD. Some tell us they have a need to withdraw from their typical daily activities because they are exhausted or overwhelmed; this withdrawal may last for a period of hours or days. During this time they tend to isolate themselves in a room or in their home and avoid external stimulation. We have heard these periods referred to as "healing," "repairing," "nesting," and "tree days." Sometimes these individuals have seen practitioners who viewed this behavior as part of a bipolar cycle. We do not agree. Typically, these individuals are in jobs or educational settings where they not only work hard, but do so with the anxiety and sensory difficulties experienced by those with AS. The individuals typically show no other sign of a BD, and we see it as positive that they recognize the need to get "rest and relaxation."

Several years ago we worked with a person who had autism and who had his own cycle of sleep and wakefulness. As long as this person could live according to his own circadian rhythm, he did well, but if he had to conform to the routine of those around him, he deteriorated and engaged in dangerous behaviors. Some practitioners might interpret his fluctuation in mood, sleep, and behavior as signs of BD or as disordered sleep. Since that time, we have seen other clients in our practice with similar individual sleep–wake cycles. We believe that their particular cycles are a disturbance only because they must conform to the schedule of someone else if they are attending work or school. Intervention should address these individuals' need for flexibility in their daily schedule and/or assist them during the period when they find nighttime sleep difficult. Some individuals have responded well to the hormone melatonin, which can be taken as an over-the-counter supplement, as a method to promote sleep.

We also see individuals who show such intensity in relation to their special areas of interest that they appear to be manic, and this has again led to queries regarding BD. Often, the discussion in the clinical interview appears "manic" when observing the degree of detail, perseveration, and affective response about their specialized areas of interest, in comparison to other topics discussed in the interview. It is important to monitor moods, sleep, and behavior, as well as drug and chemical (e.g., caffeine) intake and changes in medications, to determine what, in fact, the clinician is seeing. We feel it is also important, when looking at a possible BD, as with any other mental health disorder, to consider other possible explanations (specific to ASDs) and rule these out systematically. For example, excessive laughing or giggling in the interview (we have noted especially by females) may indicate anxiety, an inability to appropriately exhibit nonverbal communication, or the tendency for individuals with ASDs to "get stuck" in emotional states. Others may laugh, smile, or giggle spontaneously in responses to repetitive thoughts about a favorite interest (e.g., a situation comedy, cartoon, or movie), which, if left unexplored by the clinician, may lead to unfounded concerns about mood dysregulation or even psychosis.

Frazier, Doyle, Chiu, and Coyle (2002), in reporting the treatment of a child with AS and a comorbid BD, noted that the coexistence of a DSM-IV-TR Axis I diagnosis may intensify core features of AS; in this case perseverativeness, ritualistic behavior, social intrusiveness (during the hypomanic/manic phase of a BD), and social withdrawal (in the depressed phase of a BD). The existence of a comorbid, potentially treatable, disorder was therefore discussed.

Assessment and treatment issues regarding adults with AS unfortunately are not addressed in practice guidelines for the treatment of patients with BD. The "Texas Medication Algorithm Project: Development in Feasibility Testing of a Treatment Algorithm for Patients with Bipolar Disorder" (Suppes et al., 2001) or the "Community Network for Mood and Anxiety Treatments (CANMAT) Guidelines for the Management of Patients with Bipolar Disorder: Consensus and Controversies" (Yatham, Kennedy, O'Donovan, Parikh, & Mac-Queen, 2005) are useful resources.

PSYCHOTIC DISORDERS

Psychotic disorders include schizophrenia, schizophreniform disorder, schizoaffective disorder, delusional disorder, brief psychotic disorder, and other psychotic episodes that may be related to medical conditions or substance abuse. These are defined in DSM-IV-TR (American Psychiatric Association, 2000). Only those identified in the literature in association with, or as a possible differential diagnosis with AS are discussed in this chapter. The literature also makes reference to the "schizophrenia spectrum," referring to schizophrenia, schizoptypy, and schizotypal personality disorder, which are hypothesized to be genetically related (Nylander, Lugnegard, & Hallerback, 2008).

Understanding the history of the association between ASDs and schizophrenia is important to practitioners. The term autism refers to "pathological selfdirectedness and introversion" (p. 44) and was seen as a symptom of schizophrenia (Nylander et al., 2008). When children began to be identified with the symptoms we now associate with the label of autism, they were given the diagnosis of childhood schizophrenia or childhood autism. In the early 1970s the terms were interchangeable, much as the terms pervasive developmental disorder and autism spectrum disorder are today. The separation of autism from psychotic disorders took place during the 1970s, when childhood schizophrenia and autism were seen as different entities. Occasionally, we will see an individual with an ASD who received the diagnosis of "Childhood Schizophrenia" prior to the mid-1970s. Family or professionals sometimes believe the person has received a diagnosis of schizophrenia as we know it now, but it frequently meant what we now call an autistic disorder.

Schizophrenia

As is illustrated in the introductory case example, it can be extremely challenging to diagnose the presence of a comorbid psychotic disorder, particularly schizophrenia, in an individual with AS. The core symptoms of this disorder, as outlined in the DSM-IV-TR, are heavily reliant on verbal descriptions of internally felt (subjective) emotional, cognitive, and perceptual experience. Various methods of subtyping those who have schizophrenic disorders have been attempted. DSM-IV-TR refers to the subtypes as Paranoid, Disorganized, Catatonic, Undifferentiated, and Residual (American Psychiatric Association, 2000). Historically, much attention has been given to the identification of positive and negative symptoms in the diagnosis of schizophrenia. Although practitioners utilize DSM-IV-TR subtypes in applying a diagnosis, many continue to use the concept of negative and positive symptoms in identification of the disorder.

Negative and positive symptoms are those behaviors and internal experiences that vary (due to their presence or absence) from what would typically be seen in the normal population. Negative symptoms are those behaviors that appear absent in someone who has a psychotic illness. These might include lack of motivation, flat affect, and reduced speech and social interaction. Positive symptoms are those behaviors and internal experiences that are present in a person with schizophrenia, such as hallucinations or delusions, disordered thoughts/speech/behavior, and the presence of affect that is inappropriate in terms of intensity or context. The term *Mixed Schizophrenia* is applied when individuals "do not meet criteria for either positive or negative schizophrenia, or meet criteria for both" (Andreasen & Olsen, 1982, p. 790).

Individuals with AS sometimes evidence behaviors that would seem odd or bizarre to others. It is important for clinicians to be aware of the various features of AS that might otherwise account for these to ensure that misdiagnosis does not occur. For example, a person wearing sunglasses indoors may be doing this for sensory reasons. In discussion with those who have AS, we have been told that sometimes memories flash in their minds as visual captions. One man described a horror film that, when he thought about it later, came to him in large and frightening images. This experience corresponds to Grandin's (1995) descriptions of thinking in images. In discussion with adults who have AS, some have reported to us that they began to think verbally in adolescence or later, although this is not their predominant means of processing. This man's description also reflects the kind of sensory memory that is reported in those who have been traumatized (Kristiansen, Felton, Hovdestad, & Allard, 1996).

In diagnostic sessions, the question of hearing voices is often posed to assess for auditory hallucinations: "Do you hear voices?" Given that those with AS tend to be literal, this question might elicit an affirmative response, when, in reality, they are experiencing only their internal train of thought. If there is a suspicion that an individual is having auditory hallucinations, this needs to be explored in detail. In our experience, auditory, tactile and visual hallucinations are rare in this population.

Raja and Azzoni (2001) reported on five adults who were admitted to an emergency psychiatric setting and received a diagnosis of AS. Previous diagnoses had been given to them, including early-onset psychosis, paranoid disorder, residual schizophrenia, disorganized schizophrenia, and undifferentiated schizophrenia. All displayed violent behavior. When other symptoms were examined, some reflected characteristics of AS, whereas others were indicative of a psychotic disorder. The authors stated that "comorbid schizophrenia is difficult to rule out in these patients. Psychotic symptoms should not be overvalued in making the diagnosis when specific features of AS are present" (p. 285). In our experience, schizophrenia is overdiagnosed in individuals who have not been identified as having AS, and also in those who have been diagnosed with AS, although to a lesser extent.

Dykens, Volkmar, and Glick (1991) found evidence to suggest that thought disorders exist in adults with ASDs, though it was not clear if these were indicative of a schizophrenic process. We have recently diagnosed an individual with AS and schizotypal affective disorder because the individual was experiencing delusional thinking (i.e., ideas of reference) and paranoid ideation with severe depression and anxiety. There was no indication of other traits of schizophrenia.

Fisman and Steele (1996) point out that negative symptoms of schizophrenia (e.g., withdrawal, apathy, and lack of motivation) appear to parallel core deficits in the lives of individuals with ASD. Berney (2004) discusses the diagnostic confusion between schizophrenia and AS; he suggests this confusion has occurred because the developmental path of symptom presentation has not been considered. He reviews a number of features of AS that may be observed by the clinician and mistaken for a psychotic disorder, including incomplete answers, slow responses to requests, pragmatic difficulties, a lack of emotional awareness, unusual mannerisms and posturing, and improvement with the use of antipsychotic medications.

In spite of the similarities thought to exist historically between psychotic disorders and ASDs, and the research into similar features, at the current time, ASDs and psychotic disorders such as schizophrenia are considered to be distinctly different. Perlman (2000) has cautioned that social withdrawal and depression in response to individuals' with AS awareness of their differences from peers place these individuals at risk of misdiagnosis of chronic undifferentiated schizophrenia.

Although we typically think of schizophrenia and ASDs in terms of differential diagnoses, it is important to be aware that it is possible for individuals with AS to receive a diagnosis of schizophrenia or another psychotic disorder. Gillberg and Billstedt (2000) reported the onset of psychotic symptoms in adolescents who had received a diagnosis of an ASD disorder in early childhood. Ryan (1992) has also suggested that AS be considered in cases of apparent treatment-resistant mental illness, noting the possibility of misinterpreting emotional lability, eccentricities, anxiety, poor social skills and re-petitive behaviors as signs and symptoms of other chronic psychiat-ric illnesses. Leask and coauthors (Leask, Done, & Crow, 2003) re-port that those with schizophrenia present with premorbid features such as disconnectedness and motor clumsiness, which are also symptomatic of individuals with ASDs. They suggest that the similar features may provide some insight into the neurological underpin-nings of the two disorders. The author notes that although the simi-larities do exist, in those with schizophrenia the disorder is progres-sive, whereas in those with ASDs these features are present from childhood.

Anecdotally, many individuals with ASDs, particularly those with histories of institutionalization and trauma, have been prescribed traditional sedating antipsychotics that may compound deficits in social relatedness when removed. Challenging behavior may be re-vealed as consistent with mood or anxiety disorders (particularly PTSD). These behaviors can then be misdiagnosed as disorganized behavior due to delusional thought content and hallucinations symptomatic of a primary psychotic disorder.

Several articles have reviewed the diagnosis of catatonia (the ab-sence of speech and movement and the maintenance of posed pos-tures) in individuals with AS. Wing and Shah (2000) used a semis-tructured interview to determine that 17% of 506 individuals with AS, referred to a specialty clinic, exhibited catatonic features. Rea-sons for this high prevalence remain unclear; however, the authors concluded that catatonia should be included in the differential diag-nosis when a deterioration in adaptive living skills is noted in per-sons with AS, and that AS should be considered as an underlying diagnosis in individuals presenting with catatonia. Neuroimaging studies have shown similar alterations in cerebellar structure in both of these disorders.

Paranoia

Individuals with AS may present with symptoms of paranoia. A model of paranoid delusions has been developed by those doing re-search on psychosis. Research suggests that theory of mind (ToM) may be involved in the presentation of paranoia (Blackshaw, Kin-derman, Hare, & Hatton, 2001). When tested, individuals with AS received a higher score on paranoia and a lower score on ToM when compared to controls. Attwood (2007) relates the paranoia seen in those with AS to social experiences, where hostility/negative interactions can lead to feelings of rejection, causing later interactions to be viewed with suspicion by the individual. According to Attwood, "This can eventually lead to long-term feelings of persecution and the expectation that people will have malicious intent" (p. 341). Those without AS would be better able to interpret events in light of the social context. In our practice, we have witnessed this type of global suspicion in those individuals with AS who have been exploited or abused.

Delusional Disorder

We have met individuals with AS who also meet criteria for a delusional disorder, generally of the grandiose type: That is, these individuals have an inflated sense of power, identity, or of having a special relationship with someone of esteem. We have observed that these individuals also tend to be highly anxious and have poor understanding of boundaries. Abell and Hare (2005) investigated delusional beliefs in those with AS and suggested that those individuals did appear to have a high incidence of delusional belief associated with anxiety and self-consciousness. Whereas others have suggested that "mentalization" may be a factor in the delusional beliefs of those with AS, these authors disagree. They propose that delusional beliefs may be a prominent feature in those with AS. Attwood (2007) discusses delusional beliefs in those with AS and suggests that if a person's special interests relate to areas of fantasy, such as superheroes, he or she may take on this role to achieve social success. He states that "this adaptation to having AS can be of clinical significance when the person cannot separate from the alternative persona and may consider him- or herself to have special or magical powers or omnipotence" (p. 191)

PERSONALITY DISORDERS

Personality develops throughout childhood and adolescence through the interaction of the child with his or her environment. When difficulties are encountered and the person's resulting personality is in some way dysfunctional, this is termed a *personality disorder* (PD) in DSM-IV-TR, which identifies a number of them according to distinct sets of features (American Psychiatric Association, 2000). Gillberg and Billstedt (2000) noted that at the time of their writing, there had been no studies investigating the co-occurrence of AS and PDs. They suggested, however, that there might be an overlap of features between AS and obsessive–compulsive PD, paranoid PD, schizoid PD, and schizotypal PD. Ryden and Bejerot (2008) examined adult psychiatric patients both with and without an ASD to investigate the possible presence of various psychiatric diagnoses. Based on their screening, they found that those with ASD had a higher incidence of symptoms reflecting schizotypal and avoidant PDs.

Schizoid Personality Disorder

A person with schizoid personality disorder presents as emotionally flat, detached from the social environment and interpersonal relationships, and lacking in pleasurable outlets and activities (American Psychiatric Association, 2000). Wolff (2000) and Gaus (2007) have both reviewed the relationship between AS and schizoid personality disorders. Wolff notes that individuals with schizoid personality disorder share many features in common with individuals with AS. These similarities include emotional disturbances, a lack of empathy for others, increased interpersonal sensitivity, mental rigidity, unusual styles of communication, and overinvolvement with topics of interest. However, Tantum (2000) reminds us that the "core syndrome" of the disorders is different, with the core of Schizoid Personality Disorder lying in a "dismissive-avoidant style of attachment" (p. 52). The similarity between these disorders, again emphasizes the importance of getting a good developmental history, as symptoms of ASDs will have been present throughout childhood, while personality disorders aren't established until late adolescence/early adulthood.

Borderline Personality Disorder

Individuals with borderline personality disorder (BD) have unstable relationships and disturbed self-image. They may also be impulsive, reactive in mood, and engage in behaviors that cause self-harm (American Psychiatric Association, 2000). Ryden and colleagues (Ryden, Ryden, & Hetta, 2008) assessed women who had received the diagnosis of BPD, verified through administration of the Structured Clinical Interview for the DSM-IV—Second Edition (SCID-II). The women were then examined for symptoms of ASDs. Six of 41 individuals with a borderline diagnosis were found to meet criteria for a diagnosis of an ASD. The women with ASD had lower global functioning and higher rates of suicide attempts; they were also noted to have a negative self-image. Similarities have been found between early trauma (and subsequent PTSD) and BD (Hodges, 2003).

While little else could be found in the literature about the relationship between BD and AS, a search of the Internet found many blogs, testimonials, and other formats of information sharing by individuals who had received both diagnoses and expressed confusion. These also made reference to the high incidence of misdiagnosis of BD in cases of AS. Therefore, although we cannot provide a credible resource, we can state that in the community of those who have received questionable diagnoses of BD and believe they may have AS or both disorders, there seems to be a sense of abandonment.

The literature has recently identified that many women with AS are being missed in diagnosis. Among possible differences seen in women with ASDs, according to Attwood (1999a), are the subtler presentation of symptoms in women, a tendency to verbalize and exhibit a more passive personality, and a tendency for females to be nurturing toward others, assisting them in situations where boys might become more "predatory." We agree that these differences may explain in part why women are being missed, and we would add that the oversight may also be due to diagnostic overshadowing by, for example, PTSD, BD, and eating disorders—our next topic.

EATING DISORDERS

In the last decade, a number of authors noted that of those individuals with eating disorders, a larger than expected number has an ASD, including AS. This is particularly so for *females* with ASDs, who meet criteria for an eating disorder (Gillberg, 2002b; Attwood, 2007). Gillberg (2002b) stated that although there is little in terms of research on the relationship between AS and eating disorders, there is substantial clinical evidence. Some studies have shown that women with anorexia nervosa had a high incidence of AS or of another ASD. As well, young men with AS who develop unusual eating habits and become thin may meet criteria for anorexia nervosa.

One study examined a group of women in a clinical setting diagnosed with eating disorders (Wentz et al., 2005). The authors reported that 53% had a minimum of one childhood-onset neurological disorder, 27% had tic disorder, 23% had an ASD, and 17% had ADHD. Kalyva (2009) looked at adolescent females who had a diagnosis of AS, as well as those without a diagnosis. Both the girls and their mothers were asked to report on the girls' eating habits and attitudes. Results suggested that adolescents with AS were at greater risk for eating difficulties than those without AS.

In our practice, we have seen a number of women who have experienced periods of excessively low weight with a resistance to altering this state. Although some may present with a more traditional eating disorder, in a number of cases, the low weight appeared to be related to obsessive–compulsive behaviors. For example, some women monitored their food intake and food types excessively, and others engaged compulsively in high levels of physical exercise without compensating with increased calories. One woman with previously undiagnosed AS and anxiety disorder had been fed through a G-tube for 10 years and was treated successfully through a combination of medication, recognition of the sensory components of eating, behavioral, and psychotherapeutic interventions. We have also seen individuals, both men and women, who have expressed that eating is an "unpleasant task."

GENDER IDENTITY DISORDER

We have often met individuals with AS in our practices who have experienced confusion over their gender identity with a frequency that seems unusually high, leading us to an exploration of characteristics typically associated with a gender identity disorder (GID). GID is "characterized by a strong and persistent cross-gender identification, and a persistent discomfort with the assigned natal sex and its associated gender role, which causes significant distress and the wish of a cross-gender life" (Kraemer, Delsignore, Gundelfinger, Schnyder, & Hepp, 2005; p. 292).

In the literature, a few case descriptions can be found of individuals with concurrent gender identity disorder and AS (Gallucci, Hackerman, & Schmidt, 2005; Kraemer et al., 2005; Tateno, Tateno, & Saito, 2008). Locally, a woman has written about her life with AS and "gender identity conflict" (Stonehouse, 2004). Kraemer et al. (2005) report the case of a 35-year-old woman (biological) who received a diagnosis of both GID and AS. The case review indicates that the woman had always wanted to be a boy beginning in early childhood. Her behavior was consistent with this desire in terms of preferred activities and style of dress. As well, she met clinical criteria for a diagnosis of AS in terms of history and presented at age 35 with cognitive, social, and emotional factors consistent with AS.

We have been told by many women with AS that their early childhood interests were not typically "girlish" and that they often felt more comfortable playing with boys. These women most often do not develop gender dysphoria. Many men with AS tell us that they were bullied by boys as children, that the girls were more kind to them, and that they therefore gravitated to females socially. It is often difficult to determine whether strong interests that are more typical of the opposite sex are suggestive of ASD-related "restricted range of interests" or interests relevant to gender dysphoria. Sometimes, there is a hint of both. It is also important to note that the clothing worn by some individuals with ASDs may be suggestive of a GID, but may also relate to specific preferences as to fit and feelings of certain material. One young man wanted to wear female stockings under his pants. When this preference was explored, he explained that had no desire to be female or change gender, nor did he have fetishistic interests in women's clothing—he merely liked the sensation of wearing tight-fitting and smooth, layered clothing.

Henault's (2006) discussion of sexual diversity and gender identity is an excellent resource for clinicians because it provides clarification regarding sexual preferences and identifies and reviews existing literature in relation to ASDs and AS. She discusses current controversies regarding aspects of the GID construct, including time of presentation and its relationship to AS, and the need for a positive approach to individuals possibly struggling with their gender identity and AS.

METHODS TO ASSESS CHALLENGING BEHAVIOR AND MENTAL HEALTH

As discussed in the following section, a variety of rating and assessment scales have been developed to evaluate symptoms of mental health disorders. Some of these are self-report and others require reports by informants. Some measures have been designed to objectively document response to treatment and the emergence of adverse medication effects. These scales have been designed to focus on specific challenging behaviors, such as impulsivity, overactivity, poor sleep, and other symptoms of comorbid mental health concerns. To date, none of these scales is specific to those with ASDs.

Many adults we see who have AS are functioning reasonably well in relationships and are competent in their employment and in other areas of life, just as their non-AS peers would be. They may, however, encounter episodes of depression, anxiety, or other mental health concerns that inhibit their ability to function on a daily basis. Most of these individuals are able to respond adequately to assessment measures that would be administered to others in the general population. An observation we have made is that if a measure is too long, as are some of the popular personality inventories (e.g., Minnesota Multiphasic Personality Inventory [MMPI]; Butcher et al., 2001), or if questions are too vague or response options limited, the individual with AS has more difficulty. Therefore we prefer to use briefer scales and those with several response options.

Another assessment difficulty we have encountered is in the attempt to use projective measures. Burke (2005) observed that when using the Thematic Apperception Test (TAT; Murray & Bellack, 1973), the individual with ASD tends to have "difficulty projecting backward or forward in time or organizing thoughts, or perseverates on previous answers" (p. 220). Such difficulties in processing limit the usefulness of many tests that are often used in the assessment of mental health disorders. Whereas the individuals we see are typically able to respond to questionnaires and semistructured interviews, we sometimes see those whose ability to function is impaired not only by the symptoms of AS, but also by symptoms of one or more mental health disorders that are severe. At these times, the person cannot respond to self-report scales and may require reports by others or observational measures. Very rarely, if the person is extremely incapacitated, we may resort to measures used more often by those with an intellectual disability.

In a practice such as ours, which involves a group of clinicians offering private services, disorders such as depression and anxiety would be identified and treated. However, for disorders such as schizophrenia (which might require more intense intervention or, at times, inpatient treatment) a screening for a suspected mental health disorder would be completed and then the person would be referred for appropriate treatment in a more specialized mental health facility. The measures discussed below support this practice.

Self-Report Questionnaires

• *Beck Anxiety Inventory* (Beck, 1990) provides a list of 21 physical symptoms of anxiety and is recommended for individuals 17 years and over. The person being assessed is asked to rate his or her experience of those symptoms. In our experience, many individuals with AS seem to be better able to respond to this measure versus instruments that ask about their emotional or behavioral response in situations. However, there are individuals who are less aware than others of their physiological responses. For example, others may see the person "flushed," but the person does not understand what this means and, even if explained, cannot recall having noticed such a sensation.

• *Multidimensional Anxiety Questionnaire* (Reynolds, 1999) is a 40-item self-report measure, recommended for persons 18 and older, that we have begun to use regularly in both assessments and in programs designed to address anxiety in this population (Stoddart & Duhaime, 2011). The subscales include Physiological-Panic, Social Phobia, Worry-Fears, and Negative Affectivity. Given the presence of both social phobia and negative affectivity subscales, we feel that this measure is highly appropriate for use with our clients because of the frequency with which we see these symptoms in practice. High scores on either subscale may suggest the need to further explore these symptoms in assessment and treatment.

• *Beck Depression Inventory–II* (Beck, Steer & Brown, 1996) is often utilized in our assessments. It provides four options for the individual to choose from in rating different characteristic symptoms of depression. It is recommended for use for those between the ages of 13 and 80 years. We have found that some individuals with AS have more difficulty responding to the Depression Inventory than to the Anxiety Inventory. This may be due to the need to discriminate between the four sentences provided for each symptom area in the depression inventory, as compared to simply ticking the presence and severity of the symptom in the anxiety inventory.

• *Hamilton Depression Inventory* (HDI; Reynolds & Koback, 1995) is a contemporary self-report format of the clinician-administered Hamilton Depression Rating Scale (Hamilton, 1960, 1967) and assesses both frequency and severity of symptoms. The construct measured is consistent with DSM-IV (American Psychiatric Association, 1994) definitions of depression. The scale is a 23-item measure (consisting of 40 questions) that has been extensively tested. We are currently using it in assessment and also to determine treatment effectiveness, especially when pharmacological interventions are involved.

• *Clark–Beck Obsessive–Compulsive Inventory* (Clark & Beck, 2002) is a brief self-report instrument that screens for symptoms of obsessive and compulsive behaviors and their intensity. It was developed for individuals 17 years of age and older. As with the Beck Depression Inventory–II, respondents choose from four statements the one that best describes their thoughts and behaviors. We have found this measure helpful when attempting to determine if the obsessive and compulsive behaviors we see are related to the ASD or if they represent a true OCD.

• *Paranoia Scale* (Fenigstein & Vanable, 1992) is a 20-item scale of symptoms of paranoia, with ratings on a 5-point Likert scale. It was originally developed for the nonclinical population; however, others have since utilized it with clinical groups (Craig, Hatton, Craig, & Bentall, 2004).

• *Peters Delusions Inventory* (Peters, Joseph, & Garetty, 1999) is a 40-item scale that was developed to examine the tendency toward delusional beliefs across various dimensions (distress, preoccupation, conviction). The authors suggest the usefulness of this tool in clinical settings to identify psychotic features that may indicate that individuals are at risk of more serious mental health episodes, and they also note that their tool may be useful in measuring therapeutic change.

Report by Self and Others

The ideal situation is not only to have the individual report on his or her own experiences of mental health difficulties, but also to have someone who knows the person rate his or her emotional experience based on observed behavior. Although instruments that can do this are not readily available, we use the Emotional Problems Scales (Prout & Strohmer, 1991) developed for individuals with a mild intellectual disability. It is available in both "Self-Report" and "Behavior Rating" (by others) formats; we use both formats for comparison.

Sometimes we see individuals who appear to have BD. In order to determine if this is, in fact, the case, or if it reflects other issues that have been described in the bipolar section above, the clinician should have the person complete bipolar mood charts. A search of the Internet provides access to a variety of charts, developed by pharmaceutical companies and clinics, which can be used as models. They can be daily, weekly, or monthly charts. To us, the most important aspect is that the chart is individualized to reflect the person. Many individuals with ASDs have their own words to describe mood or emotions. For example, one man who had manic phases, referred to them as times when "everything goes fast" and "I talk loud." If clients are doing their own charting, they need to use their own language to understand what they are charting. Sometimes the description needs to be in terms of actions. As well, these individuals often recognize only the extreme highs and lows. It is helpful if they live with a parent or spouse to have the other individual also complete the mood charts.

Interview and Observation Measures

Earlier it was stated that one method of classifying symptoms of schizophrenia was to label them as either positive or negative. In considering a diagnosis of schizophrenia, Andreasen and Olsen (1982) published the Scale for the Assessment of Negative Symptoms (SANS) and the Scale for the Assessment of Positive Symptoms (SAPS). Although these scales were developed some time ago, they continue to be cited in the literature. The scales are completed through interactions/interviews with the client, supplemented by observational information. These scales have been used for many years, and they are appropriate for screening individuals who present with possible symptoms of schizophrenia. In a practice such as ours, if it appears that an individual may have a psychotic disorder, we would refer him or her to an appropriate mental health service.

The Positive and Negative Syndrome Scale (PANSS) was developed by Kay and his associates, integrating items from two previous scales (Kay, Fiszbein, & Opler, 1987; Kay, Opler, & Lindenmayer, 1988). The resulting 30-item scale is rated on 7 points. Items represent positive and negative symptoms as well has subscales for general psychiatric conditions. Mortimer (2007) reviewed the PANSS, comparing it to other instruments. She reports that it shows consistency over time and course of illness. A review of the literature also suggests that there are a number of brief measures appropriate for the screening of psychosis.

For those working within psychiatric services, a more in-depth and up-to-date method of diagnosis is required. For individuals who have symptoms of a clinical disorder described in DSM-IV-TR (American Psychiatric Association, 2000), such as schizophrenia, the Structured Clinical Interview for DSM-IV (SCID-I; First, Spitzer, Gibbon, & William, 1996) provides an interview format to gather relevant information regarding symptoms of clinical disorders and assist the clinician in making diagnosis. A similar format is available for those who present with symptoms of personality disorders (SCID-II).

Some individuals with AS and other ASDs may engage in extreme behaviors due to their inability to regulate their emotions or the overwhelming impact of mental health symptoms. As well, they may be unable to report what they are experiencing. Crosland et al. (2003) described the use of functional behavioral analysis methodology in the evaluation of medication effects. This study was based on previous work by Mace and Mauk (1995). It was suggested that the results of a functional analysis of a behavior—allowing the behavior to be categorized as learned or biological, or both—could assist in the selection of a treatment modality.

Others (e.g., Sovner & DesNoyers Hurley, 1990) have summarized assessment tools facilitating psychiatric evaluations and treatment in individuals with DD. They emphasize the need to use objective behavioral measurements in supporting individuals who have both DD and mental health concerns, recognizing that multiple variables contribute to the challenge of identifying specific mental illnesses in these individuals. This point would seem to apply equally to those with ASDs who are experiencing serious mental health issues. These variables include (1) the fact that client self-reports were often unreliable due to cognitive and communicative impairment; (2) the challenge of obtaining a longitudinal perspective on changes in behavior and correlate these changes with what is known about the natural history of formulated mental health concerns; and (3) the difficulty of obtaining consistency in reporting from across environments in which the individual is engaged.

Five assessment tools were reviewed by these authors (Sovner & DesNoyers Hurley, 1990): (1) a biological time line, listing in chronological order important events in the individual's life; (2) a sleep chart, which the authors consider "a biological vital sign" (p. 92); (3) a behavioral incident chart, measuring frequency of major and minor challenging behavioral incidents per week (this chart is designed to measure the severity of the presenting problem and the efficacy of treatment); (4) a bipolar chart, recording mood state on a daily basis; and (5) a psychotropic drug profile, detailing dates of medication initiation, the disorder being treated, target symptoms being monitored, the highest daily dose of medication achieved, the highest serum medication level achieved, and the reason and date of any medication discontinuation.

CONCLUSION

Despite the paucity of evidence-based research to guide clinicians in assessing and treating individuals with AS, it is clear that mental health concerns are prevalent in this population. Emerging resources and processes have allowed researchers to operationally define signs and symptoms of DSM-IV-TR Axis I and Axis II diagnoses in adults with AS and to begin to demonstrate that these disorders are both identifiable and treatable. While awaiting further evidence-based literature, it is important to acknowledge and implement a value-based best practice that emphasizes the establishment of therapeutic alliances based on trust and respect; includes care providers, families, and the individual with AS in the assessment and decision making process; and effectively utilizes the interdisciplinary team to generate biopsychosocial formulations and resulting treatment goals in order to optimize individual quality of life.

Chapter 4

NEURODEVELOPMENTAL, GENETIC, AND MEDICAL ISSUES IN ADULT ASPERGER SYNDROME

CASE EXAMPLE: UNEXPLAINED ACADEMIC DIFFICULTY AND ASPERGER SYNDROME

A school counselor referred Janet, a theater arts student in college. She was experiencing difficulty with her courses and the counselor was concerned about her attitude toward her studies and her social life. Janet had difficulty relating to others in her class; she was rigid and did not acknowledge the views of others. She had problems with starting tasks, making transitions, and getting organized.

We discovered that when Janet was a child, she rarely interacted with children outside the family. She was rigid and argumentative when she played with others and preferred to spend time alone. She acted out scenes from cartoons and movies and memorized songs. As she got older, her sisters found her behavior increasingly difficult but tolerated her, thinking her behavior was because of her age. Janet had worn hats as a little girl, and as a teen, developed an obsession with hats. In fact, she was always wearing one. If the hat she wanted was missing, she would become inconsolable. Although she had always been a fussy eater, in her teens she became conscientious about diet: She became vegetarian and lectured people on what they ate. Janet appeared capable in her schoolwork, but she had problems organizing her projects and getting started: her sisters always came to her rescue. She has never been a good math student; she makes errors in calculations, but does adequately as long as she has her calculator. Before college, her teachers told her she was careless. She has also been criticized over the years for her sloppy and slow writing, so she does most of her schoolwork on the computer. As her sisters moved off to college, Janet replaced the time with them by watching soap operas. She began to show symptoms of anxiety and her schoolwork deteriorated.

Now, Janet is an attractive and articulate young woman. She wears long cotton dresses and large hats, looking a bit like a "hippie" of the 1960s. She does not enjoy reading, but is passionate about storytelling and theater. Since Janet began college, she has had difficulty mixing with classmates. She asserts her opinion strongly and does not give others a chance to talk. Janet has been known to comment on classmates' diet or weight; others see her as eccentric. In her courses, she excels in acting and in subjects requiring memorization or rote actions, whereas she struggles with movement-related classes and visual arts.

Janet was assessed at our center. She was found to have strong verbal skills, except for comprehension; she could understand math problems but not do calculations; both fine and gross motor skills were awkward; and she did well with rote memory tasks and verbal memory, but her processing speed was slow. Janet was diagnosed with a nonverbal learning disorder (NLD). She also has symptoms suggestive of executive dysfunction and AS. Although the diagnosis of NLD could aid her in obtaining educational supports, aspects of her personality, including the restricted range of interest and obsessions, were not explained by NLD. Therefore, she was given a concurrent diagnosis of AS. The college has provided suitable accommodations, and Janet is doing better in her course work. Her counselor at the college's disability office has helped her develop strategies to compensate for her executive functioning issues. At our center, she is seeing a therapist for social issues and anxiety. Psychoeducational sessions have been held with her family members so that they can understand and support her through her difficulties.

The previous chapter addressed comorbid psychiatric difficulties often seen in adults with AS. This chapter provides information on other disorders that may coexist with AS. The first section deals with learning, neurological, and perceptual exceptionalities, and the second half addresses medical and health concerns. Although this book focuses on adults with AS, much of the research cited in this chapter refers to children because the disorders are typically identified in childhood. Despite limited research and understanding of these difficulties in adulthood, it is important for the clinician to be aware of the possibility of these coexisting with AS in adults. Further, these disorders are potentially an important aspect of the clinical formulation for adults seeking treatment, and may require focused assessment and specialized remediation.

LEARNING, NEUROLOGICAL, AND PERCEPTUAL PROBLEMS

Several learning, processing, and perceptual exceptionalities have been identified in those who have AS. These may coexist not only with AS, but may also be considered in differential diagnosis. Among these exceptionalities are learning disabilities; giftedness; executive dysfunction; semantic pragmatic disorder; hyperlexia; problems with attention; sensory, processing and perceptual differences; central auditory processing disorder; dyspraxia; motor difficulties; prosopagnosia; synaesthesia; and scotopic sensitivity. We review each of these issues and their possible contribution to the overall clinical picture in adults with AS. It should be noted that whereas some of these disorders are considered to be "mental" in nature and fall within the DSM-IV-TR (American Psychiatric Association, 2000) classification of psychiatric disorders, others are neurological, communication, or sensory processing conditions. Although not included in the DSM-IV-TR, this latter group of disorders is reported extensively in the literature and causes significant challenges for the individuals who experience them. Therefore, we have included them in this chapter.

Learning Disorders

Learning disorders (LDs; also known as learning disabilities) create challenges to learning in specific areas of information processing. Individuals who have LDs present with average intellectual abilities and problems in specific areas of processing that affect learning (Muskat, 2005). The general criteria for the diagnosis of an LD are stated in the DSM-IV-TR (American Psychiatric Association, 2000) and identify three specific learning disorders: reading disorder, mathematics disorder, and disorder of written expression. In addition, there is a fourth category: learning disorder not otherwise specified. This category is used when disorders of learning do not meet the criteria for one of the specific learning disorders. Although the DSM-IV-TR (American Psychiatric Association, 2000) provides a general description of the difficulties, specific criteria or procedures for determining if someone has a learning disorder have not been agreed on and are not in standard use. For example, the criteria for a mathematics disorder states: "Mathematical ability, as measured by individually administered standardized tests, is substantially below that expected given the person's chronological age, measured intelligence, and age-appropriate education" (American Psychiatric Association, 2000, p. 54).

Because of increased understanding and recognition of LDs in the general population, children who have LDs are typically identified in elementary school in response to the struggles they have in reading, writing, or mathematics. Although they may present as intelligent, the work of these children is not at expected levels. Assessment resulting in the diagnosis of LD generally reveals a significant difference or discrepancy between their intellectual ability and their school performance, as well as between their verbal and nonverbal abilities. This model of assessment and diagnosis has been criticized, but it is still prevalent in policy and practice (Lyon et al., 2001; Siegel, 2003). If individuals with AS meet this learning profile, they may also receive a diagnosis of a specific learning disorder (Frith, 2004).

Individuals who have a learning disorder that is not verbal in nature may not be recognized as having an LD in their early school years. Individuals affected by nonverbal LD (NLD) may be aware that they have limitations in visual and spatial tasks, but these problems are less obvious either in a classroom or at home. Strengths accompanying NLD include strong rote verbal abilities and good verbal memory skills. Challenges include difficulties with tactile perception, psychomotor coordination, visuospatial perception, interpretation and organization of visuospatial information, adapting to change, time concepts, mathematics, verbal memory for complex stimuli, organization, nonverbal problem solving, pragmatics, social perception, and social interaction (Muskat, 2005). NLDs are not among the specific learning disorders addressed by the DSM-IV-TR (American Psychiatric Association, 2000). As with LDs in general, there are no broadly accepted criteria in use at this point in time. However, some researchers have developed rules based on their research to guide diagnosis (e.g., Harnadek & Rourke, 1994; Pelletier, Ahmed, & Rourke, 2001).

Rourke has discussed the difficulties with nonverbal processing for two decades. He suggests that children who have sustained damage to, or have atypical white matter of the brain, show profiles of functioning comparable to those with NLD. He has therefore hypothesized that NLD is a consequence of atypical white matter (Rourke, 1995; Harnadek & Rourke, 1994). Rourke (1995) has suggested a relationship between NLD and a number of other genetic and neurodevelopmental disorders based on the "white matter model."

Some authors have identified similarities in the cognitive profiles of those with AS and NLD (Klin et al., 1995; Rourke et al., 2002), and suggest a different and opposing profile in those with high-functioning autism (HFA; Klin et al., 2005). In a comparative study of individual profiles of those with AS and those with HFA, differences were found in that those with AS in that they presented with characteristics indicative of NLD, while this was not the case in those with HFA (Klin, Volkmar, Sparrow, Cicchetti & Rourke, 1995). Another study, conducted specifically to examine the similarities between features of AS and NLD "confirmed the close similarity in the neuropsychological profiles of NLD and AS" (Gunter, Ghaziuddin & Ellis, 2002, p. 263).

Considering the similarity between NLD and AS in terms of the "white matter model," a case was reported in the literature in which a young man presented with neuropsychological and social-emotional features consistent with a diagnosis of AS. Upon neuro-imaging, a white-matter lesion was identified which was believed might relate to his symptom profile (Volkmar, Klin, Schultz, Rubin & Bronen, 2000). In another study, including 14 individuals with AS, atypicalities were found in the white matter of those with AS compared to controls through the use of quantitative magnetic resonance imaging (MRI; McAlonan et al., 2002). These early MRI studies would appear to lend support to Rourke's hypothesis.

In spite of the developing body of literature suggesting similarities in those with AS and NLD, there are others who maintain that profiles of those with NLD and AS are distinct (Barnhill, Hagiwara, Myles, & Simpson, 2000). Currently, there appears to be no conclusive evidence that NLD and AS are in the same family of disorders, despite their similarities. DSM-IV-TR (American Psychiatric Association, 2000) currently places AS within the family of ASDs, and does not include or make reference to NLD. Therefore, individuals with AS who also present with symptoms of an NLD may receive a concurrent diagnosis of AS and NLD. Clinically, we have assessed adults who have previously received a diagnosis of NLD, and we have made an additional diagnosis of AS. However, the opposite scenario is probably more common in our experience.

Giftedness

When students are labeled as *gifted*, it suggests that they have exceptional cognitive or learning strengths that demand stimulation beyond that which is typically available in the classroom. Frequently, these children are identified so that the school can provide them with more challenging academic work and keep them interested in their studies. If they are required to work at the pace of their non-gifted peers, they often become bored and disinterested in schoolwork. As with learning disorders, although there is a general understanding of what defines a gifted child, individual school boards may use their own criteria to determine who is identified as gifted within their system.

Neihart (2000) suggests that children with AS may be among the gifted in an educational setting, but may not always be identified as having AS. She suggests several ways in which children with AS are like other gifted children, including having excellent memory, strong interests in specific areas, sensory sensitivities, and difficulties in peer relationships. However, there are potential differences between children who are gifted, children who have AS, and children who are gifted *and* have AS. The literature related to education and the gifted child suggests that there are concerns in identifying these differences, so that appropriate curriculum and compensatory strategies can be developed for the child (Gallagher & Gallagher, 2002; C. Little, 2002).

Gallagher and Gallagher (2002) discuss the qualitative differences between those with AS and the gifted, such as the difference in social isolation of some gifted children compared to the social ineptness of those with AS, and the deeper level of understanding concepts seen in gifted individuals compared to the extreme ability to memorize in those with AS. C. Little (2002) also points out the literal interpretation of the child with AS compared to the greater ability to abstract by the gifted child. Burger-Veltmeijer (2007) proposes that "ASD in gifted individuals can be defined by means of a relative comparison between the level of cognitive and social intelligence" (p. 118). Neihart (2000) recommends a list of characteristics that can be used to differentiate a gifted child with AS from one without AS. Burger-Veltmeijer (2007), in a similar vein, has proposed that a dimensional discrepancy checklist be done as part of the assessment of the child.

Those with AS are often bullied or teased because of their intellectual presentation or their intense interest in certain topics. In our experience, they sometimes perceive that they are better accepted by peers who are gifted and who share their academic focus, as well as enjoying similar interests.

Executive Dysfunction

Executive functions (EFs) include mental skills that direct and organize complex behavior. Among EFs are the abilities to plan, organize, self-monitor, manage time, inhibit and control emotions and impulses, use working memory, change set, use new strategies, and understand complex concepts (Ozonoff & Griffith, 2000; Roth et al., 2005; Attwood, 2007). Individuals who experience EF difficulties independent of any other disorder are said to have an executive dysfunction (ED). However, ED may coexist with other learning and processing problems and can severely compound the experiences of an adult with AS.

Hill and Bird (2006) report that empirical evidence for ED in those with AS has been inconsistent. However, when they employed newer tests for EF, they found significant impairments in those with AS. In our practices, we have observed ED reflected in problems with starting an activity or project, estimating time, disengaging from an activity, performing a task that has been observed but not performed, budgeting and planning finances, and controlling anger. EF difficulties in adults may be very difficult to treat (especially if there is limited motivation to employ recommended strategies such as an organizational calendar) and may necessitate prolonged support from professionals to minimize the effect of these problems on daily life. We have begun to employ a hands-on "life coach" or "organizational coach" model with some of our clients (discussed further in Chapter 7) due to the difficulties in remediating these problems unless a practical and behavioral approach is applied. Assisting with organization of tasks related to completing school assignments may be the major role of a disability counselor in the post-secondary education setting.

As noted in Chapter 2 on assessment and diagnosis, ED is not included in the diagnostic criteria for AS. However, the literature has repeatedly identified comorbid EF difficulties in many individuals who have AS (Goldstein et al., 2001; Szatmari et al., 1990). These difficulties may become more apparent in adult life with less support from people (other than family members), who have expectations for more independence. This is often a presenting issue for parents who are concerned about the ability of their young adult to cope with daily organizational demands. Not surprisingly, it is also a common presenting problem raised in marital counseling with this group, as the nonaffected spouse is often left to organize the household, appointments and other events on his or her own.

Semantic Pragmatic Disorder

Semantic pragmatic disorder (SPD) refers to difficulty in how an individual "acquires and uses language" (Dodd, 2005, p. 57). SPD is a developmental language disorder in which an individual has acceptable vocabulary and appropriate grammar and phonology. However, the way language is used in conversational links and content, as well as comprehension of speech, is abnormal (Szatmari, 1998). The pragmatic feature implies difficulties in socially based communication (Bishop, 2000). The person with SPD may have problems with social interactions such as turn taking, staying on topic, and use of body language—all common features of individuals with AS. Speech in individuals with SPD may sound repetitive and reflect preferred topics. The person who has SPD may also have trouble understanding the communication of others and with using his or her own language with clarity (Dodd, 2005). Bishop (2000) questions the support for SPD being viewed as a "coherent" disorder and argues it should be viewed within the larger context of specific language disorders. Fitzgerald and Corvin (2001) have also queried whether SPD should be seen as distinct.

Although symptoms of SPD are present in those with ASDs, including AS, these symptoms also occur in other individuals. Bishop (1989) suggests that individuals with autism would not meet criteria for SPD. Szatmari (1998) has pointed out that children with SPD typically have delayed milestones in speech. This would imply, under current diagnostic criteria, that individuals with AS would not have SPD.

Shields (1991) provides an interesting view of SPD by comparing the impact of a right-hemisphere brain lesion with the speech patterns of those with SPD. She indicates that in both, the speaker may be grammatically correct and fluent in speech, yet produces statements that are not suitable to the context. She further relates these difficulties to those reported in individuals with ASDs.

Hyperlexia

Hyperlexia is an advanced ability to read by decoding; however, individuals who are hyperlexic may be unaware of the content or meaning of what they have read. Many parents report in clinical assessments that their children with AS were able to read by decoding at an early age. Shields (1991) identified similarities between those with SPD and those with ASDs in terms of hyperlexia. She noted that children who ignore the semantic context, which would provide understanding, are known to ignore context in other areas of functioning.

Chaing and Lin (2007) reviewed the literature on reading comprehension in those with ASDs and identified that individuals who showed poor comprehension and had an ASD were not always hyperlexic. These authors' concerns about hyperlexia and reading understanding were in relation to the educational context. As clinicians, we are concerned beyond the scope of education, into the adult world settings where poor understanding presents a significant barrier.

Attention-Deficit/Hyperactivity Disorder

Attention-deficit/hyperactivity disorder (ADHD) is defined in DSM-IV-TR (American Psychiatric Association, 2000). Individuals who have ADHD may present primarily with difficulties in either attention or hyperactivity, or with both. ADHD is a neurobiological disorder that affects behavior and learning and was initially thought to be a disorder exclusively of childhood. Starting in the early 1970s, clinicians and researchers acknowledged that the difficulties associated with ADHD in childhood continue into adulthood. There are estimates that 30–70% of those with this disorder in adolescence are also affected in adulthood (Quinn, 1997; Weiss, 1992). Difficulty with attention was one of the features of AS that was originally documented in the work of Hans Asperger, and studies of those with AS have continued to identify this concern. Attwood (1998) stated that children with this disorder also appear to have features of AS, and "although they are two distinct disorders, they are not mutually exclusive" (p. 22). Therefore, individuals with AS may qualify for the additional diagnosis of ADHD.

The presence of undiagnosed ADHD can be painful and destabilizing for an adult. The associated stress may lead to addictions (e.g., to stimulating substances such as cocaine), or related impulsivity may lead to illegal or inappropriate actions. Employed individuals may have difficulty sustaining their jobs due to absenteeism and poorly considered behavior (Weiss, 1992). Moreover, when an individual experiences both AS and ADHD, we would expect their difficulties to be greatly compounded. Little information is available on treatment for the adult with these coexisting difficulties, although pharmacological intervention has been suggested as providing benefits, as discussed in Chapter 6. Many of our clients have reported remarkable changes in their lives because of an appropriate ADHD diagnosis and medical intervention. Psychotherapeutic interventions can also be invaluable for both disorders in adulthood as a way to address psychosocial problems that might arise.

Sensory Integration Dysfunction

"We experience the world through our senses" (Smith & Gouze, 2004, p. 27). What we know of our surroundings enters our awareness through sight, sound, smell, taste, and touch. Our senses provide the context which gives meaning to our experiences in life, to our memories, and may drive our actions. If we were consciously aware of every aspect of the environment perceived by our sensory system, we would be overwhelmed and likely immobilized by the extent of the experience. The body, however, has the ability to "edit" less important sensory input before it reaches the brain.

It appears that in some individuals, the ability to filter these sensory experiences may be impaired. Although sensory-processing impairments are not diagnostic for AS, Dunn, Saiter, and Rinner (2002) remind us that Hans Asperger provided descriptions of sensory-related behaviors in the children he observed. The literature contains early evidence of differences in sensory-processing patterns seen in those with AS. Some believe it is an underlying feature of AS. In 1979, Ayres proposed that, in some people, sensory processing was less efficient than in others. When the sensory-processing system breaks down, the individual may experience behavioral and learning difficulties. Ayres called this sensory integration dysfunction (SID), and suggested that it could affect one's ability to attend, coordinate motor functions, perceive the environment, and regulate emotions and activity level.

Besides the five senses we are usually aware of, Ayres suggested two additional systems of note: vestibular and proprioception. The vestibular system is related to balance and movement issues, and proprioception allows our body to know and respond to its position in space. When we refer to sensory integration difficulties, the focus is on three of our senses: vestibular, proprioceptive, and tactile (Dodd, 2005). These senses are inter-connected and through our interpretation of experience, allow us to respond to the environment.

People with ASDs, including AS, may have extreme responses to sensory input, at either the high end (hypersensitivity) or the low end (hyposensitivity; Aquilla et al., 2005). The term *sensory modulation dysfunction* is sometimes used to describe these extremes of sensitivity and response (Reynolds & Lane, 2008). We have previously referred to this problem in Chapter 2 and noted measures we recommend to assess it.

A person who is hypersensitive to some sensory aspect of the environment may be highly distracted and unable to attend. He or she may even become anxious or frightened and engage in problematic behaviors or display a panic reaction. At times, anxiety can be anticipatory in nature, as with the woman we see who is extremely sensitive to sounds. In environments where she anticipates that there *could* be a high-pitched noise, she sits with her fingers poised near her ears. Hypervigilant behaviors can also be expected in other situations, such as when individuals have to visually scan a park to ensure that there are no dogs around, and thus no loud barking. Alternatively, others may find the response stimulating and become obsessed with accessing that sensation. An example is the man who became sexually aroused to the noise of vacuum cleaners. In contrast, people who are hyposensitive may be unaware of sensory features in their environment and miss information that is important for social or safety reasons. As well, those who have AS often have problems with motor planning and appear clumsy or uncoordinated (Dziuk et al., 2007; Szatmari, 1998).

There is a broad range of sensory responses in adults with AS, as well as possible solutions and resulting consequences. We have worked with individuals who are so overly aware of the labels in their shirts or a fabric they dislike, they are unable to concentrate on a task; in this case, it is important to be aware of clothing texture. We have also worked with those who have difficulty attending to auditory input because they have trouble filtering out irrelevant or insignificant sounds in the environment; in this situation, managing extraneous noise is important. Adults with AS have told us that they have behaved inappropriately in an effort to get near a smell that is appealing (e.g., sitting too close to a female to enjoy her perfume). One man had an agreement with one of his female coworkers that he could touch her hair (if he asked) at his smoking break, as he found this behavior relaxing. In the latter two examples, there may be significant consequences for students or employees if the intent of these behaviors is not understood.

Central Auditory Processing Disorder

Central auditory processing disorder (CAPD) has been implicated in a variety of disorders, including ADHD, learning disabilities, specific language impairment, and ASDs (Levy & Parkin, 2003; Kwon, Kim, Choe, Ko, & Park, 2007), although it is not recognized by the DSM-IV-TR (American Psychiatric Association, 2000). Levy and Parkin note, however, that there has been considerable controversy as to the scope and definition of CAPD and its existence as a "standalone entity," as part of a larger disorder, or even as a disorder at all (Wilson, Heine, & Harvey, 2004). Those who do support its existence argue that despite performing normally on hearing assessments, individuals with CAPD have problems processing auditory information. We explain CAP to clients as "how the brain hears"; others have described CAP as "what we do with what we hear" (Katz & Tillery, 2003, p. 191).

The American Speech–Language–Hearing Association (ASHA) identified central auditory processes as the auditory system mechanisms responsible for sound localization and lateralization, auditory discrimination, auditory pattern recognition, temporal aspects of audition (including temporal resolution, temporal masking, temporal integration, and temporal ordering), auditory performance decrements with competing acoustic signals, and auditory performance decrements with degraded acoustic signals (American Speech–Language–Hearing Association, 1996). If an individual is found to have CAPD, the audiologist will provide suggestions as to how the listener can perform optimally in the processing of sounds. Such recommendations may include being close to the speaker, utilizing visual cues, working or interacting in a quiet environment, recording a communication such as a lecture, or obtaining an individual's attention before speaking. Similar to the current understanding of many of the comorbidities present in ASDs, the treatment for CAPD is not well researched or established.

Dyspraxia and Motor Problems

The term *dyspraxia* refers to problems in planning and performing learned motor actions. Individuals with ASDs, including those with AS, experience a variety of motor-functioning and motor-planning difficulties (Dziuk et al., 2007). Although dyspraxia is often reported in those with ASDs, clumsiness or problems with coordination is repeatedly identified as a characteristic of AS, and some suggest that it is one trait that differentiates AS from autism (e.g., Szatmari, 1998). Brasic and Gianutsos (2000) suggest that topography and incidence of neuromotor disturbances are not the same in all individuals with autistic disorders. The authors reviewed the literature and hypothesized that the type of neuromotor difficulty may assist in distinguishing between types of autistic and other neurodevelopmental disorders.

Dyspraxia can have a strong impact on an adult in his or her daily life. Kirby (2002) pointed out the difficulty a person with dyspraxia has in driving and parking a car. She also discussed the constraints of dyspraxia on a person attempting to obtain or keep employment. These situations are already areas of concern for the adult with AS. In our practice, we have witnessed many motor-functioning and planning difficulties. Often, individuals report that they are uncoordinated and do not engage in sports. As with Kirby's example, we saw one individual who had been in over 20 car accidents. We have also seen people who have difficulty climbing stairs, writing, and assembling items.

Prosopagnosia

Prosopagnosia, or "face blindness," is the inability to recognize familiar objects or faces. This condition can occur following brain trauma, either acquired or congenital, and is often associated with a syndrome or disorder such as AS. The congenital condition, referred to as developmental prosopagnosia (DP), is believed to occur in as many as 2% of the general population (Kennerknect et al., 2006). Individuals with ASDs, including those with AS, have been identified as having difficulties in face recognition.

Duchaine and Nakayama (2005), testing recognition of faces compared to other objects, found that individuals who were impaired in face recognition were able to recognize other classes of objects. The authors suggested that different mechanisms are in play when an individual looks at faces as opposed to objects. Another study examined gaze patterns in children with autism and those without the disorder. Researchers found that when the children with autism looked at fixed images of a face, they were able to perform comparably to nonautistic peers, but when the image was dynamic, they did more poorly (Speer, Cook, McMahon, & Clark, 2007).

The impact of prosopagnosia on an individual's daily life and activities can be severe and compound the existing difficulties of those with AS. One study examined the psychosocial impact of this condition and found that subjects with DP did not recognize family members, friends, or coworkers (Yardley, McDermott, Pisarski, Duchaine, & Nakayama, 2008). Of course, this was problematic at family gatherings and business meetings. These individuals experienced anxiety and tended to avoid situations where it would be important to recognize others. The authors proposed the presence of long-term risks, including overdependence on a few select people, fewer employment options, and less involvement in social activities. (Prosopagnosia is included in Table 3.2 in Chapter 3.)

Synesthesia

Synesthesia occurs when one sense that is stimulated causes a second sense to be activated (Baron-Cohen et al., 2007). For example, an individual may see a color in response to hearing a sound. As with other conditions, "acquired" synesthesia may result from a trauma; however, for some individuals this condition is present from early childhood. Referred to as developmental synesthesia, it is characterized by (1) early onset (before age 4); (2) involuntary and unlearned acquisition; and (3) clear dissimilarity from other phenomenon such as hallucinations, delusions, or imagery. Bargary and Mitchell (2008) suggest that developmental synesthesia may be an inherited condition that is believed to occur more commonly in women than men (at a ratio of 6 to 1). They suggest that usually, the activation of one system by another is unidirectional. Although originally thought to be extremely rare, estimates now suggest prevalence in the general population at between 1 and 4%. Baron-Cohen et al. review models to explain this condition, questioning whether it results from differences in brain structure or function, and argue for the former.

Baron-Cohen et al. (2007) reported on a man with AS, synesthesia, and savantism. This individual was noted to be exceptional in his abilities in mathematical calculations and in numerical memory. The authors pointed out the potentially superior ability of those with ASDs to systematize and they suggest that the combination of AS and synesthesia in an individual may increase the probability that the person is savant. Savant syndrome occurs when a person who has some cognitive limitations shows exceptional abilities that are superior to what is seen in others and inconsistent with his or her own general abilities (Bolte & Poustka, 2004).

Scotopic Sensitivity

Individuals who we have seen in our practices have often reported discomfort because of glare and light. Some tell us that the discomfort is specific to certain kinds of light, others report seeing halos, many indicate headaches and twitching from glare or fluorescent lights. They also report extreme eyestrain and headache from reading. Additional difficulties found in the literature include movement or blurring of letters and perceptual distortion (Ludlow, Wilkins, & Heaton, 2006). The authors also refer to a preference for certain colors by some individuals with ASDs.

Irlen (1991) proposed that color processing could affect one's ability to perform. The term *Meares–Irlen syndrome* or *scotopic sensitivity syndrome* has come into use to refer to the difficulties individuals experience when they read or perform vision-related tasks. This problem is dealt with by applying color overlays to eyeglasses. Ludlow et al. (2006) found that when wearing Irlen lenses, 79% of children who had autism and were tested on reading speed showed at least a 5% improvement. In 2007 the same authors replicated their results and also reported individuals' improvement in discriminating objects presented in pictures when the overlays were used (Ludlow, Wilkins, & Heaton, 2007).

Deficits in Attention, Motor Control, and Perception

Some individuals experience concurrent deficits in attention, motor control, and perception (DAMP; Gillberg, 1995; Fitzgerald & Corvin, 2001). While DAMP can occur independent of other disorders, this group of difficulties is sometimes seen in those who have neuro-developmental disorders including ASDs (Gillberg & Billstedt, 2000). The term was initially used in Scandinavia but is beginning to be seen more often in the international literature.

MEDICAL AND HEALTH PROBLEMS

Any medical problem can coexist with AS. We frequently see individuals who have diabetes, high cholesterol, arthritis, and other medical disorders to which individuals in the general population might be susceptible. However, some medical issues coexist with ASDs at a higher rate than would be expected by chance. Before the inclusion of AS in DSM-IV (American Psychiatric Association, 1994), Gillberg (1992) identified several medical conditions that appeared to co-occur with autism. These included fragile X, tuberous sclerosis, neurofibromatosis (which will be discussed later in this chapter), hypomelanosis of Ito (a disorder of pigmentation), and Moebius syndrome (persons experience paralysis in portions of their face and impairing eye movement). Gillberg and Ehlers (1998) stated that in all probability, fewer than 15% of those who have AS or HFA will present with a comorbid medical condition. Among those most likely comorbid medical conditions is fragile X, neurofibromatosis, and tuberous sclerosis. Gillberg and Billstedt (2000) suggest the following prevalence rates for some disorders seen in ASDs: epilepsy, 30%; anorexia nervosa, 28%; thalidomide syndrome, 4%; tuberous sclerosis, 2–9%; fragile X syndrome, 2–10%. Roberts and Kagan-Kushnir note: "While in most cases AS and other ASDs are not associated with any underlying syndromes or genetic disorders, there are conditions that carry a higher risk of developing ASDs, including fragile X, neurofibromatosis, microeodeletion 22, and tuberous sclerosis" (2005, p. 143).

There is little research on the rates of occurrence of medical and health issues specifically in adults with ASDs, and for those with ASDS at the "mild" end of the spectrum. Two of the studies located combined adults at various functioning levels, making it difficult to determine if severity of ASD traits and other variables, such as intellectual ability, are significant predictors of certain medical or health-related disorders (Stoddart, Burke, & Temple, 2002a; Seltzer & Wyngaarden Kraus, n.d.). Other factors such as age, income, genetics, dietary habits, addictions, level of support, and presence of co-morbid mental health problems need to be considered as additional potential determinants of health-related conditions in this population.

In a large U.S. study on the health needs of youth and adults with ASDs ($N = 286$), 16% of parents reported their son's or daughter's heath as "poor" or "fair," whereas the remaining 84% gave ratings of "good" or "excellent." The six most common health symptoms reported (in descending order) were sleep difficulty (70%), gastrointestinal problems (58%), anxiety (34%), breathing problems (32%), depression (25%), and seizure disorder (25%). Fifty-five percent of the individuals who had sleep difficulty reported that it occurred once a month or more (i.e., once a month, a few times a month, once a week, a few times per week, or daily). Of those who reported gastrointestinal problems, 35% indicated that they occurred once a month or more (Seltzer & Wyngaarden Kraus, n.d.).

In our review of 100 clinical files representing adults with a range of ASDs and intellectual functioning in Toronto, we found that 11 individuals sought our assistance with medical issues. Of these, seven were "higher functioning" (i.e., IQ > 70) and four were "lower functioning" (i.e., IQ < 70). This did not include needs related to anxiety or depression, which were considered separately. Of the 100 individuals, 32 had an identified chronic medical issue, including epilepsy ($n = 9$), cerebral palsy ($n = 5$), fragile x syndrome ($n = 5$), hearing/vision impairment ($n = 4$), head trauma ($n = 2$), and neuroleptic malignant syndrome ($n = 2$). Single cases were identified with diabetes, asthma, hydrocephalus, a thyroid condition, ulcerative colitis, organic brain disorder, physical mobility problems, and temporal lobe dysgenesis. One individual had three medical issues, and a second had two (Stoddart et al., 2002a).

Another Canadian study examined the quality of life of 19 "high-functioning" (i.e., IQ > 70) men ($M = 30.8$ years old) with ASDs by administering measures of physical and medical well-being (Mousseau, Ludkin, Szatmari, & Bryson, 2006). The total number of long-term physical problems reported ranged from none to six ($M = 1.47$). Only one subject smoked cigarettes daily, and one reported having used illegal drugs. None of the men reported having an alcohol or drug dependency. The number of times per year that individuals contacted health care professionals ranged from 4 to 67 ($M = 24$ times). Body mass index (BMI = weight divided by height) was calculated; the average BMI score was 28.21, putting the average total BMI of the subjects in the "overweight" category. The average time in physical activity per month was 14.29 hours (Mousseau et al., 2006).

Much of the research into coexisting medical disorders refers to ASDs generally rather than specifying if subjects have autism or AS. In the following discussion, we have excluded those disorders that co-occur primarily in those who have an ASD and a severe intellectual disability. Others, however, which are seen in those who are not intellectually disabled, are being included in this chapter because the clinician working with this population is likely to see individuals with these disorders, and it is important to recognize that they may present concurrently.

For difficulties that are related to health rather than a medical diagnosis, we have found the Internet to be overwhelming in terms of information; furthermore, much of what is available is not from credible sources. Individuals and their families are often desperate for help and may fall prey to fads and expensive "cures" that may not only be unhelpful, but may actually be harmful. We therefore encourage caution: Individuals should discuss all decisions to engage in an alternate therapy with a licensed practitioner who, ideally, is experienced in treating ASDs.

As reviewed in Chapter 1, there is strong evidence that ASDs, including AS, have a genetic etiology. Early evidence and interest in genetics as a causative factor came from studies that showed the recurrence of an ASD in families where it already existed, from twin studies, and from case reports of coexistence of ASDs with other genetic disorders. As well, the higher incidence of ASDs in males suggests a relationship to sex chromosomes. These factors have led to broad spread genome research (Klauck, 2006). We do not review this research further in this chapter. However, we do discuss some of the genetic disorders that are found to coexist with ASDs.

Tic and Tourette Disorders

The association between ASDs and Tourette disorder (TD) or tic disorders is becoming well established in the literature (Marriage et al., 1993; Sverd, 1991; Kerbeshian & Burd, 1996; Baron-Cohen, Mortimore, Moriarty, Izaguirre, & Robertson, 1999; Ringman & Jankovik, 2000; Epstein & Salzman-Benaiah, 2005). According to the DSM-IV-TR (American Psychiatric Association, 2000), diagnostic criteria for TD include the following:

> (A) Both multiple motor and one or more vocal tics have been present at some time during the illness, although not necessarily concurrently . . . ; (B) The tics occur many times a day (usually in bouts) nearly every day or intermittently throughout a period of more than 1 year, and during this period there was never a tic-free period of more than 3 consecutive months; (C) the disturbance causes marked distress or significant impairment in social occupational, or other important areas of functioning; (D) the onset is before age 18 years; and (E) the disturbance is not due to the direct physiological effects of a

substance (e.g., stimulants) or a general medical condition (e.g., Huntington's disease or postviral encephalitis). (p. 114)

Epstein and Salzman-Benaiah (2005) note that there is some controversy in the diagnostic community as to the suitability of the DSM-IV and DSM-IV-TR (American Psychiatric Association, 1994, 2000) criteria and prefer to use the DSM-III-R (American Psychiatric Association, 1987) because it does not have the requirement that the tics be intrusive or impairing and that there not be a tic-free period for 3 months. They also argue that it is important to recognize the considerable overlap of symptoms in AS and TS based on their clinical experience and on empirical evidence. Baron-Cohen and colleagues (1999) reported that tic disorders were present in 6–8% of their ASD sample, and Freeman's group (2000) reported 4.5% prevalence in an ASD sample. No known prevalence studies have addressed the prevalence of tics or TD in adults with AS or ASDs.

Fragile X Disorder

Fragile X disorder (FraX) is the most common inherited disorder that leads to developmental challenges. It is caused by a mutation of the *FMR1* gene on the X chromosome that impairs the gene from producing adequate amounts of FMR protein (FMRP; Denmark, 2002; National Institute of Child Health and Human Development, 2003; Garber, Visootsak, & Warren, 2008). The less FMRP produced, the more severe the symptoms of FraX. Prevalence is estimated to be 1:3,200–4,000 males and 1:6,000 females (Sherman, 2002). As it is carried on the X chromosome (thus, often referred to as an X-linked disorder), females who are affected show less severe symptoms because they typically have a normal X chromosome as well (National Institute of Child Health and Human Development, 2003). Males may be carriers of the disorder, but females transmit FraX. Carriers sometimes present with some features of the disorder. However, the gene can be passed on without individuals showing symptoms, and so families may be unaware that they carry the disorder.

FraX has been associated with ASDs (Denmark, 2002). Many behavioral features of FraX are also symptoms of autism. The noted author indicates that one study showed as many as 47% of those with FraX disorder displayed symptoms of autism. Johnson and Myers (2007) suggest that 30–50% of those with FraX will show features of ASDs. FraX carries with it both behavioral and physical/ health characteristics. Those with both FraX disorder and an ASD may also have learning or intellectual challenges. Denmark (2002) notes both groups can fall anywhere along the intellectual spectrum, including those with an intellectual disability as well as those with average (or above) IQs.

Physical and health characteristics of FraX include a long face with course features, high palate, prominent jaw, large ears, increased head circumference, hypotonia, disorder of the connective tissue, scoliosis, orthopedic problems, heart murmur, seizures, vision problems, otitis media, gastroesophageal reflux, and epilepsy (Roberts & Kagan-Kushnir, 2005; National Institute of Child Health and Human Development, 2003; Garber et al., 2008).

Behavioral and learning characteristics include hyperactivity, gaze aversion, shyness, repetitive behaviors, hand biting, repetitive and/ or odd speech, conversational difficulties, distractibility, social interaction difficulties, obsessive–compulsive behaviors, social withdrawal, stereotypic behaviors, sensory sensitivities, good visual memory, unusual environmental responses, strong responses to change, and tremors as the person ages (Mahoney, 2002; Denmark, 2002; National Institute of Child Health and Human Development, 2003).

Individuals with FraX may receive concurrent diagnoses of psychotic disorder, ADHD, OCD, anxiety disorder, intellectual disability, and ASD (National Institute of Child Health and Human Development, 2003; Denmark, 2002; Garber et al., 2008). Approximately 30% of those who have FraX syndrome also have a diagnosis of an ASD (Holden & Liu, 2005). Although most of the literature related to FraX and ASDs discusses the relationship to autism, there has been some suggestion of AS occurring in association with X chromosome atypicalities (Searcy, Burd, Kerbeshian, Stenehjem, & Franceschini, 2000).

Tuberous Sclerosis Complex

Tuberous sclerosis complex (TSC) is an inherited disorder in which a gene mutation reduces the availability of proteins that act to suppress tumors. The tumors contain an overgrowth of nerves or connective tissue. Individuals with TSC have skin-related symptoms, such as light patches and growths. The impact of the resulting tubers

145

is dependent on where they develop. For some, growths develop on the kidney, eye, heart, or lung (Yates, 2006). Cortical tubers are related to epilepsy. Cortical tubers that grow in the temporal lobe appear to be present in some individuals with ASDs (Bolton, Park, Higgins, Griffiths, & Pickles, 2002). Behaviorally, individuals with TSC are prone to hyperactivity and sleep disturbance (Mahoney, 2002). Although less than 4% of individuals who have autism are diagnosed with TSC, as many as 50% of individuals with TSC present with features of an ASD (Wiznitzer, 2004). Depending on the degree of impairment, this may include those with AS.

Neurofibromatosis

Neurofibromatosis (NF1) is a genetic disorder caused by mutations on the 17th chromosome (17q11.2). The gene involved in NF1 regulates the protein neurofibromin, which is believed to suppress development of tumors. In neurofibromatosis, benign tumors develop on the skin and nerves. As well, abnormalities in skin pigmentation occur on numerous parts of the body. Additional features vary and may include a large head, learning difficulties, hyperactivity, seizures, and skeletal problems such as scoliosis (Mouridsen & Sorensen, 1995). Dodd (2005) contends that there is a slight increase in occurrence of neurofibromatosis in those who have AS, as compared to the general population.

Duchenne's Muscular Dystrophy

Duchenne's muscular dystrophy (DMD) is an X-linked disorder in which a gene mutation reduces or prevents the production of the protein dystrophin, which provides some stabilization of the skeletal muscles. As well as the impact on the body's physical structure, research has shown that there are neurological effects as well with DMD. Dystrophin is typically found in various parts of the central nervous system. In males who have DMD and have learning challenges, dystrophin was not found in the cerebrum and cerebellum. Various authors have identified concurrent diagnoses of ADHD, ASD, dyslexia, and OCD in males with DMD (e.g., Hendriksen & Vles, 2008). Poysky (2007) suggests that the incidence of DMD in those with ASDs is higher than found in the general population.

146

Fetal Alcohol Syndrome/Spectrum Disorder

Fetal alcohol syndrome (FAS) is a nongenetic disorder that reflects the neurological impact of prenatal consumption of alcohol. Clinical symptoms are behavioral, physical, and learning. Fetal alcohol spectrum disorder (FASD) refers to a broader group of characteristics seen in those whose mothers drank prenatally, but for whom the specific diagnosis of FAS may not apply (Chudley et al., 2005). Individuals with FAS or FASD present with similar behavioral and learning symptoms as those with ASDs; these symptoms include sensory sensitivities and executive functioning difficulties.

When it is known that an individual's mother ingested alcohol prenatally, often a diagnosis of FAS is given in infancy or early childhood. However, there are situations, such as when children have been adopted, that the prenatal history is either unknown or undisclosed. When those children experience behavioral or learning difficulties, diagnosis is based on current observable or testable criteria. Diagnosis of ASDs, including AS, is currently based on clinically observed behavioral indicators. We are aware of situations where a diagnosis of autism or AS has been applied to individuals rather than a diagnosis of FAS/FASD, because their prenatal history wasn't available at the time of the original diagnosis.

As with many other disorders, the literature reflects the possibility of the co-diagnosis of ASDs (including AS) and FAS. Johnson and Myers (2007) state there is a higher risk of ASDs in those with prenatal exposure to alcohol. However, few studies provided specific information. In their review of 100 cases of AS, Cederlund and Gillberg (2004) identified only one of the 100 as having FAS. In our practice, we have seen individuals with a diagnosis of an ASD who have been brought by their adoptive families for services. They know little about their child's early history, although the adoptive families have sometimes been told there is a suspicion of maternal drinking. Some of these individuals show physical features of FAS. However, without substantiation prenatal drinking occurred, the diagnosis cannot be pursued.

Thalidomide Syndrome

Thalidomide exposure in utero has long been identified with limb deformities (Annas & Elias, 1999). More recently, some individuals

147

whose mothers took thalidomide prenatally have been diagnosed with ASDs. Depending on when the drug was ingested, the impact on development differs (Rodier, 2000). A Swedish study of those exposed to thalidomide in utero showed that 4% met diagnostic criteria for an ASD (Gillberg & Billstedt, 2000). Further, it is suggested that thalidomide may create a stronger risk in utero than alcohol (Medical Research Council, 2001). One individual whom we saw in our practice, who was exposed to thalidomide in utero, has strived not only to overcome his symptoms of an ASD, but also to inform himself about the impact of thalidomide syndrome.

Epilepsy

The occurrence of epilepsy in those ASDs was identified early in the research on autism. It is estimated that 40% of those with an ASD will develop epilepsy (D.C. Taylor, Neville, & Cross, 1999). Although little research into the coexistence of AS and epilepsy has occurred, Berney (2004) suggests that the risk is probably lower in AS than in autism, estimating between 5 and 10% in AS and with a later onset. In our review of the literature, several single case studies were found in which the person of interest had comorbid epilepsy and AS (Burgoine & Wing, 1983; Jones & Kerwin, 1990; Warwick, Griffith, Reyes, Legesse, & Evans, 2007). In D.C. Taylor et al.'s (1999) study of individuals with ASDs who were being considered as candidates for epilepsy surgery, 8 of the 19 had AS. Cederlund and Gillberg (2004) reviewed 100 males with AS; clinical epilepsy was found in 4, and an additional 20 showed atypical electroencephalograph (EEG) results.

Diet and Health

There has been substantial discussion over the years in the field of ASDs about diet, food sensitivity, vitamin therapy, and many other issues related to diet. Some of these reflect serious health issues or medical disorders. As well, issues of diet are often an obsessive interest for individuals who have AS. One woman who came to our center was so immersed in this topic that she monopolized conversation at mealtimes by lecturing family members on what they should eat and what supplements they should take. Family members ultimately stopped sharing meals with her. In many cases, families who are desperate for solutions have become caught up in the excitement

148

about a new dietary or supplement treatment, often spending large amounts of money, then experiencing disappointment when the intervention fails, and sometimes putting the individual with AS at risk. Clients have become toxic on vitamin therapies after unknowingly taking large quantities of the same product under different names or feeling that because the supplement is "natural," it is therefore safe. In this discussion, we attempt to review diet-related health issues that have been evaluated and reported by credible sources.

Food Allergies and Sensitivities

Although some individuals with AS may be allergic to some foods, the incidence is not believed to be greater than that seen in the general population. However, those with AS do appear to have a higher rate of food sensitivities. According to Lawton and Reichenberg-Ullman (2007), when a person has food sensitivity, there may be an observable behavioral reaction, but a conventional test will not confirm an allergy. They discuss ways to test the possibility a food is influencing behavior, including withdrawing the suspected food item from the individual's diet.

Research beginning in the 1990s suggested that individuals with ASDs were particularly sensitive to foods containing gluten and casein. Gluten is found in grains such as wheat, and casein, in dairy products (Lynch, 2004). Reactions to these products may include hyperactivity, diarrhea, constipation or gas, and either red face or pallor. Although the literature varies on the impact and on the incidence of food sensitivities, we hear many individuals and their families providing anecdotal accounts of the positive effects on behavior when gluten and milk products are withdrawn. As well, probiotics are reputed to increase positive bowel function and reduce discomfort. Probiotics are the "good bacteria" that maintain balance in the bowel (Lawton & Reichenberg-Ullman, 2007). As well as reducing bad bacteria, increasing food breakdown, they also may decrease food sensitivities.

Gastrointestinal Disorders

The prevalence of gastrointestinal symptoms presenting in children and adults with ASDs, including AS, has led to a belief that there is a co-occurrence of ASDs and gastrointestinal (GI) disorders.

As noted above, some food sensitivities can lead to GI symptoms. These symptoms, described in children with ASDs, have included heartburn, gastritis, abdominal pain, bloating, food intolerance, chronic constipation, and diarrhea (Erickson et al., 2005). Upper GI tract difficulties include reflux esophagitis, chronic gastritis, and chronic doudenitis, and lower GI problems include chronic ileonic and/or colonic lymphoid nodular hyperplasia (LNH: abnormal rapid increase in cells in lymph nodes of the intestinal system) and inflammation (Horvath, Papadimitriou, Rabsztyn, Drachenberg, & Tildon, 1999; Krigsman, Boris, Goldblatt & Stott, 2010).

In one study, 143 children who had an ASD and experienced symptoms of gastrointestinal difficulties underwent colonoscopy. More than 75% of those examined were found to have ileocolonic inflammation. The authors noted most of these also showed concurrent LNH (Krigsman et al., 2010). In another study of 172 children and youth diagnosed with ASDs, researchers found that 22.7% experienced GI problems. No differences in rate of GI problems were discovered based on intellectual levels or ASD severity. Not surprisingly, those subjects with GI problems were more irritable, anxious, and withdrawn (Nikolov et al., 2009).

One theory that has been suggested is that those with ASDs have "leaky gut," and this belief has led to a number of dietary interventions. Because of leaky gut epithelium, contents of the intestine leak through the intestinal wall and enter the bloodstream. Opioid-like proteins may be absorbed that may affect neurological development. In response, dietary interventions have become popular and include gluten- and casein-free diets, which are believed to assist in reducing core GI symptoms as well as behavioral difficulties (Sicile-Kira, 2004; Roberts & Kagan-Kushnir, 2005). However, more contemporary research specifically investigating intestinal permeability (leaky gut) found no difference between children with ASDs and controls (Robertson et al., 2008).

Many individuals present in our practices have experienced GI disorders, sometimes associated with anxiety and stress. It has been unclear whether this occurrence is related to the notably poorer eating habits in many individuals who have ASDs, including AS, or if this is related to a specific medical difficulty. Individuals with AS experience the same range of GI difficulties as anyone else, and their experiences will be affected, in part, by their diet. In many individuals we have seen, no specific diagnosis was given, and intervention was based on acute symptoms.

Celiac Disease

Celiac disease is an inflammation of the small intestine caused by an immunological inability to tolerate gluten (Murray, 1999). It has been noted to be at higher than normal incidence in some groups, such as those with Type 1 diabetes and thyroid disorders (Murray, 1999). As well, it occurs at high frequency in those with Down syndrome or ASDs (Percy & Propst, 2008). Percy and Propst (2008) note that in North America, it is one of the most prevalent medical disorders, with an incidence of 1/133 and report anecdotal information that individuals with ASDs may benefit from a diet that is free from gluten and dairy products. In our practice, we have seen individuals with ASDs who received a diagnosis of celiac disease. Suitable dietary intervention was reported to not only decrease discomfort but also positively impact behavioral issues.

Yeast

The literature suggests that individuals with ASDs, including AS, may experience a higher level than normal of yeast in their system (Shattock & Whiteley, 2002; Lynch, 2004). Although the reason for this high level is unclear, it appears to be reflected in behavioral and physiological symptoms. This condition may result in headaches, GI discomfort, rashes, hyperactivity, or states of irritability or confusion. Yeast may also lead to behaviors specifically focused on the area of discomfort (Sicile-Kira, 2004). We have seen individuals with yeast overgrowth in our practices, and often their discomfort is extreme. Based on this experience, an immediate referral to a physician for a yeast swab is made if the person is referred for behaviors such as rubbing the genital area or engaging in acts such as fecal smearing. Sometimes dietary interventions are adequate. If stronger intervention is needed, some antifungal treatments may be effective in reducing problematic symptoms (Shattock & Whiteley, 2002).

Hypoglycemia

Hypoglycemia occurs with some frequency in the general population. It results from an imbalance in blood sugar levels, causing individuals to feel lightheaded and anxious (Lawton & Reichenberg-Ullman, 2007). We are including it in this chapter, as individuals with ASDs, as noted, tend to have poor eating habits. Often the person with an AS is already anxious and is sensitive to the environment. The signs of hypoglycemia in someone with AS might include hyperactivity, anxiety, mood swings, problems with speech, and apparent confusion. The ultimate impact of hypoglycemia on someone with AS, besides the discomfort, might then present as oppositional behavior or a major behavioral outburst (Lawton & Reichenberg-Ullman, 2007).

Eating Preferences and Disorders

Individuals with ASDs are noted to have atypical food preferences (texture or type of food) and behaviors (e.g., rituals influencing eating behavior; Attwood, 2007; Dominick, Davis, Lainhart, Tager-Flusberg, & Folstein, 2007). The authors just cited identified some of the reasons it is believed that those with ASDs exhibit these atypical food-related behaviors; these include GI problems that cause an avoidance of the food causing the difficulty, sensory sensitivities, and features of autism related to a restricted range/desire for sameness. Eating habits may not only indicate sensory preferences (taste, smell, texture) or habit. At times, they may reflect a fad, hoarding behaviors, or pica (eating nonfood material; Gillberg & Billstedt, 2002). Sometimes the atypical eating habits may signal a food sensitivity or allergy (Sicile-Kira, 2004). Some individuals crave foods to which they are allergic, causing physiological discomfort and behavioral challenges. Others will avoid foods to which they know they respond negatively.

We have noted that many of the individuals we have seen who have AS have food preferences that tend to be bland, and they do not include highly textured items that we typically rely on for fiber and nutrition. This kind of bland diet is sometimes referred to as a "white diet" and includes pasta, rice, processed chicken, white bread, and "junk food." Such a diet may lead to elimination problems and will affect the balance of vitamins and minerals available to the body. Individuals with AS who have poor eating habits should consult with their physician about vitamin supplements, food restrictions, allergies, and the intake of bioactive cultures (e.g., cultures found in yogurts). We regularly include questions about eating habits and GI health (i.e., constipation, diarrhea, and elimination frequency) in assessments of adults with AS, which they may be too embarrassed to raise with their general physician. They are often relieved to discuss their symptoms and discover that others on the autism spectrum experience similar problems.

In the last decade, reports have focused not only on eating preferences in those with ASDs. A few authors have noted that of those with eating disorders, a larger than expected number has an ASD, including AS. This is particularly so for women with ASDs, who meet criteria for an eating disorder (Gillberg, 2002b; Attwood, 2007). Gillberg (2002b) stated that although there is little research on the relationship between AS and eating disorders, there is substantial clinical evidence. He indicated that some studies have shown that women with anorexia nervosa had a high incidence of AS or of another ASD. As well, young men with AS who develop unusual eating habits and become thin may meet criteria for anorexia nervosa.

We have seen cases of food refusal, excessive exercise, and bingeing and purging in adults with AS. Bingeing has been seen primarily in males, but also in females. Parents report that the adult does not seem to have a sense of how much food to take, and eat, in a socially acceptable manner. Others have reported that they do not realize that they have eaten enough until they feel unwell. Overeating can also be understood as a response to anxiety or depression or as a sensory-seeking behavior (e.g., in the case of sweet/salty/spicy foods or carbonated beverages). In males, obsessive concern about weight, BMI, and muscularity, coupled with repetitive exercise, may indicate body dysmorphic disorder.

One study examined a group of women at a clinical setting who were diagnosed with eating disorders (Wentz et al., 2005). The authors reported that 53% had a minimum of one childhood-onset neurological disorder, 27% had tic disorder, 23% had an ASD, and 17% had ADHD. Kalyva (2009) studied adolescent females who had a diagnosis of AS, as well as those without a diagnosis. Both the girls and their mothers were asked to report on the girls' eating habits and attitudes. Results suggested that adolescents with AS were at greater risk for eating difficulties than those without AS. In a systematic review of 46 articles that described 22 studies of individuals with anorexia nervosa, affected individuals were more likely to have mood and anxiety disorders and an ASD (including AS) than comparison groups. Low body weight in those who have autism or AS has also been examined independent of known eating disorders (Bolte, Ozkara, & Poustka, 2002). Results did not show a consistent relationship, and the authors suggested that hyperactivity could be partly responsible for the low body weight.

Sleep Disorders

Individuals with ASDs, including those with AS, frequently experience sleep difficulties that begin early in life and last through their adult years. Gillberg and Billstedt (2000) suggest that sleep difficulties during infancy may be the earliest indicator that there is something of concern. Lack of sleep affects a person's daily functioning, including his or her level of alertness and activity and ability to cope with stress and to concentrate. As well, individuals who do not sleep at night may disrupt the sleep of those with whom they live.

The issue of sleep abnormalities in those with autism has been researched and reported for many years. Ornitz (1985) found that those with autism showed differences in rapid eye movement (REM) patterns. Stores and Wiggs (1998) reviewed the literature on sleep difficulties in individuals with autism and suggested various possible reasons for such abnormalities, including those that are neurologically or biochemically based, those related to other underlying medical difficulties or cognitive and psychological impairments, and those with an emotional or behavioral cause. Hypersomnia and behavioral and mood problems have been reported in two cases of adolescents with AS (Berthier, Santamaria, Encabo, & Tolosa, 1992). The cases also suggested the presence of Kleine–Levin syndrome (a rare sleep disorder experienced by male adolescents and characterized by hypersomnia and disturbances in cognition, behavior, and mood; Berthier et al., 1992). A recent survey of parents of children with autism or AS found that sleep problems were common (73% in both groups), and children with AS were more likely to be sluggish and disoriented after waking. These children had higher total scores on the Behavioral Evaluation of Disorders of Sleep (BEDS) compared to typically developing children, indicating more symptoms of sleep disturbance (Polimeni, Richdale, & Francis, 2005).

A laboratory study of sleep compared high-functioning individuals with ASDs who did not experience sleep issues or coexisting psychiatric difficulties with a control group of healthy adults (Limoges, Mottron, Bolduc, Berthiaume, & Godbout, 2005). The results showed that those with an ASD had longer sleep latency, awakened more often during the night, had longer Stage 1 sleep, fewer eye movements during REM sleep, and showed fewer EEG spindles during Stage 2 sleep. They also found some differences between those with AS or HFA in terms of "morningness–eveningness preference" (p. 13) and in density of EEG spindles. The results suggest that there are inherent differences in the physiological aspects of sleep in those with AS compared to other individuals. Limoges et al. compared their findings for those with AS to a study reported in 2003 (Tani et al.). The research by Tani et al. found less restfulness or satisfaction with sleep in the participants than did the participants in the Limoges et al. study. However, the 2003 study included participants with concurrent psychiatric disorders, which may have added to their sleep difficulties.

Roberts and Kagan-Kushnir (2005) addressed sleep issues in those with ASDs, including AS, and suggested that poor sleep hygiene and anxiety may be contributing factors. They also indicated that seizures may occasionally disrupt sleep. Individuals we have worked with also appear to be aroused by distracting events in the environment, such as sounds in the house (e.g., furnace motor going on and off) and other sensory responses (e.g., the feel of the sheets, temperature of the room). We encourage maintaining an optimal sleep environment for the person. Often fans or white noise machines are utilized to decrease distractions.

In our practice we see sleep problems as a major concern for individuals with little structure in their lives. The most common and serious problem seen in these cases is the tendency to sleep during the day and be awake at night. Even those struggling to complete postsecondary education or attend employment can struggle with sleep hygiene. The interaction between mood and anxiety disorders, repetitive behaviors/activities/thoughts, and sleep problems requires further investigation in this population. We have noticed that many individuals who have too many items in their bedrooms are distracted by them and feel an obsessive need to utilize these items when they should be sleeping. We often recommend that items in their bedroom be kept to a minimum.

In terms of pharmacological interventions, Furusho et al. (2001) presented a case report of an 8-year-old boy who responded positively to the SSRI fluvoxamine, with an attenuation of initial insomnia and a decrease in repetitive behavior. The value of melatonin in addressing sleep disturbances in children with AS, as well as guidelines regarding its use, was noted by Panksepp (2005) and Sloman (2005). Insomnia that begins subsequent to the introduction of an SSRI, however, may require morning administration, a dosage change, or a trial of another antidepressant. We tend to discourage the use of benzodiazepines for long-term sleep regulation. However, the sedative effects of antipsychotics such as respiridone, initially prescribed to reduce anxiety or address behavioral dysregulation, can also be advantageous in assisting with sleep.

SUMMARY

Individuals who have AS have the same likelihood of having any medical diagnosis compared to those in the general population. However, there appears to be an increased risk of learning, processing, and perceptual difficulties and of some medical and health problems. Individuals with AS should be assessed for learning difficulties and receive thorough medical examinations and tests to ensure that any coexisting difficulty is treated. Singly, these disorders affect the daily life of the individual; when they are combined, they can be overwhelming and substantially incapacitate the individual.

Currently, research is examining the genetic component of ASDs and progress is being made. However, there is still much confusion and disagreement about learning, medical, and health issues. This state of affairs leaves individuals and their families without adequate guidance about, and confidence in, intervention. Rigorous and ongoing research is required to resolve these issues, so that we add to our knowledge base of the disorders themselves and have a range of empirically based interventions at our disposal.

Chapter 5

PSYCHOSOCIAL ISSUES IN
ADULT ASPERGER SYNDROME

CASE EXAMPLE: LIVING WITHOUT
HOUSING SUPPORTS

I was meeting Edward and a potential new support worker for him at his new apartment. In the last several years, Edward had made several suicide attempts because of untreated anxiety and depression. He had lived in a few apartments on his own in the past, but for various reasons, including nonpayment of rent and conflict with his neighbors, he was never able to keep them for any significant length of time. Despite being in his late 30s now, he continued to rely on his retired parents for support. We had agreed that I would knock two times on his apartment door and identify myself as the Superintendent, as he didn't want his neighbors to know that he was receiving professional help.

As I entered the basement apartment of the large old house, my hopes sank. The room was no more than 12 by 12 feet. His windows were covered with aluminum foil so that the neighbors would not "spy on him." Under the window stood his large TV, piled high with pornographic DVDs and copies of "The Sopranos." His futon mattress was lying on the floor, and empty beer cans were strewn everywhere. His kitchen counter was covered with pizza boxes, take-out food containers, and dirty coffee mugs. His fridge was empty save for several frozen dinners provided by his mother, now entombed by ice in his freezer. I casually remarked on the glaring bare lightbulb hanging precariously by a few exposed wires from the ceiling. Edward began pacing anxiously. We agreed that we would write a note together asking the landlord to fix it, but he was clearly anxious that the landlord would "kick him out" because of it. He dictated. I scribed.

The community worker arrived. She identified herself to Edward as a caseworker who supported individuals with "dual diagnoses." She explained that this meant her clients had developmental disabilities and mental health problems. Edward, who was intimately familiar with local social service policies and clinical nomenclature, began arguing that he did not have a developmental disability and did not want help from anybody who worked with "retards." Although she proceeded to describe the services she provided and offered in-home support with bills, grocery shopping, and household chores, I knew that continuing the interview would be pointless.

A few months later, Edward moved back in with his parents.

The intent of this chapter is to review the most common psychosocial concerns that we have seen in clinical practice; these are reflected in clinician writings and the research literature (e.g., Engstrom, Ekstrom, & Emilsson, 2003; Hofvander et al., 2009; Stoddart, 2006a). If they are to be addressed successfully, many of the issues highlighted here will require the cooperation and combined expertise of multiple service providers who may come from many service sectors. Unfortunately, some of these psychosocial problems occur, or are not well managed and treated, because of the lack of collaboration and knowledge dissemination between service sectors. The clinician working with this population can play a key role in ensuring that there is necessary expertise on the team, advocating for the client (and others similarly affected) and ensuring that team members are working in tandem. Here, we discuss behavioral problems and legal involvement, finding and keeping intimate relationships, expression of sexuality, parenting, employment, postsecondary education, and aging. We begin by highlighting housing and life skills.

HOUSING AND LIFE SKILLS

The dearth of supported living choices is a universal concern among individuals with AS, their families, and service providers. Seventy percent of parents of individuals with ASDs surveyed by the National Autistic Society in the United Kingdom said that their children would not be able to live independently without ongoing supports in place (Barnard et al., 2001). This concern was echoed by parents and service providers in Canada and led to policy recommendations by a provincial advocacy group (Ontario Partnership for Adults with Aspergers and Autism, 2008), which points out: "Individuals [with ASDs] often require long-term support throughout their life and rarely move 'out' of their support system. . . . There are limited support structures [e.g., lack of affordable housing] in generic services once individuals are ready to move towards more independence" (p. 16). This advocacy group recommended that government "ensure sufficient and regulated services for adults with ASD in the adult/child mental health, social service, colleges/universities and developmental sectors through an Ontario-wide cross-sector policy framework and devoted funding based on a provincial needs assessment. Specifically, this policy framework would ensure . . . a range of supported living options" (Ontario Partnership for Adults with Aspergers and Autism, 2008). From a policy standpoint, it was noted by this group that adults with AS fall between government departmental responsibilities because of reliance on outdated classification systems and lack of recognition of the effect of poor functional abilities. Rather, current governmental responsibilities are defined by an individual's intellectual ability, which is not necessarily reflective of functional capacity, especially when supports and life skills training are lacking. Further, they note:

> Although their symptoms and characteristics change over time, the approximately 50,000 adults with ASD in Ontario need a range of supports for their whole lives. Housing is an important part of that support structure, and one that is particularly troubling for aging parents and overly stressed families. For many individuals with ASD, the only thing standing between them and homelessness is their family. However, families are not always able to safely cope with the

behavioural challenges of their loved ones. (Ontario Partnership for Adults with Aspergers and Autism, 2009, p. 1)

Because of this experience of many parents in Ontario, Canada, a housing committee was formed by a local group of parents that was concerned about the lack of supported housing choices for their young adults with AS (Asperger Society of Ontario, 2006). The committee concluded that rather than risk an unsuccessful independent living situation, they preferred a supported living arrangement:

> To successfully meet the needs of individuals with Asperger Syndrome living semi-independently in the community, or wishing to, they will need to be supported and advocated for by professionals who have knowledge of their unique needs. A supported independent living program specifically for individuals with Asperger Syndrome would address such challenges. (p. 5)

Poor performance in life skills may reflect many possible precipitants, such as depression and other mental health problems, lack of interest in the activity, lack of motivation, rejection of socially derived notions of the importance of cleanliness and organization, poor executive functioning, collecting/hoarding behaviors, sensory sensitivities, or an inability to generalize learned skills from one environment to another. Adults may report that their living environment is clean or organized in the clinical interview, yet a visit by the clinician to view their home or apartment may provide a very different perspective. Clinical contact with other family members also provides an additional opinion about the individuals' ability to maintain a clean living environment and live self-sufficiently. An objective indicator of the cleanliness or organization of the home environment (e.g., via a digital picture or home visit) is often called for in cases when the adult engages in repetitive and circular arguments that his or her parents' expectations for cleanliness are unreasonable.

A picture of one of our client's apartment was e-mailed to us. After viewing the picture in the office, we discussed the health hazards in the living environment, and as a consequence the young man moved back to the parental home. Other behavioral characteristics of AS were noted by the parents, and he was diagnosed with AS, anxiety, and depression. Another man with AS denied that there were any problems with his hygiene or living situation in individual office-based interviews. However, a call from his mother and his house cleaner revealed that he was having bowel accidents and had begun hoarding his feces. Often, the lack of cleanliness and the inability to cope with the demands of independent living call for further assessment or intervention, whether medical, psychological, or cognitive in nature.

Clinical experience suggests that occasionally, adolescents with AS are able to move out of the home and live successfully with few or no supports, whereas for others this same transition is disastrous. In the latter case, it becomes clearer to service providers and family that the person lacks the requisite life skills to live independently. Lack of community supports sometimes results in excessive isolation, increased addictions, mental health problems, unclean living situations, poor hygiene, and financial problems. These difficulties, in turn, lead to moving back to the parental home either for a specified period of time or indefinitely.

It is therefore vital to have a realistic understanding, via the assessment process, of individuals' life skills and abilities to cope with the varied demands of living on their own. This assessment might be performed at the point of diagnosis if it occurs in late adolescence or early adulthood. Alternatively, it might be part of a discussion with the young adult about future goals, or moving out of the family home. If individuals with AS are not able to accomplish basic life skills under the supervision of parents as adolescents and young adults, it is unlikely that they will be able to do so as adults, living on their own. For those families with younger children that we support, we stress the cultivation of life skills as a developmental task to be practiced and used in early adolescence. Regular expectations, scheduled household duties, and rewards such as an allowance serve an essential forerunner to managing independent living in adulthood.

Through a detailed discussion with the young adult and their parents, an assessment of these skills can occur in the clinical interview and with the administering of standardized functional assessment tools. These measures might include the Vineland Adaptive Behavior Scales, Second Edition (VABS-II; Sparrow, Cicchetti, & Balla, 2005) and the Adaptive Behavior Assessment System, Second Edition (ABAS-II; Harrison & Oakland, 2003) or online checklists such as the Adolescent Autonomy Checklist (Youth in Transition

Project, 2010). Often, the functional life skills or activities of daily living of adults with AS are surprisingly poor, given what might be expected with average to above average intellectual abilities. Powell (2002) notes 11 areas in which individuals with AS might need help: (1) financial, (2) morning routines, (3) organization and reminder systems, (4) food hygiene, (5) diet, (6) avoiding loss of personal possessions, (7) home safety, (8) home skills and maintenance, (9) personal care; (10) community skills, and (11) understanding and applying for welfare benefits (p. 31). Also relevant to this list are leisure skills.

For some individuals with AS, moving out of the family home may be precipitated by conflict in the home between the adolescent and his or her parents, or other members of the household. Alcohol/drug use or inappropriate behaviors such as stealing may also be antecedents to leaving the home, as parents feel that they can no longer tolerate their adolescent's behavior. In these punitive situations, we have seen adolescents "couch surf" with a series of friends, leading to more instability in their lives. However, we are also supportive of parents enforcing "house rules" by evicting their older adolescent or young adult children if other, less intrusive measures have been unsuccessful.

Generally, both the typically developing young adult and their parents may feel the event of leaving the family home provides a clear demarcation of responsibility: The young adult is now responsible for paying the bills, getting up in the morning on time for work, feeding him- or herself, and other similar tasks. However, this simple "division of responsibilities" is not always what occurs in reality for young adults with AS. Even if the individual with AS does move out of the family home, parents may continue to be responsible for supporting the young adult. Tasks such as paying bills, shopping for groceries, keeping their apartment clean, and being a "responsible tenant" are all skills that may need to be taught and monitored. Although these tasks may not always be carried out by family members, *arranging for others* to deliver groceries, help with paying bills, or do laundry may be left to the parents. A candid discussion between parents and the young adult is important; this might need to be facilitated by a helping professional when these issues are a point of conflict in the family. Other possible housing supports for adults with AS include a life skills coach, a house cleaner, a case manager, and a visiting nurse or mental health worker.

Infrequently, we support individuals who "hyperfocus" on issues of cleanliness and organization in their home setting. These clients may insist on ordering their belongings, be vigilant to any changes to their environment made by others, or clean repeatedly. These behaviors or routines might interfere with their ability to engage in routines that are functional. Although some of these behaviors are symptomatic of AS (i.e., repetitive behavior), they also suggest OCD and might be diagnosed and treated as this. A clinical determination therefore needs to be made about the intensity and severity of the behaviors, their impact on daily functioning, and whether the behaviors are beyond that which would commonly be seen in adults with AS.

The risk of developing a mental illness or experiencing a worsening in mental health may also be associated with independent living and the lack of supports available to this population. The supported living model proposed by the Asperger Society of Ontario (ASO, 2006) addressed this: "In supportive housing, individuals with Asperger Syndrome would be connected with staff that would be aware of the increased risk of mental illness, identify the signs of a developing illness earlier, and ensure that the individual with Asperger Syndrome is connected with the necessary supports" (pp. 5–6). The ASO suggested the follow features for shared living units: individualized units with shared living areas (e.g., kitchen, TV area), on-site security, mixed-use housing attracting a cross-section of the local population, affordability, accessibility of public transit, and community amenities within walking distance (e.g., gym, recreation center, and movie theaters).

BEHAVIORAL PROBLEMS AND LEGAL INVOLVEMENT

Increasingly, adults with AS who have been charged with criminal offenses are seen in clinical practice settings—a trend that is reflected in the recently published clinical and research literature. The prevalence of criminal activity in this population may be surprising to some, given that most individuals with ASDs are strictly law-abiding and cognizant of rules and laws, sometimes to an obsessive extent. Early reports summarized by Ghaziuddin, Tsai, and Ghaziuddin (1991) suggested that individuals with AS may engage in violent acts, but the frequency with which the violence comes to the attention of the authorities is limited. In contrast, more contemporary reports have made the case for a high risk of violence (Silva & Haskins, 2006) and other crimes. Cases in the media have also highlighted the possible connections between AS/ASDs and criminal behavior. One of these cases involved a man who impersonated transit authorities in New York City (Tietz, 2002); another involved Gary McKinnon, an individual with AS in the United Kingdom who hacked into U.S. military and NASA computers (Hirsch, 2009).

We have seen adults with ASDs who have been charged with the following criminal offenses: possession of marijuana, public intoxication, theft, fraud, identity theft, attempted murder, driving while impaired by alcohol, physical assault, sexual assault/interference, possession and distribution of child pornography, dangerous driving, and stalking. The literature contains case reports of violence (Baron-Cohen, 1988; Kohn, Fahum, Ratzoni, & Apter, 1998; Mawson, Grounds, & Tantam, 1985), murder/attempted murder (Murrie, Warren, Kristiansson, & Dietz, 2002; Newman & Ghaziuddin, 2008; Schwartz-Watts, 2005; Silva & Haskins, 2006), theft (Chen et al., 2003), sexual offenses (Barry-Walsh & Mullen, 2004; Murrie et al., 2002), and arson (Barry-Walsh & Mullen, 2004; Haskins & Silva, 2006; Murrie et al., 2002).

Although the contributors to illegal/criminal behavior in adults with AS are not yet well understood, there are several emerging theories. Many of the legal issues that confront adults with AS relate to their poor grasp of social skills and social boundaries, their social naïveté and ability to be influenced by others, and their inability to make or keep friends or engage in intimate relationships (Murrie et al., 2002; Stokes, Newton, & Kaur, 2007). The lack of a social network or affinitive group may lead individuals to join groups that are involved in risky or illegal activities. Involvement in a youth gang that engaged in petty criminal acts is one example seen in practice. Some people with AS crave group membership and are easily drawn into illegal behaviors (sometimes naïvely) in order to feel a sense of belonging.

Stalking behaviors might be reframed as the failure to decode the social cues, often nonverbal, the subject of affection is communicating. The pursued individual may not want to "hurt the person's feelings" and so provides artificial or trivial explanations for his or her lack of interest. For example, a woman may claim that she is "busy" on a given day or days and is not able to go on a date. In turn, the man with AS might continue to pursue her with other possible days for a date. The woman's communications might not be understood as intended, and so the pursuit may continue. This behavior may also be fuelled by the individual's sexual frustration, concern over not having met a woman, loneliness, belief that it is unusual not to have had a sexual experience, and past romantic failures.

Public concern over stalking behaviors has increased over the past few decades. In Canada, recognition of stalking as a criminal behavior took place in 1993 with Section 264 of the *Criminal Code of Canada* (Dept. of Justice, 1993). Many of the repetitive behaviors that males, especially, with AS engage in while expressing interest in a person may look like stalking, although the intent to harm or intimidate is not usually present. Attwood (1999b) has noted: "There can be a developmental progression from collecting objects, to a topic, to a person and there can be an infatuation with an individual. They are besotted by that person, they can follow that person, they want to be with that person and it's a degree of adulation or crush which is quite considerable" (p. 1).

Eye gaze toward the person of interest may be unusually intense, and affected individuals may need to be taught that this appears threatening or impolite. We have also seen individuals who have misinterpreted innocent situations with serious consequences. For example, one man saw himself in pictures (taken at social events) with a woman in whom he had an interest. His parents had similar pictures taken, as did people in the media who were in relationships. He therefore misinterpreted having his picture taken with this woman as an indication that they were a couple. This situation ended in a violent confrontation and a restraining order was issued against him. Many clinicians describe, to us, adults with AS who are at risk of being charged with (sexual) harassment because of their tendency to ask personal and intrusive questions to relative strangers.

One young man that we were seeing in treatment expressed a romantic fixation about a young woman whom he had known in high school a few years prior. This woman acted in a friendly way to the young man during their school years together (although they were not close friends), and a few years after leaving high school he decided to pursue her, despite not having any social contact with her since their association in school. Individuals in the community, such

165

as storeowners, provided him with information about the young woman's whereabouts (probably as a rouse) when he expressed his affection for her to them, and he gradually gained detailed knowledge of her whereabouts. He began leaving her notes and flowers and traveled to another city to see if he could find her at her university dormitory. Discussion of his behaviors occurred in therapy; he was clearly unaware of the potential impact of his behaviors on this young woman. His romantic fixation was reframed by his therapist as a byproduct of his loneliness, social isolation, and interest in sexual activity. Other avenues to pursue relationships and sexual activity were therefore explored.

In our practice, two clients became caught up in incidents that resulted from their lack of understanding about inappropriate social behaviors through social networking sites and electronic communication; their behaviors led to police investigations. In both of these instances, the young men sent inappropriate messages by text messaging and the Internet. One sent anti-Semitic messages and threats to harm an individual; another sent inappropriate sexual messages to a minor. In both instances, the perpetrators claimed that they did this "as a joke"; however, both threats were taken seriously by the recipients of the communications and the police.

Besides poor social skills, repetitive thoughts or a restricted range of interests may precipitate illegal or inappropriate behavior (Murrie et al., 2002). For example, a man in his mid-30s was prevented by family members (with whom he resided) from watching violent movies because they felt that this led to inappropriate thoughts and behaviors. Subsequently, he began stealing videos from stores and was charged with theft. Often, interests of adults with AS are not inherently illegal or troublesome, but the means by which they exercise the interests can become problematic. Conversely, it should be understood that potentially harmful interests do not necessarily lead to criminal activity. An interest in firearms and the military, for example, may be troublesome to family and the community, however. Understandably, the intensity with which interests are pursued and the time engaged in certain interests can be worrisome to many. A young man who drew sexualized cartoon pictures in a Japanese anime style was suspected by his coworkers to be a sexual risk to others in the community. However, he has not attempted to act on his sexualized artistic interests.

166

A third possible risk factor contributing to illegal behavior is substance abuse, which is now being recognized in individuals with ASDs (Santosh & Mijovic, 2006; Stoddart, 2006a; Tinsley & Hendrickx, 2008). The abuse of drugs or alcohol is sometimes a means of self-medication without proper pharmacological, behavioral, or psychotherapeutic treatment for anxiety, mood, or sleep disorders. It is probable that adults with AS are at risk of substance use because of lack of other coping mechanisms, the presence of addictions in their families (Miles, Takahashi, Haber, & Hadden, 2003), their repetitive thought patterns, their difficulty with regulating mood, the effect of environmental stressors, and the absence of other socially protective influences. Use of addictive substances can be extreme and may result in offending behavior, decreased ability to anticipate the consequences of their behavior, and decreased ability to conceal illegal activities or inappropriate behaviors from the public or police. We discuss treatment of addictions in the context of AS in chapters 6 and 7.

Other factors have been proposed as possible contributors to criminal behavior in individuals with ASDs. These include poor ToM (see Chapters 1 and 2; Haskins & Silva, 2006), the inability to control impulses, problems considering the future stress an act may cause (Chen et al., 2003), and deficits in empathy (Murrie et al., 2002; Wing, 1981). We suggest that many of these variables would not necessarily be problematic, or could be remediated if there were better access to early diagnostic services, greater awareness of ASDs in forensic services, better screening of psychiatric and cognitive comorbidities, and more general support services for adults with AS.

In cases of serious crimes such as serial murders, Silva and colleagues (Silva, Ferrari, & Leong, 2002; Silva & Haskins, 2006; Silva, Leong, Ferrari, 2004) have suggested several neuropsychiatric developmental reasons individuals with ASDs might be involved in such destructive behavior, including the possible overlap between AS traits and schizoid personality disorder. As well, early life stressors, left unmanaged and unaddressed, may place these individuals at risk of chronically using maladaptive coping mechanisms/behaviors. It has been recognized in a few case reports, that early experiences of bullying and social isolation were evident in the childhoods of offenders.

Individuals with ASDs may also experience paraphilic pathologies of a fetishistic nature (Murrie et al., 2002). Silva et al. (2004) note:

> These paraphilias are characterized as involving a strong tendency to experience the object of erotic interest as physical hyper-representations of the body either by focusing on body parts (i.e., partialism) or physical symbolic extensions of the body proper (i.e., Fetishism), or exclusive focus on the physical make-up of the body (i.e., necrophilia). . . . We hypothesize that among autistic serial sexual killers this deconstructive paraphilic pattern is a partial, but intrinsic, outcome of the tendency of autistic persons to focus on physical objects and their component parts with a relative neglect for their mental qualities. (p. 790)

Problems with anger management in adults with AS is also pertinent to this discussion of criminal behavior. In this group, anger often reflects underlying anxiety, rigid and inflexible thinking, poor theory of mind, inability to see the gestalt, and poor problem-solving abilities (Channon, 2004; Channon et al., 2001). The difficulty of displaying proper reactions to stressful situations (that require thoughtful-proactive responses versus impulsive-reactive reactions) is often reported in clinical interviews. The cognitive resources that are necessary to negotiate stressful social situations successfully may not be available to the individual in the moment, and he or she may revert to inappropriate social behaviors such as yelling, threatening, destruction of property, name-calling, swearing, or other behaviors that are seen as developmentally immature. Understandably, in adults these are seen as threatening to members of the public, and police involvement is sometimes the result.

We have seen many cases in which individuals were involved in violent acts (i.e., assault) or illegal activity but were not charged. In many situations, although there is chronic aggression in childhood, it subsides in later years because of pharmacological, behavioral, or cognitive–behavioral interventions (Smith Myles & Southwick, 1999), or simply maturation. Pharmacological interventions can be used for aggressive behavior (Weller, Rowan, Elia, & Weller, 1999), as reviewed in Chapter 6. It is also important to consider how anger is displayed and disagreement is managed in the home setting. Often, we see individuals with anger management issues (and aggression) who have been raised with ongoing conflict in the home that has not been managed or addressed adequately. Managing conflict may require a family intervention, a series of marital counseling sessions, and/or individual therapy (Stoddart, 1999). Problems with anger management can be a major obstacle to keeping employment and experiencing success in a postsecondary setting, despite possessing the essential skills or knowledge (Stoddart, 2005c).

Considering the literature reviewed, reported cases of crimes by individuals with AS involving mental health professionals (Barry-Walsh & Mullen, 2004; Murrie et al., 2002), and our own clinical experiences, it is paramount that safety issues be considered for clinicians who assess or treat adults with AS. This is especially critical if an individual has a recent history of aggression or violence. Proper assessment of risk should occur through a review of clinical information and reports in the patient chart, information and discussion with other service providers, family members, or the individual him- or herself. It is ill-advised to see previously offending individuals alone or without the suitable security measures in place in a clinical setting. We have witnessed the violent destruction of property and been threatened and assaulted, even with the exercise of caution and fitting protocols in place. Careful management of risk is also essential while engaged in the clinical interview and while in the clinical setting. This management might include setting up a behavioral contract with the individual, deescalation of anger in the clinical interview, avoidance of difficult topics until the therapeutic relationship has been well established, and involvement with the individual at lower-stress/anxiety times only.

The question of criminal responsibility is often raised in legal cases involving individuals with AS (Haskins & Silva, 2006). Specifically, do individuals with AS understand the law or rule that they broke and do they appreciate the potential negative impact of their offending behavior on the alleged victim(s)? Understandably, parents of individuals with AS are reluctant to have adults with AS be involved with the legal system, feeling that it will not be helpful, will not lead to better or effective treatment, will further stigmatize them, and worsen their chances of finding employment. Legal and pathological labels can also be inappropriately applied and misunderstood: In one instance, a man who had a costume fetish was caught in a costume store touching his genitals through his pants;

although he was not arrested or charged, the incident was recorded on the local police records as "possible sexual offender," and this designation prevented him from obtaining employment where a police record check was mandatory.

Despite this concern, the lack of consequences for illegal behavior by individuals with AS is also sometimes problematic. Conflicting social and institutional messages are, not surprisingly, confusing for these individuals. Despite discussion and controversy in the media and the legal profession about the culpability of individuals with AS, the use of the defense of AS may contribute to a lack of remorse in these individuals, an absence of punishment or consequence, poor or limited understanding of the seriousness of the behavior, and subsequent recurrence of the activity or behavior. This opinion is based solely on clinical experience, as there are no known outcome studies of the effect of criminal punishment on the remediation of offending behavior in this group.

Though a previous AS diagnosis may provide access to appropriate services, misapplication of this diagnostic label has also been problematic in our experience. In one instance, for example, behavioral observations and documentation of self-centeredness, grandiosity, poor peer relationships, fire setting, risk taking, extreme impulsivity, and aggression before and during an admission to an adolescent mental health facility by an adolescent diagnosed at age 4 as having AS challenged an experienced interdisciplinary team. A sense of purpose in his antisocial actions, a sense of entitlement, the use of intimidation, the "deliberateness" of his sexually inappropriate behavior, and his strong rationalization of his antisocial behavior led the team to question whether a diagnosis of AS was sufficient to formulate an optimal understanding of his behavior. Although aware of the possibility of mind-blindness and a lack of knowledge of social mores and skills, ultimately a retrospective, comprehensive developmental history and review of previous assessments failed to support a diagnosis of AS. Disclosure by the youth and his mother and father of significant family dysfunction and multiple exposures to trauma led to the brief formulation of a diagnosis of a conduct disorder and ADHD. This was accompanied by a recommendation for treatment in a secure facility to address the imminent danger of his proclivity for fire-setting and impulsive, aggressive behavior.

FINDING AND KEEPING INTIMATE RELATIONSHIPS

> One cause of my depression is my need for intimacy—that which I feel I am sorely lacking. I have a deep-rooted need for intimacy, specifically romantic intimacy, that I feel is not being fulfilled in my life. (Jansen, 2005, p. 317)

When we think of the challenges that are inherent in AS and the social demands of intimate relationships, we might conclude that they are an insurmountable obstacle for these adults. However, adults with AS who are involved in intimate relationships are increasingly seen in clinical practice (Myhill & Jekel, 2008), and it is likely that this trend will continue as individuals with milder forms of AS are identified—by themselves, by partners or family members, or following the diagnosis of a child. Despite this increase however, other adults with AS may remain single for extended periods or may never meet a partner. We have little knowledge of the frequency of marriage for individuals with AS, or of marital "success rate." Much of the evidence from our practice with children affected with ASDs would suggest that the combination of AS traits in one of the parents *and* the stress involved in raising a child with exceptionalities, results in a high rate of divorce. Some of the outcome studies of adults on the spectrum have suggested that marriage in this population is rare; however, it is essential to note that the subjects in these studies are individuals who have been diagnosed, often as children, and comprise a clinical sample, as opposed to those who have not accessed services, as noted in Chapter 1.

We now understand that more than ever, adults are being diagnosed with AS precisely because of their difficulty in engaging in intimate relationships (Myhill & Jekel, 2008), as discussed in Chapter 2. Some individuals with AS have a limited need for close personal relationships, although this varies widely. Jansen (2005), above, described his need for intimacy and its lack in his life as a significant contributor to his depression. A limited desire for intimate relationships in individuals with AS may relate to past (unsuccessful) relationships, social anxiety, a need to control their environment and routine, and a sense of comfort and ease with their own company.

171

One of the few empirical investigations of marriages involving men with ASDs discovered that for these men, "marital adaptation was significantly associated with more received and perceived social support from the spouse and from family, friends and acquaintances," but that avoidant types of coping were associated with more psychosocial distress for them (Renty & Roeyers, 2007, p. 1250). For the women, "individual adaptation was strongly related to received social support from family, friends, and acquaintances, such that women with higher levels of psychosocial distress received more support. Marital adaptation of the women was inversely related to the degree of autism-specific traits of their husband, while perceived and received supports from their spouse were positively related to marital adaptation" (p. 1250).

A major contribution to the literature on intimate relationships in this group is by Maxine Aston, who provides therapy for couples in which one partner is affected by AS. Among her books is the summary of a study that she carried out (Aston, 2003). Subjects included "forty-one adults with Asperger Syndrome, all with current or previous intimate relationships, and… thirty-five of their partners. The adults with AS had either been officially diagnosed or self-diagnosed" (p. 14). Although this work was presented in a non-peer-reviewed and nonscientific format, this study provides some of the most valuable insights into couple relationships in this population that the current literature offers.

It should be noted that, in the majority of heterosexual couples we have seen, the man has AS. In our experience, the men that are seen with AS often need unusually long periods in which to "decompress" after work, or engage in their particular interests. One husband with AS refers to his basement apartment in the house, equipped with big-screen television and comfortable leather recliner, as his "man-den." Such reclusive behavior can be likened to the teen with AS who needs to have "his space" when he returns home from high school. He has been asked to perform socially and academically all day, process overwhelming sensory input, and do things for which he is neither well equipped, nor for which he has any interest. After a day of interacting socially and managing the demands of work, adult males also need respite. It is important for the partner to not interpret her spouse's reclusive behaviors as a response to her (or her behavior), but as symptomatic of AS. Some men explicitly discuss the need for this solitude, especially if there are children in the household. Interestingly, women we have worked with who have AS tend to have more stamina around the daily schedule, but hit periods when they totally shut down, requiring hours, days, or longer to reenergize.

Although the degree of isolation needed by adults with AS is often a problem for the spouse who is caring for the children and coordinating the household tasks, acceptance of this need can also be seen as a functional manner of coping. It has been suggested that some intimate relationships between an individual with ASD and a "neurotypical" individual may be most successful if the couple does not cohabitate (Engstrom et al., 2003; Moore, 2008). We have seen situations in which the husband has a separate self-contained apartment in the house—which is another less costly solution to the affected partner's need for solitude.

An ability to engage in various activities, interests, and pastimes and discuss those interests is part of developing and preserving relationships. A "restricted range of interests" (American Psychiatric Association, 2000) can limit opportunities for social interaction/ intimacy, because an excessive amount of time is spent on the activity—and often these activities are not "social" in nature, conversation is restricted to these topics/interests, and the interest limits opportunities for social skill rehearsal. Isolating preoccupations may be the precursor or result of increased social anxiety or agoraphobia.

Alternatively, special interests can provide opportunities for social interaction. Many individuals tell us they feel more confident socially when they are with others who share similar interests. We have worked with individuals who were environmental activists or had interests in specific types of collections. When they were with others who shared their interests and experiences, they found a social fit that was lacking in other situations. Because of the inherent capacity of many of those with AS to use technology, social networking, and online dating, many of these adults attempt to communicate with others online. For many, communication online is slower-paced and visual—which are preferred learning and communication attributes for many individuals on the spectrum. Interfering sensory comorbidities (e.g., central auditory processing disorder) and the pressure to interpret facial expressions or other nonverbal communications are not an issue online.

Both Attwood (1999b) and Aston (2003) note that some adults with AS are attracted to individuals who have similar interests or like to engage in similar activities. We know of one couple, (both have an ASD), who met at an Asperger social group. The "match made in heaven" was apparent when we realized that they were both Sesame Street fans, both had a collection of Sesame Street puppets, and both could provide convincing impressions of all the characters! Aston (2003) pointed out that strong interests in music, the theatre and the arts, and animals as well as shared beliefs were common among her couple participants. In cases where couples do not share strong interests or beliefs differ, the relationship can become contentious. The partner without AS may feel abandoned or that the partner is having "an affair" with the hobby or interest, to the exclusion of their relationship or tasks and activities around the house. Romantic affairs with other individuals, either online or in person, and sexual activity (both romantic and nonromantic in nature) outside the relationship are also reported.

Individuals with AS struggle with various social–communication concerns that have been described elsewhere in this book. As one might expect, the problems arising from poor reading of nonverbal communication and slow or inaccurate processing of verbal communications are often raised in marital sessions with these couples (Myhill & Jekel, 2008). For example, the woman (without AS) may go through a ritual of preparing herself for a night of passionate lovemaking, putting on sexy lingerie and lighting candles in the bedroom. Not noticing the nonverbal cues, the husband with AS may enter the bedroom, fall into bed, and go straight to sleep. Other detrimental influences characteristic of adults with AS in relationships include poor repair strategies, a lack of interest in or ability to meet the partner's needs (especially through "mind-reading"), an inability to recognize social patterns and problems in previous relationships, and suspicious views of others' intentions.

Other issues are commonly observed in clinical work with couples when one partner is affected by AS. Partners often complain about their affected partner's lack of involvement and interest in running the household, that they must always plan the family vacation, enroll the children for sports events (and go to watch), plan for seasonal events (e.g., Thanksgiving dinners with extended family), and so on. Many unaffected partners report that they are the "glue" holding the family together and that if it were not for them, appointments would be missed, homework would not be done; overall, the house would not run as smoothly as it does. Many of these problems reflect the husband with AS not having an interest in these things, not devoting proper time to them and not seeing himself as a part of a household and family (i.e., having capacity to see the "bigger picture").

In relationships in which the woman has AS, the problems in these cases tend to be more about the "way" a woman does things than about her isolation or lack of involvement. In most situations, we have found that the woman with AS is excessively focused on the details of the tasks being done. For example, she is obsessively organized, preparing lists, manuals, color-coding items, and alphabetizing clothing or food. Frequently, she can't tolerate her husband or children leaving anything out of place, or doing a task in a different way than she did. However, we have also seen women presenting with disorganization. For example, one woman had difficulty completing household tasks and went through the house doing steps of one task, steps of the next, and then cycling around several times before each task was completed. Although the tasks were eventually done, her husband found her method very distracting.

Comorbid mental health conditions, including addictions, depression, and anxiety, are sometimes issues in the relationship. Anger management may be problematic, and partners have alleged physical, verbal, and emotional abuse in the worst of these situations. For example, when individuals in the household do not comply with the rules that the adult with AS feels are important, emotional "meltdowns" may occur. In one family, in which the husband and a son both have AS, the wife complained that the husband and son frequently raged at each other, and it was "like having two 12-year-olds in the house," rather than a parent and child. Many individuals with AS who have anger issues within the family acknowledge that they do become angry, but they appear to not understand the impact of their outbursts on family members.

Some women realize soon after the courtship period or early in the marriage that "something is terribly wrong," and they begin to notice problems in communication, emotional and sexual expression. At times, these problems become even more obvious when children arrive.

Despite the challenges we have discussed, marriage to a man or woman with AS is positive for many spouses. Partners seen in practice talk about the engaging and positive qualities of the individual with AS that led to their courtship and marriage or cohabitation. In many instances, even in the midst of considerable marital conflict and poor dyadic adjustment, spouses bring the "positive" to our attention. Myhill and Jekel (2008) have led support groups for spouses of individuals with AS and report that participants have noted: "Some people with AS have traits that attract partners, such as being intelligent, gentle, appreciative, loyal, receptive of caretaking, well-read, interesting, creative, unusual, or quirky" (p. 2). Many women, after finding out that their ex-partner has AS (even when divorce and separation have occurred or are occurring) continue to seek out services for their ex-partner because of their concern and appreciation for their ex-partner and their relationship, despite its problems.

EXPRESSION OF SEXUALITY

Issues relating to sexuality are a common presenting problem in clinical practice with adults with AS and other ASDs. Unfortunately, we know little about the sexual practices of adults with AS through research, and knowledge of intervention programs and approaches is lacking (Hénault, 2005, 2006). Both group education (Hénault, 2005, 2006) and individual counseling (Stoddart, 1999, 2006a) can present fitting venues in which to discuss sexuality and AS. The older adolescent or young adult often has a basic knowledge of sex, but, as could be expected when a social–communication disorder is present, has difficulties with expressing his or her sexuality; understanding and knowledge can be naïve or shallow (Stoddart, 1999). As discussed further in Chapter 6, before individuals with AS utilize sexual outlets in the community and on the phone or the Internet (such as strip bars, sex shops, bathhouses, prostitutes, or pornography sites, or participate in phone sex, "sexting," or cybersex) candid discussions are necessary to ensure that their physical and sexual safety are maximized and that financial expense is lessened.

Sexual identity (and gender identity; see Chapter 3) may be in question and is another potential issue for psychotherapy and psychoeducation. Clinical experience shows that individuals with AS may be more open than the general population to identifying themselves as gay, lesbian, bisexual, or "questioning"; although clinical and research evidence are limited, the prevalence of homosexuality or bisexuality in the ASD community may be higher than in the general population (Hénault, 2006). We have seen individuals who talk about their marriage, separation, engagement in same-sex relationships, and then again dating in heterosexual relationships as if these shifts were typical and in no way unusual. On the other hand, some individuals can have rigidly moralistic views of sexual practices, based on their subjective worldview or religious upbringing. Feelings of guilt for having homosexual fantasies or engaging in homosexual behavior, extramarital affairs, masturbation, or viewing pornographic materials are potential sources of anxiety to be sensitively discussed in individual therapy.

Understanding and adhering to social rules around sexuality may be difficult for the individual with ASD and lead to illegal sexual activity, as discussed previously. Reading subtle social cues and signals often presents problems. Appreciation of "risky situations" is also a concern for many parents of young adults with AS. A young woman with AS met men online and had sexual liaisons with them in remote but public locations of her town. A few young men with whom we have worked, who identified as gay, have spoken openly about their wish to go to local bathhouses upon turning 18 to have anonymous sex with men. They also perseveratively discuss their sexuality and search for other gay men online and through newspaper or Internet personal advertisements. The quest for sexual activity in public locations may lead to criminal charges (Haskins & Silva, 2006). The undiscussed rules for social–sexual conduct in gay or lesbian bathhouses can be confusing to this group and might require candid discussion with a counselor from a knowledgeable gay-positive organization. Regular and effective condom use, especially among young adults, cannot be assumed. Sex education and information to the gay community is now being offered in bathhouses and is another potential information resource for gay men with AS (Tivey, 1989; AIDS Committee of Toronto, 2008). We recently heard of a group in a small town for gay, lesbian, bisexual, transsexual, and queer (GLBTQ) youth, many of whom are also on the autism spectrum. Programs such as this, however, are sorely lacking.

It is well known that individuals with developmental disabilities are at higher risk of sexual victimization than is the general population. Individuals with AS are no exception. Because individuals with AS have poor social perception, they may be vulnerable to, and oblivious of, the harmful intents of others. Asking about any previous experiences of sexual exploitation by peers and adults should be part of a clinical sexual history-taking. Sadly, this kind of abuse can sometimes date back to childhood, as children with AS are often not understood by school and community personnel and may therefore be at greater risk of abuse and sexual bullying in unsupervised settings, such as school washrooms and swimming pool or gymnasium changing rooms.

Some individuals with AS describe themselves as asexual (Hénault, 2006). This self-perception may raise the possibility of low estrogen or testosterone, and this should be ruled out medically. When desirable, the effects of psychotropic medications in reducing sexual impulses may be of benefit in some cases, but may also result in sexual disinhibition, priapism, anorgasmia, erectile dysfunction, and sexual frustration (Hénault, 2005).

In our experience psychopharmacological interventions, including antilibidinal agents, to treat sexually inappropriate behavior have been used unnecessarily with this population in forensic psychiatric settings; however, this misuse can be understood in relation to the absence of specialized services for individuals with ASDs and the use of less intrusive interventions such as psychoeducation, psychotherapy, and risk prevention methods. Long-term side effects with the use of antilibidinal agents can be a concern based on our experience and that of others (Gordon & Grubin, 2004). One man with ASD we treated was unable to achieve an erection for many months after the (inappropriately prescribed) antilibidinal agent was withdrawn. There are concerns about the reliability of self-report for sexual offending behaviors and the intrusiveness of penile plethysmography (i.e., measuring blood flow to the penis) in assessment of risk of sexual offending in the general population (Gordon & Grubin, 2004). These methods have also been used in assessing risk by individuals with ASDs seen in our practice.

Considering the tendency toward repetitive thoughts and behaviors and focused interests in ASDs, hypersexuality, cognitive fixation, and sexual rumination can present as a clinical concern (Hénault, 2005). The clinician needs to consider the risks and benefits of addressing this area by providing psychoeducation, because such an approach may increase sexual fixation. Excessive masturbation can be physically damaging for those who fixate on masturbation (especially for men who are treated with SSRIs or other medications that can delay or prevent ejaculation and arousal), and for those who use harmful methods of self-stimulation (e.g., rubbing against hard or abrasive surfaces). Both men and women may need education on safe and effective self-stimulation and masturbation.

Hénault (2005, 2006) has proposed a social–sexual group education program that addresses the areas of communication, love and friendship, the sexual response cycle, sexual intercourse and other sexual behaviors, emotions, sexually transmitted diseases and prevention, sexual orientation, drugs and alcohol, abuse and inappropriate behaviors, sexism and violence, and theory of mind (Hénault, 2005, 2006). Excellent resources are available for individuals with developmental disabilities that we have used with "high-functioning" youth and adults with ASDs. An example are the videotapes and booklets produced by Hingsburger that depict actual male and female masturbation and condom use, and provide clear and accurate instruction about privacy, safe sexual practices, use of pornographic material, and methods of masturbation and hygiene (Hingsburger, 1995, 1996; Hingsburger & Haar, 2000).

Even with masturbation, tactile issues (e.g., touching their own penis) may be troublesome for males with ASDs, and manual stimulation may be replaced by rubbing genitals against objects (e.g., towels, bed sheets, mattress, or pillows) and other forms of self-stimulation. The sexual educator, health practitioner, or clinician should ensure that physical damage or self-harm is not occurring in these cases. Penetration of the urethra and anus may be part of sexual self-stimulation; however, this practice can be indicative of a medical issue such as the presence of a sexually transmitted disease, constipation, hemorrhoids, or yeast overgrowth. Clients may need information about the use of artificial lubricants for masturbation and objects such as dildos and other sex toys that can be safely inserted into the anus or vagina. We have worked with individuals who, without this type of information, have engaged in unsafe self-stimulatory practices, inserting large, sharp, or toxic objects/substances into rectal or vaginal orifices due to a sensory- or obsession-related need.

When the individual with AS does have a long-term partner, problems of sexual expression are often raised in couples counseling (Myhill & Jekel, 2008). Problems here relate to how often the partners have sex, how they have sex, and how sexual activity is negotiated in the relationship. Some adults with AS make "appointments" to have sex with their partner. Although all sexual spontaneity would appear to be lost in this approach, communication and planning can also lead to much more mutually satisfying expressions of sexuality. This is another arena in which the partner often feels that her needs or sexual wishes are not met, and certainly not *intuitively* met, often because they are unknown and/or misunderstood. Sensory sensitivities, particularly tactile and olfactory sensitivities, can create obstacles to establishing healthy, mutually reciprocating sexual relationships. One woman told us how aversive it was when her husband gently stroked her leg. What he interpreted as an expression of affection was a clear "turn-off" in her mind. The reluctance to share information, which we often see in those with AS, increased the emotional distance because he didn't know his expression of affection was not interpreted as such by his partner.

Finally, diverse sexual interests are an important aspect of sexuality to assess; sexual fetishism (e.g., shoes and boots) has been reported by adults with ASDs. We have seen sexual interests in typically nonsexual body parts (e.g., noses, arms, feet), sexual arousal through viewing cartoons and movies, arousal associated with sensory-seeking experiences (e.g., amusement park rides), and sexual experimentation with animals.

PARENTING

After Hans Asperger, Christopher Gillberg (1989, 1998) was another clinician to point out that we need to consider the issues and concerns that arise for parents with AS, and some of the problems and benefits of the day-to-day presentation of AS in relation to parenting. He suggests:

> It would not be unreasonable to assume that poor empathy in the parent might contribute to some behavioural/psychological problem in the child quite apart from any genetic influence.

However, one might equally argue that a parent with similar but milder problems would be better able to understand and cope with some of the child's problems because they may be perceived as personality style rather than "disorder." Future studies should seek to explore these issues and try sensibly and sensitively to avoid the mistake of the past regarding the scapegoating of parents. (Gillberg, 1998, pp. 204–205)

Aston (2005) also points to the problems that are inherent in raising a child when parental empathy is lacking and understanding a child's thoughts, needs, and perceptions is difficult. We have also seen this in clinical practice. For example, partners often report that fathers with AS are unable to connect emotionally with their children, express and display interest in what they are interested in, and successfully predict and respond to their needs. An often reported example occurs when the father with AS may not know what grade his child is in, or he may buy the child Christmas or birthday presents that *he* likes, versus those that *the child* would want. An egocentric perspective, without theory of mind, is prominent.

Another issue is that fathers with AS often do not value their children "for who they are, but rather for what they achieve" (Aston, 2005, p. 8). The potential effect of this attitude on any child's self-esteem is significant. Sensory sensitivities of the parent with AS may also present difficulties; demonstrations of physical affection may be limited or occur only when the parent initiates them. "For some AS parents, women in particular, there can be an extreme reaction to their child's vomit, soiling, smell, crying or, in some extreme cases, their physical contact" (Aston, 2005, p. 8). One mother who had AS ran to the basement each time there was a thunderstorm, leaving her children upstairs unattended. Management of children's behavior may be inflexible and rule-bound. Further, undiagnosed AS in parents may lead not only to confusion and anxiety for the partner, but also for the children. Lack of recognition of comorbid mental health issues and executive functioning deficits may create added difficulties for the family.

Given that parenting is "an intensely social activity" (Spicer, 2004), the inability of parents with AS to socialize and play with the child (especially if the child's play interests are different from theirs) may be problematic. A recent clinical observation of a play session with a family illustrated this point: While children, the clinician, and mother were on the floor playing together, the father with AS, sitting in the corner of the room, provided occasional direction from a chair when behavior needed attention, but otherwise read work material pulled from his briefcase. We have coached affected parents in understanding how to interact with their young children, taught them how to "play," and helped them understand that they can engage in household activities in addition to interacting with their child.

Both unaffected and affected parents describe difficulties with co-parenting and with the "executive functioning" of the parental subsystem. Consistent with this perspective, parents with AS may be unable to establish suitable boundaries between themselves and their child; therefore, boundaries are either too flexible or too rigid. This may result in their being perceived by the child as more of a peer in the former case, or as an authoritarian acquaintance in the latter.

Finally, problems are often expressed about affected parents' inability to recognize basic physical and safety needs of their children and to know how to prevent accidents or attend to children when they do occur. Because some parents with AS do not eat a healthy diet, nutrition also becomes an issue of concern, and these parents may need encouragement to provide healthy foods for the family that aren't their preference. Treating all the children equally and fairly, as opposed to favoring some over the others, may also require explicit discussion in some families (Aston, 2005).

EMPLOYMENT

Many individuals with AS can work well in both unsupported and supported work environments. However, supportive environments are often not available for individuals, and unemployment rates are high among individuals with AS and high-functioning autism (Järbrink, McCrone, Fombonne, Zandén, & Knapp, 2007). We have suggested previously that preparation for employment should start in adolescence and that participation in high school work co-ops, volunteering, and summer jobs can contribute important information about the individuals' understanding of appropriate behavior in their work setting, the skills required for ongoing and long-term work, and the field(s) of employment which are of interest (Stoddart, 2005c). We are often struck by our clients' inability to "imagine themselves" in a particular job or field of work because they have not had any experience in the setting. It is therefore important that they experience a trial or temporary work situation so that they can judge this accordingly.

Many problems in employment may relate to problems with anger management and to the challenges of working in teams of people, multitasking, following directions, and abiding by the policies and regulations of the employer. As discussed elsewhere in this book, work performance is one of the developmental challenges of adulthood that might be addressed in the diagnostic assessment process and may lead to clues that a yet-undiagnosed individual has symptoms of AS.

Individuals who are not diagnosed until mid-career demonstrate that they have been able to find employment and maintain it for some time. However, difficulties have arisen in the absence of an understanding of their strengths and areas of need, by both the employer and the individuals themselves. Subsequent to diagnosis, we may work with individuals and their employer to ensure that employment can be continued through a range of supports and accommodations. Bissonette (2009) points to the importance of disclosure that also includes a potential solution: "Saying something like, 'I have Asperger's Syndrome and can't multi-task' is not a good approach because it puts the burden on the employer to find a solution. If you are proactive in suggesting reasonable accommodations there is a greater likelihood that your employer will implement them" (p. 6).

A collaborative approach to resolving performance issues that includes the clinician is optimal in that he or she can obtain information from the employer that the person themselves has not brought to the clinician's attention. Written performance appraisals from the employer provide concrete, behaviorally defined and specific data on which to base employment-related interventions. The clinician can also get a sense from the employer of his or her degree of commitment to keeping the employee, or whether he or she is moving toward dismissal. It is important to know (1) if the employer has made a commitment to hiring a diverse cohort of employees, (2) policies that the employer espouses to support individuals with disabilities, and (3) actions that the employer has taken in the past with respect to employees' work performance. As noted in Chapter 6 and 7, employment may be an ongoing issue for individual counseling sessions. Once an individual is diagnosed, or if he or she enters the workforce with a diagnosis, disclosure of the person's difficulties can be a concern. Some considerations are offered in the literature (Bissonnette, 2009).

Autism Society Canada's Advisory Committee of Adults on the Spectrum recommends that potential employers be educated about the positive aspects of individuals with ASDs in employment settings. These characteristics include logic, attention to detail, punctuality, honesty, reliability, and attention to routines (Autism Society Canada, 2007). We have witnessed firsthand the benefits of employing adults with AS. One of the local real estate companies boasts about how accurate and detailed their company databases are because an individual with AS is responsible for maintaining it. There has been wide acceptance of this individual, despite his eccentricities, because of the significant contribution that he has made to the overall good functioning of the corporation.

POSTSECONDARY EDUCATION

It is now common to hear of students with AS entering postsecondary education, either at the college or university level. It is likely that more students with ASDs will be entering postsecondary education in the future as we identify children with ASDs earlier, implement better interventions in school leading to better adult outcomes, and more frequently identify individuals with milder forms of ASDs (Adreon & Durocher, 2007; Farrell, 2004; Smith, 2007). It is our experience and others' (Dillon, 2007) that many students with AS (diagnosed and undiagnosed) seek out community or mental health supports after a difficult first or second year at college or university. This challenging experience may have involved dropping out of the program, increased mental health or addiction problems, or social and behavioral problems (e.g., isolation, inappropriate behaviors, and problems getting along with dorm mates).

The college experience can be positive for individuals on the spectrum (Shore, 2001), as individuals with ASDs often experience great pleasure and are highly motivated to gain further knowledge of their area of interest(s). Despite this apparent fit, many have reported in personal biographies by people on the autism spectrum, various psychosocial difficulties related to college or university. Fortunately, requisite "survival skills" for individuals in these settings have been offered by some and are a positive outcome of these experiences (Willey, 1999). Increasingly, resources are available on the Internet for students with ASDs (Al-Mahmood, McLean, Powell, & Ryan, 1998) and their professors (Organization for Autism Research, 2009a), which help to ensure that the postsecondary experience is positive.

Colleges and universities have resources, practices, and policies in effect to support the inclusion of individuals with disabilities. Although people with AS can benefit from being identified as having exceptionalities at the postsecondary level, the willingness of these individuals to disclose their AS diagnoses varies. This variation may reflect their acceptance of the diagnosis and their experience with disclosure in secondary school (Humphrey & Lewis, 2008). Because familiarity with the term *Asperger syndrome* is not widespread, or the term may have pejorative connotations, some students prefer to reframe their social difficulties as a "social disability" or "social learning disability." Others do not disclose any diagnosis and therefore may not receive accommodations or support. Disclosing one's disability is analogous to "outing oneself," a term typically associated the experiences of gay, lesbian, bisexual, or transgendered individuals. This is neither a simple nor insignificant disclosure. The Organization for Autism Research (2009b) advises parents:

> Your young adult is an expert on being a person on the spectrum and has a unique opportunity to let others know, to the extent possible and appropriate, what it is like. In addition, it is important for him to understand that disclosure is not an "all or nothing" proposition. Each individual will need to learn both how and when to disclose, in addition to how much information he needs to disclose, in what format, and to what end. Disclosure is a much more complex and personal process than simply saying, "I have autism spectrum disorder."

Some authors have pointed out that even though college and university students with AS have a diagnosis in common, they may display problems in the postsecondary context in idiosyncratic ways, thus necessitating accommodations that are specific to each individual with AS and distinct from those with other types of disabilities (Dillon, 2007; Smith, 2007). For example:

> One person may talk in class all the time preventing discussion, while another might never speak up at all. One person might miss most classes, not due to lack of interest, but rather poor planning and organization of time and self. A third might arrive at class an hour early to make sure he will acquire his favourite chair. Another might get lost crossing the campus or be late waiting to park in his preferred parking spot rather than taking an available spot. (Dillon, 2007, p. 501)

Parents of adults with ASDs may be surprised to find that colleges and universities are not necessarily used to working with parents of students with disabilities. Although many parents of children with AS have advocated for them throughout their grade school and high school years, because their children are now adults, the school is often reluctant to engage parents, and in fact, sometimes refuses. Although the importance of the parental role in the transition to postsecondary education cannot be underestimated for this population, this typical postsecondary culture reinforces the need for students to learn some degree of independence in advocating on their own behalf in this setting. This practice is the exception rather than the rule most of the time, since adolescents with AS are often excluded from meeting with their high school teaching/individualized education plan (IEP) team. If parents are invited to work collaboratively with the disability adviser in the college or university setting, together with their son or daughter, a plan should be put in place to fade their involvement throughout the course of the first year.

Many variables might be considered in choosing a (community) college or university for a student with AS. Some of these might include the program of study, the cost of the program, the size of the college or university, the layout or size of the campus, the presence of supportive faculty, and the location of the campus relative to home. Many students with ASDs choose to enter smaller community college programs as opposed to larger university programs. Typically, shorter community college programs are more applied and less theoretical, community college diplomas may lead directly to a vocational activity, academic demands in college programs are usually less rigorous, the classes are smaller, and students tend to receive more individualized attention from their professors than in a large university setting. It is important to be familiar with the program of study, tour the campus, see available housing, meet with disability services personnel, and investigate the availability of supports for exceptional students before applying to any college or university program. There are some helpful guides online for assessing the student's options (Wheeler & Kalina, 2000).

A challenging issue for college and university students is deciding where to live if the campus is far from home. We have had both positive and disastrous experiences with students (especially in their first year) living in a student residence or an off-campus student housing situation. Given their difficulties in social interaction, the social issues of students with AS are often magnified in these settings, which typically lack parental supervision and regular schedules. Add to this many life changes, the ever-present opportunities/requirements to meet new people, and the newfound freedom to engage in young adult "rites of passage," which may include alcohol, drugs, and sexual activity. Some have suggested that students with AS should live at home, if possible, in the first year of their college or university experience to defer the need/pressure to adjust to social and living challenges while they are acclimating to the academic demands (Perner, 2003). In situations where the student cannot live at home, regular visits to home on the weekend may provide respite from the relentless social demands of dormitory life and prove comforting to parents, who are concerned about their young adult's performance away from home.

AGING

Older individuals with ASDs, including AS, have received little attention in the research literature or in clinical practice (Gold & Whelan, 1992; Stoddart 2006b). However, there are some reports of older individuals identified as having AS. For instance, 14 parents of patients with ASDs were diagnosed as a result of their children's diagnoses. It is of note that 10 of the 14 parents had more than one child with autism. At the year of publication, the parents were ages 37–77 years old; six individuals were over 50 years old (Ritvo, Ritvo, Freeman, & Mason-Brothers, 1994).

Similarly, others have presented a case series of five elderly adults who met criteria for AS (James, Mukaetova-Ladinska, Reichelt,

Briel, & Scully, 2006). The authors stressed the importance of getting a detailed developmental history focusing on social development, interpersonal and communication skills, and information on repetitive and observed behaviors of interest. All five cases were males who had a chronic history of interpersonal problems, obvious from early school years, and all had a history of interpersonal difficulties throughout adulthood. They were initially referred for treatment-resistant mood disorders and anxiety. The authors concluded that "... there is a great need even for elderly people to receive an appropriate diagnosis of AS, because this may ensure that they do not receive an unsuitable intervention—whether that be medication or a psychological regimen" (p. 959).

It is possible that many in the aging or elderly population who have exhibited lifelong problems in social functioning, mental health problems, or a restricted range of interests have AS or an ASD that has gone unrecognized. We have previously noted the costs of going a lifetime without an appropriate diagnosis of AS. In practice, AS and ASD traits of parents, aunts, uncles, or grandparents of individuals who have been diagnosed with an ASD or AS are often discussed by the individuals themselves or by family members. Realization that an older family member may have traits of AS can lead to better or more positive understandings of his or her behaviors or personality. Older adults may come to the attention of clinicians for other comorbidities such as anxiety or depression (James, et al., 2006), which can then lead to a more comprehensive diagnosis of AS. James and colleagues (2006) explain:

> Identifying these individuals and diagnosing them correctly would benefit their treatment, especially as they were originally referred for mood disorders and anxiety. Indeed, those in our clinical sample have been thought to be 'treatment resistant', thus they had received unnecessary, lengthy medical and psychological care (in one case they had received ECT . . .), with poor results. The latter is largely due to misinterpreting some of the symptoms (e.g., restlessness, anxiety) for depressive symptoms. This also raises the need for further research into the development of pharmacological and non-pharmacological interventions for this rather neglected group of elderly. (p. 959)

With retirement often comes less structure in day-to-day living and more social isolation; both factors may have negative effects on the mental health of individuals with ASDs. With few interests and friends, retirement may be a difficult stage of life. We currently know little about the health needs of older adults with ASDs or about the life expectancy of individuals with AS, and it is important to consider the possible effects of preexisting medical conditions, poor medical attention, diet, exercise, and social isolation. It is known that fragile X can contribute to some ASDs, though a small proportion. In aging individuals with fragile X syndrome, mitral valve prolapse, musculo-skeletal disorders, early menopause, epilepsy, and vision problems may occur. The collaboration of service providers from various service sectors, including health and care services for the elderly, is essential in meeting the needs of this group.

SUMMARY

The psychosocial needs of adults with AS—including housing, behavioral and legal problems, intimate relationships, sexuality, parenting, employment, education, and aging—are receiving some attention in current research. Further study is needed to clarify the nature and extent of the issues that arise in each of these domains. However, since many of these problems and the approach(es) to them are affected by local supports and policies, research into psychosocial problems specific to countries and geographic regions is especially necessary.

Methods of intervention to address these psychosocial needs now require closer examination. Some interventions, which have been applied in other areas of the world, need to be carefully described and evaluated so that they can form the basis of evidence-based practices locally. Another source of useful practices may be those utilized by individuals with other types of disabilities, which can be adapted to the unique psychosocial needs of this group. The cooperation of service providers across funding sectors and collaboration between wide-ranging government departments is imperative if this creation of evidence-based practices is to occur. We now turn our attention to the processes of intervention in Chapters 6 and 7.

Chapter 6

PSYCHOTHERAPY AND PSYCHOPHARMACOTHERAPY IN ADULT ASPERGER SYNDROME

Considering that increasing numbers of adults are being diagnosed with AS in adulthood and the cohort of children and youth diagnosed with AS is aging into adulthood, it is disheartening to realize how few established support services and treatments exist for this population. For some colleagues and affected individuals, the lack of services for adults with AS provides a partial rationale for not providing, facilitating, or pursuing an AS diagnosis. Although the United Kingdom has shown leadership in raising awareness of the support needs of adults with ASDs through large surveys and public education, unmet service needs have also been identified there (Barnard et al., 2001; Powell, 2002; Rosenblatt, 2008). In Canada, we have contributed to similar reports and conferences voicing concern about the dearth of services for adults with ASDs here (Autism Society of Canada, 2007; Munro & Burke, 2006; Ontario Partnership for Adults with Aspergers and Autism, 2008; Stoddart, 2007a, 2007b, 2009).

Simblett and Wilson (1993) poignantly noted that adults with AS are perceived by the social and medical services system as: "(1) not autistic enough for autistic services; (2) not ill enough for psychiatric services; and (3) not learning disabled enough for mental handicap services" (p. 93). Similarly, Tantum (2003) has remarked: ". . . there is no group that has accepted that AS is part of their mission. This means that parents and sufferers are constantly the subject of turf wars in which they find themselves being referred back and forth until someone takes responsibility for their care or until they give up and break contact with services altogether. The latter is an all too common outcome" (p. 147). Munro (2010) has observed: "Across North America, there are few clinical or community services for teens and adults with AS. This leaves many bright and sensitive individuals experiencing empty and unfulfilled lives" (p. 86).

This chapter focuses on what we believe to be two core treatments for adults with AS: psychotherapy and psychopharmacotherapy. We review the literature and our clinical experience in providing individual psychotherapeutic and pharmacotherapeutic interventions to adults with ASDs, specifically AS. First, we discuss the process of formulating cases utilizing a biopsychosocial model. Common themes in individual therapy are then summarized. Following this, literature on common pharmacological interventions is reviewed. This chapter concludes by presenting a combined model of psychopharmacotherapy and psychotherapy. Complementary treatments are discussed in Chapter 7.

Whether available treatments change the core features of ASDs—specifically, deficits in language use, impairments in social reciprocity, and behavioral rigidity—has been the central question scrutinized in systematic reviews. Bodfish (2004) has addressed the depth of the intervention effect question by exploring "how deeply" established treatments impact the continuum of impairment within each of these domains. He notes that compounded claims of treatment efficacy are often made in relation ASD interventions, which create confusion about treatment choices for parents of affected children and adults. He concludes that significant issues remain regarding (1) the routine application of validated treatments for most individuals with autism, (2) resistance to treatments validated for a subtotal majority of cases of autism, and (3) the need to validate efficacy for treatments that target specific core features of autism that are the most disabling for people with ASDs and their families (Bodfish, 2004).

PREPARING FOR INTERVENTION

In Chapter 2, we emphasized the need to take a comprehensive developmental and service history to inform the diagnostic process. Obtaining a full history from various informants is also essential in devising a comprehensive and well-informed treatment approach for adults with AS. Although this is sometimes challenging because of the passage of time, key content of this history-taking is information about significant life events, health, past assessments and services obtained by the individual. This review, dating back to early childhood (if information is available), provides crucial data on previous diagnoses, assessments and their findings, and treatment approaches and their outcomes.

This historical information forms the basis of our biopsychosocial formulation. The biopsychosocial model allows a clinician to consider an individual, not only in terms of discrete areas of functioning (such as medical, learning, social or environmental issues) but also through the interactions of these areas. It further respects the individual manner in which a person understands or copes with his or her situation (Gilbert, 2002). These, in turn, influence the person's vulnerability or resilience in the face of challenges (Griffiths & Gardner, 2002). For example, if a person who has AS comes to us for assistance because he is experiencing difficulty in his work environment and his employer feels he is not able to do his job, one might initially decide that the person's skills were not suitable. But it is important to look at all potential contributors to the problem: Do they have sensory hyper-responsiveness? Do they have attentional problems? Are they experiencing social or performance anxiety? Do they have hearing or vision problems? Each of these issues considered individually, as well as the interaction and possible synergy between them, needs to be questioned before one can truly understand the person's difficulties.

Many individuals with whom we work, report that previous involvement with professionals or organizations has not been productive; others have also reported this in the professional literature (Anderson & Morris, 2006; Ryan, 1992). It is therefore important to ascertain what obstacles (whether actual or perceived) to effective treatment were experienced. Often, previous intervention attempts may reveal a lack of professional knowledge or understanding of AS in adults, or an assessment leading to an inappropriate diagnosis or intervention.

Although there may not have been an early and accurate diagnosis to guide the way for ASD-specific treatments, some approaches may have been suitable and helpful, given the individual features that *were* understood. An example is the many adults we have seen with a previous diagnosis of ADHD. Despite not benefiting from the most fitting and inclusive diagnosis of AS previously, a trial of stimulant medication to decrease inattention may have been helpful. Similarly, an individual placed on an SSRI before the diagnosis of AS may have experienced a significant reduction in symptoms of depression and anxiety because of that pharmacological intervention.

Occasionally, previous professional or therapeutic involvement has been counterproductive and even harmful. Although we have seen countless adults who have had experiences that are illustrative of this problem, the case of the man prescribed electroconvulsive therapy (ECT) for depression is likely one of the most troublesome examples we have seen. After a brief trial of two antidepressants (without the benefit of psychotherapy), ECT was introduced. The result of the ECT was a loss of skills and memory. This man was unable to continue his professional career, in part because of the impact of the ECT. It is likely that his flat affect (symptomatic of AS) and inability to describe and manage feelings of anxiety and depression were misdiagnosed as severe and treatment-resistant depression. If we had met him prior to the ECT and had been able to formulate his case using a biopsychosocial model, we would have looked at life events and aspects of his behavior and personality that might have led us to a diagnosis of AS. In considering his situation through the lens of this model after the fact, the medical treatment (ECT) led to new biological (neurological/mental health), psychological (learning/personality) and social (employment/relationship) challenges. Although we do not dispute the potential role of ECT in treating mood problems in individuals with AS (in the absence of any literature), we feel that the least intrusive approaches(s) need to be first considered carefully and attempted. The philosophy of starting with the least intrusive intervention guides all clinical decisions that we make.

Identification and understanding of comorbid issues that have been identified correctly is essential, especially if they possibly relate to the presenting issue. It is useful to question how, for example, a history of poor mental health or organizational difficulties has affected the presenting problem. Difficulty finding employment (although a common developmental challenge that many adults with AS experience because of the lack of suitable community resources) may be perpetuated by these comorbid traits.

An individual's acceptance of, and knowledge about, his or her AS traits is a central issue to be considered before engagement in treatment. This focus may yield important clues about the subjective experience of the diagnostic process and how the diagnosis was provided. The result of this line of questioning may lead to discussion of the diagnosis as the first therapeutic task. The subjective response of some adults to the diagnosis will be to eradicate all signs of AS, an attitude that may then be superimposed on therapy. For others, the diagnostic concept of AS has little relevance in their self-appraisal, and therefore little relevance in the therapeutic relationship. In the latter case, central questions include (1) whether these individuals have difficulty with insight and self-awareness (i.e., they disregard the diagnosis as relating to themselves), (2) if they have difficulty with AS because of the manner in which it was presented to them initially, (3) as communicated to them throughout their life, or (4) as a diagnostic concept generally. For instance, many adults report to us that they are not "like other people with AS" they have met. When this view is further explored, the clinician may hear of their early attendance at groups for children or adolescents on the autism spectrum and their negative experience of being placed with others who were much lower functioning than they were. This experience distorts their view of AS. Some may take the diagnostic criteria or other symptom checklists literally and feel that they do not have all the characteristics noted.

Others will express great relief at finding a diagnosis for their children and themselves, and revel in the liberation that it brings them. About the diagnostic process for her girl, Liane Holliday Willey (1999) writes:

> . . . my heart was not breaking. It was filling up with self-acceptance, it was filling up with possibilities. I knew then, that even though this was not a picture that everyone would find beautiful, or even acceptable, it was our picture and it was perfect to us. All the insecurities and frustrations that I had

195

carried for so many years were beginning to slip away. I had not imagined a thing. I was different. So was my little girl. (p. 89)

Based on the leading theories about ASDs and comorbid issues and our knowledge of the possible contributors to psychosocial difficulties, clinicians have the benefit of a list of possibilities from which to choose in formulating clinical hypotheses and the manner in which to address them. Ten key antecedents, perpetuators, or precipitators of clinical problems presenting for treatment include:

1. Poor social skills and social insight
2. Inability to understand emotions (their own and others)
3. Sensory-processing differences (seeking or avoiding behaviors)
4. Poor executive functioning/organizational difficulties
5. Idiosyncratic learning/information-processing/output profile
6. Restricted and repetitive interest-related behaviors
7. Problems with emotional regulation and mental health
8. Poor fine or gross motor development
9. Difficulty navigating transitions
10. Problems with changes/inflexible cognitive style

During clinical consultations and ongoing therapy, we are asked (either explicitly or implicitly) for our opinion about "what the cause of the problem is" in those cases where a diagnosis has been made. Occasionally, adults or their families might have their own theories, and in keeping with a collaborative treatment approach, we ask them what these are. An adolescent who presented for a consultation identified why he was having "emotional meltdowns," and together we identified several factors that might be at play. One of these included not eating any food or drinking water for the entire day! This was framed as an organizational and self-monitoring challenge (consistent with his AS), which he is attempting to address as he becomes more independent. It is important to determine the relative contribution of each of these factors. When this is established, the discussion can then turn to how they will be addressed. The input of the client in this hypothesis-generating process is crucial and provides a collaborative foundation for further treatment; it also serves as a foundation for the revision of the hypotheses as necessary. At all times, the notion of "client as expert" should be reinforced and a "cross-cultural" therapeutic dialogue nurtured.

Finally, in the context of a biopsychosocial assessment, knowledge of the individual environment is a critical, yet many times overlooked, contributor to clinical problems. Inflexible, uninformed, and restrictive environments are experienced as "disabling." For the adults with whom we work, we consider the family, school, employment, housing, and community contexts. Intervention might be directed to the individual, but should also target the context in which the problem(s) is occurring. If, for example, the individual's employer has little understanding of the difficulty an employee with AS experiences with a group of other employees during staff meetings, he or she can be educated in this regard and that aspect of the job might be modified. Similarly, an individual's lack of success in postsecondary education may be understood as the school not recognizing the student's needs for academic accommodations. We consider important features of the environment such as sensory overload, interpersonal demands, and the degree of understanding, acceptance, and knowledge of the individual's diagnosis by others. The patients' views of these issues may be distorted or imagined (e.g., "My boss feels that I am rude and is going to fire me"); nevertheless these need to be explored.

PSYCHOTHERAPY

Considering the central role of psychotherapy in treating adults with AS, it is concerning that related literature is so limited. Much of the existing intervention literature in this field is child-focused. However, in the last decade volumes have emerged that have contributed to our knowledge base about the practice of psychotherapy with individuals with AS; diverse therapeutic paradigms include the use of psychoanalytically oriented psychotherapy in children and adults (Rhode & Klauber, 2004), cognitive behavioral therapy (Gaus, 2007), and marital counseling (Aston, 2001, 2003, 2009). Publication of such clinical texts is, however, at an early stage. Moreover, the task of empirically evaluating the efficacy of these models using state-of-the art research approaches such as randomized controlled trials, has just begun.

Clearly, the use of cognitive–behavioral therapy (CBT) is leading the way with evidence-based psychotherapeutic approaches in AS. For example, CBT has been used to treat anger (Attwood, 2004; Sofronoff, Attwood, Hinton, & Levin, 2007), anxiety (Sofronoff, Attwood, & Hinton, 2005; Sze & Wood, 2008; Wood et al., 2009), social behavior problems (Lopata, Thomeer, Volker, & Nida, 2006), and OCD (Reaven & Hepburn, 2003). Although these accounts focus on the use of CBT with children, we feel the likely carryover of these positive outcomes to adults is promising (Stoddart & Duhaime, 2011) and has also been promoted by others (Donoghue, Stallard, & Kucia, 2011; Gaus, 2007, 2011; Hare & Paine, 1997; Weiss & Lunsky, 2010). It is critical to note that outcomes of CBT are not always positive, as found in our own clinical experience. One individual with AS, when completing his assigned CBT homework became extremely agitated, which led to his requiring emergency medical attention.

The lack of interest in psychotherapy for individuals with developmental disabilities may arise from lingering and problematic myths about this population. That is, individuals with ASDs or developmental disabilities are not capable of psychological insight, of using a therapeutic relationship to effect change in their lives, or of thinking reflectively about themselves and their goals for the future. A case example illustrates this point: A young man with high-functioning autism and near-average intellectual ability was seeking counseling for the impending loss of his mother from lung cancer. After a brief assessment by a professional in the community, the mother was told that the young man was not able to engage in counseling, and the intervention would not be productive. One of the authors has since seen this individual; he has been able to greatly benefit from psychotherapy before the death of his mother and following the loss.

Although the merits of psychotherapy in individuals with developmental disabilities have been debated in the literature (King, 2005; Sturmey, 2005; Taylor, 2005), the consensus is that many can benefit from psychotherapy. In our own research and practice evaluation, we have found that even individuals with cognitive delays have benefited from both group and individual psychotherapy to address men's issues (Stoddart & Ratti, 1999), grief and loss (Stoddart & McDonnell, 1999; Stoddart, Burke, & Temple, 2002b), and various psychosocial problems in a brief, solution-focused format (Stoddart, McDonnell, Temple, & Mustata, 2001).

The field of ASDs itself has not been immune from a reluctance to support psychotherapeutic interventions. Early in the literature, Gillberg and Ehlers (1998) argued that usually psychotherapy is not warranted in individuals affected with AS. However, others have noted that the poor outcome of psychotherapy with autistic individuals may reflect the psychoanalytic and nondirective approach used in the past (Mesibov, 1992). The process of understanding an individual's worldview; developing rapport and trust; helping them understand their thoughts, feelings, and perceptions; facilitating understanding of the impact of their behaviors on others; and helping them deal with day-to-day situations are all potential outcomes of counseling (Mesibov, 1992).

The challenge for many adults and caregivers is to find a therapist who is able to adapt the psychotherapeutic skills developed for the general population to meet the needs of clients with AS. Experienced psychotherapists in this field of practice are limited. In a U.K. survey of 1,400 individuals, many reported unmet needs for counseling services for adults with ASDs (Rosenblatt, 2008). These unmet needs may reflect both lingering historical myths and the lack of current knowledge about the benefits of psychotherapy for this clinical group.

Brief Review of Current Psychotherapy Literature

A search of the peer-reviewed literature found few discussions of psychotherapy or evaluations of interventions used with adults who have AS. Much of the psychotherapy literature in adulthood remains at the level of a single case description and analysis in adulthood. For instance, CBT was used to target social anxiety in a young adult male with AS (Cardaciotto & Herbert, 2004). Using a single-case analysis, data collection during and after treatment, and multiple measures, a 14-week social anxiety protocol was found effective in reducing the man's depression and social anxiety (Heimberg & Becket, 2002; Herbert, Rheingold, & Goldstein, 2002). "Treatment focused on the reported feared and avoided social situations, including initiating, maintaining, and ending conversations, meeting new people, dating, assertiveness, and job interviewing. Intervention techniques included cognitive restructuring, role-playing, and weekly homework assignments" (Cardaciotto & Herbert, 2004, p. 75). The CBT protocol was adapted to address the individual's difficulties with verbal, nonverbal and paralinguistic skills, deficits typical of individuals with AS. Eye contact was taught in this example.

Similarly, an early case was presented that used CBT in a young man with AS who presented with cutting behaviors, excessive drinking, and depression (Hare, 1997). Hare used a nonspecific CBT approach (Fennell, 1998) for 10 sessions. Adaptations included the avoidance of metaphorical concepts and language, maintenance of clear boundaries, and use of a "concrete but logical approach." Hare points out that the use of visually presented material was the preference of this man; since this preference is common in individuals with ASDs, this approach might be successful with other individuals. It is promising that these single-case studies have been effective with adaptations. Others have suggested that CBT for individuals with AS include an emphasis on affective education, a more directive approach, and involvement of a family member or cotherapist to promote skill generalization (Anderson & Morris, 2006).

A cognitive–behavioral approach was also reported in treating OCD in a group of high-functioning adults with ASDs (Russell, Mataix-Cols, Anson, & Murphy, 2009). Russell and colleagues used a nonrandomized, nonblinded controlled trial comparing CBT with treatment as usual in 24 patients. The CBT group ($n = 12$) attended an average of 27.5 treatment sessions. Using the Yale–Brown Obsessive Compulsive Scale—Severity Scale (Y-BOCS; Goodman et al., 1989), a significant group x time interaction, in favor of the treatment group, was found ($p = 0.049$), although 40% of the treatment participants were considered "nonresponders."

Munro has presented what he calls "Asperger Integrated Psychotherapy" (AIP; 2010). "The AIP Model integrates features from many treatment schools of thought, respects evidence-based knowledge, and demonstrates sensitivity to the challenges and potential strengths of people with AS. Considering the complex nature of AS, it seems wise and ethical to use a treatment model that borrows from several therapeutic traditions" (p. 86). He describes the seven features of the AIP model as: (1) a supportive lifeline, (2) combining individual and family therapy, (3) cognitive-behavioral strategies, (4) recomposing the narrative, (5) prescribing physical exercise, (6) mending "broken spirits," and (7) psychoeducation.

The literature also suggests that individual treatment can be effectively combined with family-based interventions (Fidell, 2000;

Stoddart, 1999; Munro, 2010). Stoddart (1999) offered three descriptions of adolescents with AS who received individual treatment combined with systems-based and structural family therapy. The systems-based family interventions involved discussion of boundaries between siblings and between the parent and child subsystems, healthy "executive functioning" of the parental subsystem, and appropriate exchange of information with external systems. Stoddart also noted the use of communication (Bandler, Grinder, & Satir, 1976; Watzlawick, Beavin, & Jackson, 1967), role (Biddle, 1979), psychoanalytic, behavioral, cognitive, psychoeducational, and developmental theories (Carter & McGoldrick, 1980). Although the cases presented by Stoddart (1999) involved adolescent males, we believe that the model is also applicable to families of young adults. Developmentally, many of the young adults whom we see are delayed in achieving independence from their family and struggle with many of the issues that were evident in these cases. Further, the issue of their expectations and those of their families and society are contributory (Stoddart, 2006a). Family therapy is further discussed in Chapter 7.

Engagement in Treatment and the Therapeutic Relationship

Given the central role of the therapeutic relationship and its potential contribution to therapeutic change, a compelling concern is voiced by Anderson and Morris: "Difficulties forming and maintaining relationships may be particularly evident in the one-to-one therapeutic relationship in which we are attempting not only to establish a new relationship, but asking the person to discuss their thoughts and feelings" (2006, p. 294). A similar concern is raised by Ramsay and colleagues: "How does a therapist establish a workable therapeutic relationship with a patient whose fundamental problem is the inability to understand and engage in social relationships in his or her daily life?" (2005, p. 483).

Our experience suggests that, after years of not "connecting" socially or emotionally with others, individuals with AS can experience a "corrective" relationship in the course of the therapeutic encounter. This healing effect is fostered through the explicit understanding that emerges between the therapist and the client that troublesome social issues and relationships can be addressed in

201

the supportive and accepting therapeutic environment. The most important aspect of engagement is "unconditional positive regard" and acceptance (Rogers, 1951) offered by the therapist, who also encourages the client to describe the subjective narrative of his or her life. This positive relationship experience comes about not only as a part of the content of therapy, but the process of therapy, because that process is inherently a social one. Others have noted that therapy can provide a "very useful laboratory for helping AS patients to learn and practice how to better handle social situations" (Ramsay et al., 2005, p. 484).

Reluctance to engage in treatment may reflect a variety of causes: previous unproductive or destructive experiences with professionals, lack of insight, anxiety, depression, or inflexible thinking. Part of the assessment is to discover which of these issues may be contributing to the person's reluctance or refusal to participate in therapy and to treat those issues suitably. Many adults with AS not only recount difficult experiences with service providers in their adult years, but discuss significant grievances with organizations and schools in their childhood and youth. Understanding and addressing the components of this transference may play an important role in developing an alliance with the adult with AS and in understanding his or her worldview.

Often, as with other clinical issues, the "identified patient" may have a clear opinion about the presenting problem, which may be different from that of family members. In one instance, the family felt that the identified patient, a young man, was too socially isolated, and needed to perform more independently at school, whereas his complaint was that he needed to (in his words) "get laid." (He did not necessarily want a girlfriend.) The young man was willing to engage in counseling only when he was able to discuss the pros and cons of dating services and Internet websites. His forays into the local "dating scene," prostitution, meeting women online, and adult entertainment were also discussed. He was able to continue treatment as long as he and his therapist (and, to some extent, his family) had a shared understanding of the purpose and desired outcomes of the therapy.

For individuals who experience the clinical appointment as anxiety provoking, especially those with a preexisting (social) anxiety disorder, it is important for the clinician be aware of this anxiety and to engage in preventive and repair strategies throughout the therapeutic involvement to preclude the person's abrupt termination. Strategies that we have used include:

- Ensure that the appointment starts and ends on time.
- Meet at regular appointment times.
- Shorten appointments, if necessary.
- Use humor.
- Use rating scales to gauge intensity of emotions.
- Use written information such as emails, information about AS, and individual journals.
- Devise a list of topics for discussion in appointments.
- Provide a sensory-friendly therapy and waiting room.
- Give access to sensory objects (e.g., fidget toys, stress balls) during the appointment.
- Allow a variety of seating arrangements.
- Engage in relaxation techniques during the appointment.
- Limit attending collaborators (e.g., family members, case managers) if necessary.
- Slow pace of appointments and simplify speech/verbal communication.
- Engage in discussion/activities related to the individual's interests.
- Gradually introduce issues that are emotionally laden or difficult to discuss.

Social Interaction

Grandin and Baron (2005) counter the myth that individuals with ASD are not interested in social and emotional reciprocity:

"As a young adult I wanted a girlfriend more than anything and was determined to get one. While I was trying to get a grip on social relationships, I was learning how elusive they often are. The harder I tried to find my place and get firm answers, the more everything slipped through my fingers. Unwritten social rules were everywhere, written in invisible ink; if only I had the magic solution to make them appear!" (p. 273)

Given the centrality of social deficits to the presentation of AS and the resulting frustration, depression, and loneliness, it is likely that these social deficits are the major presenting concern of individuals seen in a clinical setting. The focus of intervention in this area is often to (1) increase opportunities for social interaction, (2) decrease social anxiety, (3) promote developmentally appropriate social interaction, and (4) improve understanding of social interaction, including non-verbal communication.

Once many adults with AS leave school, they have increasingly limited opportunity to interact with others. Even though grade school and high school are stressful for many children and youth with AS, they are required to interact socially and have structure in their lives. For those who cannot find employment or do not continue to postsecondary education, these positive influences end when high school ends (Stoddart, 2005c). Some young adults might have friendships that have lasted since childhood, because they have found a sympathetic individual who is accepting of their differences. They may have gravitated to, or been accepted by, a "fringe" group of peers that is diverse in their abilities, culture, or sexual orientation (Dakin, 2005). Sadly, more often, individuals with AS report that people leave their lives for reasons that are not apparent to them, and that they feel inadequate initiating a social interaction, let alone maintaining a friendship. Their experiences of being bullied and teased in childhood (Dakin, 2005; Dubin, 2007; Heinrichs, 2003; L. Little, 2002; Mishna & Muskat, 1998) have added to their anxieties and insecurities, serving as a further reason to be wary of social contact.

Sloman, Schiller, and Stoddart (2008) have proposed that a "negative cycle of social interaction" is a common experience for children with AS which is produced through the combination of the typical social and behavioral problems for children with AS (e.g., behavior regulation, misreading others and inappropriate behaviors) and lack of social opportunities, social withdrawal and isolation. This cycle of social approach, lack of social success, lack of peer acceptance, and then social avoidance can be chronic and well-entrenched. Unfortunately, this approach-avoidance pattern can be easily perpetuated well into adulthood.

Although some of the evaluations of adults with AS about their social abilities seem accurate, many of them engage in chronically and excessively negative cognitive appraisals of their capacity and ability to engage in social interaction. Thus, it is important to review past social experiences and assess the impact of these experiences on the individual's future interactions. Lerner and colleagues identified the role of "critical self-referent attributions" (CSA) "from ambiguous peer cues" on outcome in a social skills group for adolescents with AS or HFA (Lerner, Spies, Jordan, & Mikami, 2009). In other words, individuals with AS can be prone toward negative self-evaluations even when peer messages were not necessarily negative. Some individuals with AS can present as if they are experiencing symptoms of a posttraumatic stress disorder if these social experiences have involved extensive failure, threats, abuse, chronic misunderstanding, or bullying. The "black-and-white thinking" that is characteristic of individuals with AS often contributes to a pessimistic social evaluation. It is important, therefore, to challenge beliefs and cognitions, when fitting, and to highlight even minimal social successes.

Problematically, in individual therapy one encounters the challenge of not having an objective observer of social interchanges, past or present. Work with couples (and other family members) can provide a solution to this dilemma. One couple we saw for marital counseling negotiated a system whereby the partner was to squeeze the hand of the affected partner if he spoke too long in a social situation about his particular interest. This subtle signal, not evident to others, was important to this man because he was not picking up the nonverbal signs of boredom or disinterest from his peers. Later, social scenarios were deconstructed with help of the partner, with the assumption that she would give honest and constructive feedback about the affected partner's performance. This feedback could occur in the counseling room, or if suitable, at home.

We have seen individuals with anxiety that increases with lack of opportunity for social interaction and develops into social phobia or agoraphobia. Unfortunately, our practice suggests that extreme social isolation may be common for those young adults that have not yet found a partner, are not in work or postsecondary education, and who suffer with other preexisting comorbid issues such as anxiety and depression. They may go for days without having a conversation with somebody or leaving their apartment. It is helpful to ask adults with AS specifically about the frequency and duration of their social contact. We have been surprised to discover that the only conversation some of our clients engage in is during therapy sessions.

Given the anxiety that many individuals face, and the overlapping symptoms thought to exist between social anxieties and AS, desensitization to social contact is sometimes a priority. Gradual desensitization through exposure to social stimuli is a first step to broadening the range and quality of the person's social interaction. This is one aspect of treatment for social anxiety that is proposed in some self-help books (Antony & Swinson, 2008). Setting the person up for success at this stage of intervention is paramount. If an individual with AS has anxiety in large social gatherings, a family reunion is not the place to start this process. Some of the common negative cognitions that we hear that relate to social performance include:

- "I can't do small talk."
- "People don't like me."
- "I bore others."
- "I don't know when to stop talking."
- "I don't know what to say."
- "I'm too anxious."
- "The costs of social interaction outweigh the benefits."
- "I can't be social without alcohol or drugs."
- "People are not interested in what I am interested in."
- "Others look at me in a disapproving way."
- "I talk too much about my interests."

Often, the relative strength of "parallel play" in ASDs removes some anxiety and eases some of the pressure to "perform" socially. We encouraged one man who collected vintage Disney™ toys to join a toy collectors club so that he could share his hobby with others in the community. Similarly, a woman with AS decided to join a runners club, so she could meet others while enjoying her passion for running. Both clients found conversation with like-minded people interesting, and their audience never found their favorite topics of conversation odd or excessive. The activity involved in these social gatherings reduced their stress levels and reduced the pressure to engage in a face-to-face conversation about an unfamiliar or uninteresting topic.

If severe social anxiety continues to be present, it may need to be treated with an SSRI or other pharmacological intervention (Antony

& Swinson, 2008). SSRIs can be effective, and their use is reviewed later in this chapter. A young woman treated with paroxetine (Paxil; indicated for social anxiety) boasted about how, being on the medication for several weeks, she could approach strangers and start a conversation with them for the first time in her life.

Engaging in "social autopsies" can help pave the way for easier social interventions. Here, the therapist and the individual with AS discuss a past social event, such as being at a party, asking a woman out for a date, or attending a large family gathering, and realistically evaluate how the individual fared socially. This review provides an opportunity for the critical evaluation of social skills and behavior in the context of a therapeutic relationship; it is also helpful to use the therapeutic relationship as a platform for planning such events. For instance, instruction might be given to the man who is interested in a woman at their workplace about how to further the friendship, assess whether she is interested in him as a friend, and plan the early stages of the courtship. Of course, social autopsies might also be used in situations that have involved clearly inappropriate behavior, such as e-mailing somebody repetitively or approaching a woman when there has been legal action invoked, such as a restraining order.

As we have already pointed out, social interaction is affected by the environment—including the responses of others to the social behaviors of our client. Much of the social autopsy work involves helping the individual with AS predict how others might respond to his or her behavior and how that behavior either promotes or interferes with social interaction. The therapist's challenge here is to gauge the possible responses of others or to infer reasons for their actions. The man who is overtly friendly to a female colleague and asks her out for coffee, only to be met by a flat "No thanks!" is forced to "fill in the blanks" with the support of the therapist. Here, the man's degree of insight can be assessed by asking him to discuss the social scenario. If he appears to be missing the cues in a subtle situation, the therapist can increase the degree of guidance and interpretation provided.

Some inappropriate social behaviors or *faux pas* are more obvious. One young man who was passionate about rock music went to the local bar every Friday night wearing a "rocker wig" bought in the nearby novelty shop, with his bathrobe belt tied around his head. He felt that he received a good response from women on the dance floor because they were laughing. We explored the possibility that they may not have been laughing in a positive way. In another example, a young woman became threatening toward a parking attendant on her campus when he pointed out the "Lot Full" sign. The student could see that there was one spot available at the back of the parking lot and became verbally aggressive and threatening. Campus security was called. During the "autopsy," she was encouraged to consider the university's perspective, given increasing concerns about campus security in North America.

What sometimes arises during conversations with adults with AS is the type and difficulty of social interaction that some individuals are requiring of those with a "social learning disability." One must question if the expectations are realistic. Social scenarios may differ widely in terms of the cognitive, sensory, and emotional demands placed on an individual. Specifically, we evaluate the complexity of a social interaction in relation to an individual's (1) familiarity with and enjoyment of the social environment; (2) familiarity with the other participants; (3) number of people in the social setting; (4) levels of anxiety experienced before or during the interaction; (5) demands for processing of emotional or multimodal sensory information; and (6) whether the social interaction was planned or anticipated. This hierarchy would be different for each individual, but the greater the "pileup" of stressors or sensory/social/emotional demands in an interaction, the more difficult it might be.

It is important to emphasize that the desire for social contact varies widely among individuals with AS. Some are keenly aware of their need for social involvement, and the lack thereof causes them great distress and contributes significantly to feelings of loneliness, depression, and anxiety. For others, limited social contact or interaction within their daily environments (e.g., at school or work) is all that is necessary. Adults who were diagnosed in childhood and were forced into social interaction by parents, teachers, or therapists may feel that as adults they no longer need to engage in regular social activities (Stoddart, 2007b). The therapist's response to this concern may reflect his or her professional view of AS being either a "disability" or a "difference."

Problems with social skills may be magnified in early adulthood because of fewer supports, less structure, and the expectation for sexual and intimate relationships to develop. It may be more difficult to find opportunities for socializing, as the social opportunities provided by a daily high school routine are no longer present. Adults with AS differ widely in their comfort regarding with whom they socialize (Stoddart, 2006a). Some may be comfortable socializing with others who have developmental difficulties, such as an AS social group, whereas others prefer to relate to typically developing adults. Even at social groups intended for adults with AS, there may be a wide range of behavioral functioning and social capacity, and that range can be off-putting for some. Strong preferences and opinions about whom they affiliate with may reflect the degree to which adults with AS have accepted the diagnosis or their experience in the past with similar social groups. Whatever their choice, it is essential to discuss the desirability or undesirability of opportunities for social interaction.

Many young adults, both with and without AS, are now seeking friendships and relationships with others through the Internet. The Internet slows communication and makes it visual. Pros and cons of Internet dating must be discussed (e.g., the fantasy of the Internet girlfriend, the risks involved). Facebook, MySpace, Lavalife, and other social networking sites provide opportunities for personal web pages and advertisements. Pornography sites and phone chat/sex lines may also provide social and sexual outlets. Meeting somebody online or the online friend, can easily become "the obsessive interest."

In the therapeutic relationship, the lonely and distressed individual with AS will view the therapist or clinician as an ally; however, this can easily shift into seeing the therapist as a friend or even as a romantic interest. There is always a possibility that clients might experience this positive transference reaction and develop romantic or unrealistic expectations of their therapist. Individuals with problems interpreting social language and nonverbal communication, who are desperate for friendship and companionship, might be even more vulnerable to this transference. It is essential that the therapist be vigilant to how he or she may be contributing to this amplified transference. For example, a friendly hug on a special occasion such as a birthday (common in the field of developmental disabilities in some centers) may be misperceived by an adult as a romantic gesture. Similarly, complimenting the client on his or her appearance may be seen as helpful therapeutically if improving the client's appearance has been one of the goals of the intervention, but it can also be easily misunderstood. Such communication needs to be carefully offered and processed within the protective boundaries of the therapeutic relationship. Clarification of the role of the therapist as a professional relationship and the need for, and potential to develop other relationships can be explored (Stoddart, 2005c).

Interests

Although a "restricted range of interests" is identified as pathological in the DSM-IV-TR (American Psychiatric Association, 2000) there is surprisingly little discussion among professionals about interventions for this problem. The most common issues that arise in therapy with respect to restricted interests are (1) the appropriateness of the interest(s) for an adult, (2) the interference of the interest(s) in the necessary activities of daily living, (3) the amount of time the person spends engaging in the interest(s) and, (4) how the interests might be successfully incorporated into the individual's daily life and provide an employment opportunity.

One issue arises on occasion from family members but usually from individuals with AS themselves. They question: "Am I too old to be interested in this?" Some of the interests that may present a concern are stuffed animals, cartoons and animation, toys such as fantasy or science fiction figures, and video games. The individual may have developed an interest in these activities from childhood and has carried them over into early or even middle adulthood. Often, engaging in the interest is seen as soothing or relaxing; therefore, it would be counterproductive for the therapist to recommend relinquishing the activity entirely. However, in this case, it is important to discuss the location of the activity. For example, if a young woman who enjoys the sensory comfort of a large stuffed teddy bear takes the bear to university, this would probably lead to her being ostracized. If, however, the young woman replaced the large bear with a smaller one that could be kept within her knapsack, this would be a fitting adaptation.

The "restricted range of interests" seen in adults with ASDs sometimes interferes with activities of daily living. Most often, this interference is related to the time an individual spends engaging in the activity, such as playing computer games or surfing the Internet. Feeding this problem is the difficulty in stopping and starting a behavior, understanding and attending to the passage of time, planning (i.e., executive function), self-monitoring, and difficulty in engaging in less rewarding behaviors (e.g., homework for university).

The precursors to and consequences of computer, video game and Internet addiction are receiving increased attention in the media and professional literature (e.g., Chow, Leung, Ng, & Yu, 2009; Gordon, 2011; King, Delfabbro, & Griffiths, 2009; Liu & Peng, 2009; van den Eijnden, Spijkerman, Vermulst, van Rooij, & Engels, 2010). Individuals with AS may be especially prone to this problem, and indeed, referrals for the treatment of these repetitive and addicting behaviors are on the rise. A behavioral strategy that has been useful is to limit the activity to a certain number of hours per day, or for certain periods of the day, and to work with the client to expand their range of interests as he or she restricts the preferred activity. Time spent on the computer by individuals with AS can be limited by family members; however, this method often leads to conflict. Alternatively, a more helpful approach is to limit the time using a self-monitoring strategy. Various clocks and timers can be downloaded from the Internet and shown on the computer desktop, for example.

In some situations, the concern is not the time spent in the interest, but the disturbance that it causes in meeting other daily demands. Although a young man with AS enjoyed television cartoons shown only twice a day (and the daily time watching them was only an hour), the times at which they were shown were problematic; he had difficulty attending school or work at those times. He was later convinced that he could record the cartoon and watch it at a time that would not interfere with his daily schedule.

Despite the drawbacks of specialized interests, they also have the potential to provide enjoyment and information, increase self-esteem and social interaction, and reduce anxiety, depression, and boredom. It can also be pointed out how the special interests can (1) serve as reliable self-rewards for engaging in less desirable activities and (2) guide the individual in choosing what area to pursue for vocation or in postsecondary education (Grandin & Duffy, 2008).

Mental Health

In Chapter 3, we detailed the range and severity of mental health symptoms that can affect people with ASDs. Discussing mental health concerns is a major task in most therapeutic relationships with this population. The role of the therapist includes assessing mental health issues and the factors/interventions that may contribute to, or ameliorate symptoms, and educating the client about

211

mental health problems and interventions. Psychoeducation about mental health problems and affective education have been discussed by others in the context of a cognitive–behavioral approach (Anderson & Morris, 2006).

Four approaches are useful in overseeing mental health symptoms: self-report, reports from others, use of standardized measures, and client-specific measures. Stoddart (1999) suggested that the effects of medication on mental health symptoms can be monitored during therapy through self-report, the use of standardized measures, and requesting information from family members and others. One of the most important routine questions in ongoing therapy is to check in with the client about his or her mental health at the beginning of the session. It sometimes becomes apparent how severely the client is affected by mental health problems during the session through observation of their behaviors.

Some clients respond well to completing a self-report questionnaire in the waiting room before the appointment, and they can bring this into the therapy appointment as a means of self-monitoring and a starting point for discussion. Because clients complete the questionnaire before the appointment, therapists can feel reasonably assured that the effect of the session does not contaminate the questionnaire results, and the responses are representative of the mood in the past few weeks. We have also had clients complete a checklist or measure on a daily basis. This can be a brief standardized measure, or one that is specific to the individual's mental health symptoms and devised by the therapist and patient. This is especially helpful for those clients who have difficulty recalling their mood over a period of time, and for highlighting significant contributors to fluctuations in mood or anxiety. It is also a way to bring concreteness to feelings and is especially of interest to clients who enjoy using graphs or spreadsheets. Both the client and the therapist can then easily visualize any variations in mood and anxiety over several months using a computer-based spreadsheet program and graph. Our clients have also kept diaries (which are then brought to sessions) and used electronic/computer-assisted measures (which are completed at home or in the clinic) and e-mails as useful adjuncts to reporting on mood and anxiety between appointments.

A corollary benefit of using standardized scales or self-created Likert-type scales is that black-and-white thinking is discouraged. A client who is characteristically a dichotomous thinker might report being either "depressed" or "not depressed." The benefit of this in assessment is limited, especially when one is trying to determine the subtle effect of an intervention. Rather, if the client has access to a mood scale with 1–5 points, there are a greater number of options, and fine-tuning his or her responses is possible. Given that we are dealing with individuals who have long-term chronic mental health issues, it is important to look for those small changes in mood or other mental health symptoms, understand the source of the change, and therapeutically amplify it when possible (Stoddart et al., 2001).

One helpful self-report questionnaire we have used to determine treatment effects is the Hopkins Symptom Checklist (Parloff, Kelman, & Frank, 1954; Stoddart et al., 2002b). This checklist, if presented in a tabular format, provides a visual depiction of symptoms for both the client and the therapist. These data can also be graphed later to present a long-term depiction of symptoms. When long-term data collection occurs, both therapist and client can begin to predict potentially difficult periods throughout the year, such as the anniversary of a loss, university exams, or seasonally related mood disturbances. This kind of information can also provide important single-case data about the efficacy of specific periods of treatment (e.g., with an SSRI) and the effects on mood and anxiety. This single-system approach is discussed by others in the context of the use of CBT with individuals with AS (Anderson & Morris, 2006)

Creating client-specific measures addressing mental health problems serves multiple purposes in treatment. Primarily, it facilitates a conversation between client and therapist about the client's idiosyncratic presentation of mental illness. Symptoms or behaviors that are not typically associated with a specific mental health disorder, but that are idiosyncratic symptoms for a particular client (or for this population) can be highlighted with this approach. When asked of the effect of an SSRI on his mood, one young man stated that he knew it was good because he was now able to enjoy playing his computer games again. Other behavioral indicators, such as getting out of bed on time, feeling sexual desire, socializing with others, or completing activities of daily living may also be targeted with a checklist or Likert-type response scale. It is important to point out that alexithymia (i.e., difficulty identifying feelings) is a common symptom of individuals on the autism spectrum. Therefore, discussing emotional reactions throughout the course of therapy and reflecting on the potential causes of those feelings are important psychoeducational tasks.

Finally, an easy source of information about mood and anxiety problems is the Internet and self-help books. It is useful to note an individual's uptake of this information and incorporate it into therapeutic treatment plans, if possible. For example, many individuals with AS enjoy the concrete exercises that are provided in CBT workbooks, and completing these exercises can be used as "homework" for the client between therapy sessions.

Self-Care

Elsewhere (Stoddart, 2006a), we have discussed the possible ways in which our clients might prevent mental health problems and contribute to their overall well-being. This overseeing of social, mental health and physical needs is often a priority issue for individuals in psychotherapy. The need to address these concerns may be the result of the many intersecting challenges—mental, social, and organizational—that diagnosed adults experience.

It is also important to recognize the contribution of poor self-care to mental health and social problems. Engaging in particular self-care strategies might be assigned for homework. If the client does not have success in this, reasons for this can then be explored such as problems in planning, hyper-sensory responses or social anxiety. At times, the job of the therapist may be more of a "life coach" or mentor, whereas at other periods, teaching and helping with organization and daily living skills may be identified as therapeutic goals. One young man with AS benefited from bringing his unopened mail and bills to his therapy appointments each week. These unopened bills and calls from collection agencies meant considerable stress for him and his family. The therapist assisted him in managing his finances and paying his bills on time. The family was grateful that the therapist played this important role in aiding with these life skills, and the anxieties of the individual and family were lessened. Other self-care strategies might include:

- participation in a support group or a drop-in center
- self-management strategies (e.g., deep breathing, cognitive strategies)

- physical activities (e.g., walking, swimming)
- meditation and mindfulness approaches
- journaling and data collection on mood states
- regular physical self-care routine (e.g., showering, shaving)
- calming or relaxing activities (e.g., music, massage, yoga)
- keeping a daily schedule
- planning rewarding activities consistent with interests (e.g., travelling, photography)
- proper sleeping routines and sleep hygiene
- healthy and regular eating routines
- practice of spirituality (e.g., going to church)
- sensory activities (e.g., listening to music)
- development of friendships and social activities
- establishing new hobbies/interests/pastimes

Addictions

As discussed in Chapter 5, addictions can be difficult to address in adults with AS, and they can vary from prescription and over-the-counter drugs, to food, illicit drugs, alcohol, exercise, work, sex, gambling, and computer, video game and Internet use. It is also important to reiterate that addictions in this population can be highly destructive and chronic in nature. Possible addictive behaviors need to be assessed carefully and their impact on the individual's life considered. For many clients, AS is a secondary presenting problem to the addiction. On occasion, addictions can be addressed within the confines of the therapeutic relationship. However, given that the treatment of addictions is a complex and specialized area, our preference is to refer individuals to addiction programs whenever possible. Further discussion of inpatient treatment can be found in Chapter 7.

Whether the addiction is addressed in the therapeutic relationship, via attendance at a treatment program, or through a combination of both, it is often helpful to explore the functions(s) of the addiction for the client with AS. Some of the subjectively identified functions of addictive behavior overlap with those found in the general addictions literature, whereas others relate more closely to the psychosocial problems inherent to AS. Unfortunately, repetitive thinking and behavior (cognitive profile), mental health problems, and social isolation intersect insidiously to perpetuate addictive types of behavior in this population. Table 6.1 provides an overview of common maladaptive functions of addictive behaviors and their adaptive alternatives.

The main problem that we have encountered in accessing addiction services for individuals with AS is managing the social component of intervention, which is often a part of group treatment in a residential or community-based facility and in community supports such as Alcoholics Anonymous. We usually try to determine if there is flexibility in attending group meetings or therapy in a treatment program, depending on the individual's ability to participate in, or benefit from a group or community milieu. If, for example, the individual with AS is singled out and asked to speak in a group session by others, this type of forced involvement may be more anxiety- and anger-provoking than therapeutic and precipitate substance abuse.

TABLE 6.1. MALADAPTIVE USE OF SUBSTANCES FOR PSYCHOLOGICAL PROBLEMS AND ALTERNATIVE ADAPTIVE RESPONSES

COMMON MALADAPTIVE FUNCTIONS OF ADDICTIVE SUBSTANCES	ALTERNATIVE ADAPTIVE RESPONSES TO REPLACE ADDICTIVE SUBSTANCES
Regulates or reduces anxiety and depression	Treat anxiety proactively via CBT, medication
Helps with socializing	Assist with the formation of appropriate social relationships in treatment
Helps with insomnia	Improve sleep hygiene, use sedating medication
Provides relief from stress	Implement stress management approaches
Gives relief from boredom and isolation	Assist with scheduling a range of social activities
Increases creativity/cognitive function	Provide healthy approach to increase creativity/cognitive function
Assists in blocking memories/recall in PTSD	Treat traumatic experiences/PTSD in psychotherapy

The role that family and others play in enabling the addict is central to the addiction literature and requires special consideration for adults with AS. Research, self-help and practice literature discuss the circular trap in which some families become mired when a family member has an addiction. In an effort to care for or protect the addicted person, they inadvertently become an enabling agent in the individual's addiction. Alcoholic individuals, for example, do not experience the negative effect of their addiction because family enablers "cover" for them or unintentionally support their addiction by providing them with money, calling in "sick" to their workplaces for them, or chauffeuring them when they are too intoxicated to drive themselves.

The enabling scenario may be even more complex for addicts who have AS. Enabling behaviors of family members and spouses are driven not only by the addiction, but also by concern over mental health and traits related to the AS. For example, parents may feel guilty that they did not get help for their addicted son or daughter earlier, have their AS diagnosed sooner, or may struggle with the degree of support that they provide to their adult child who lacks life skills or "common sense." Spouses may fear that their partner will disengage from the family even further or become more depressed or even suicidal (as they may have become in the past) without their support. Many of these families have struggled for years trying to get support for their family member with both AS and addictions and have been turned away, leading them to believe that *they* are the only support available for their family member. A codependent relationship is sometimes the outcome. This belief about their dependence is perpetuated when they go to Al-Anon meetings and hear the very different stories of other families who do not have to deal with the "double hit" of AS *and* addiction.

Parents of individuals with AS may have experienced alcoholism previously in their families, as there is evidence that alcoholism has a genetic component, and families of individuals with ASDs may have a history of substance abuse. Dysfunctional patterns of coping with an addicted family member may span generations. Those factors that perpetuate codependence should be addressed by a clinician who has expertise in identifying and treating these counterproductive interpersonal and familial behavior patterns.

Postsecondary Education

In Chapter 5 we highlighted some of the difficulties that individuals with AS might face in postsecondary education. Increasingly, those who provide disability services for students with ASDs are making connections with clinicians and psychotherapists in the community who specialize in the field of AS or ASDs. Some universities are able to pay for, or at least subsidize, counseling and psychotherapy costs for students in order to augment the support that they receive directly from the university or from government programs, but in many cases payment is left to the student and his or her family (Dillon, 2007). Despite the benefits of this collaborative approach between institutions of higher learning and community agencies, it is important that there be clear delineation of roles of both agencies and a joint assessment as to whether the student is benefiting from the approach (Dillon, 2007). Therapeutic support might focus on social and mental health issues that may influence student learning, class attendance, and academic achievement. In our experience, it is especially helpful if the clinician is teaching or has worked at an academic institution so that the student is assured of the therapist's familiarity with academic demands. A therapist who is teaching at the same institution that the student is attending may have a better understanding of the institution's academic policies, the layout of the campus, academic and library supports, and dates that may be significant for the student (e.g., "drop dates" for courses). This "specialized knowledge" of the therapist can prove comforting to the student.

In a busy dormitory individuals with AS may have an acute sense of their isolation and loneliness, or on the other hand, feel overwhelmed with the relentless social demands of residence life. Sometimes, negotiating the social and life skill demands of dorm life needs to be discussed with somebody who is familiar with the student's needs. A university disability center recently had to become involved in the dormitory's monitoring and support of a student with AS when she was sexually assaulted by one of the cafeteria kitchen staff. Advocacy and planning have to occur in the dormitory or student housing as well as in the classroom. For example, how might the student best respond when he is invited to a fraternity party where there will be a demand to drink alcohol? On some occasions, we have helped the student "script" what he or she will say to roommates about the ASD and his or her reluctance to engage in certain social activities. In other instances, deficiencies in life skills might become an issue. One young man moved into a large university dorm and was coping reasonably well there until he attempted to dry his sweater in a frying pan on the stove! Dorm mates angrily complained to the manager of the dorm, and disclosure of the student's diagnosis was necessitated. However, the incident led to increased understanding of the student and eventual acceptance by the dorm mates.

Given the inherent social difficulties that students with AS face, the social experiences of these students, especially in residence, must be given careful attention, as these experiences often affect academic performance, sense of inclusion, acceptance, and mental health. In a recent investigation of broader autism phenotype (BAP) characteristics among the general population of college students, the problem of loneliness was investigated in 97 undergraduate college students in a large urban university in the United States. Using the autism quotient (AQ; Baron-Cohen, Hoekstra, Knickmeyer, & Wheelwright, 2006) as a measure of characteristics of autism, the presence of autism traits was found to be a significant predictor of loneliness ($p < .001$), even though the students were in the nonclinical range according to this measure (Jobe & White, 2007). Both the Social Skills and Communication subscales of the AQ made significant contributions to loneliness scores. The risk of feelings of loneliness developing for students with AS is likely high in large colleges and universities or in large cities where students do not have the opportunity to affiliate with others in small groups around a common interest. Moving a distance from long-time friends and acquaintances in their smaller community or high school may also give rise to feelings of loneliness. In order to address this concern, social and support groups have formed at some universities to provide a base for students with ASDs (Dillon, 2007; Farrell, 2004; Hancock, 2008; Manett, 2007; Smith, 2007), and there are reports of other universities engaging in social skills training for students (Farrell, 2004). Specific interventions for post-secondary students with AS are discussed in Chapter 7.

Trauma and Loss

The most common trauma that we have seen in our practices is sexual victimization, most frequently of adolescent and adult females with AS. In part, victimization is precipitated by the intense and unrelenting desire to find friendships, the inability to read social cues, and the difficulty in assessing risky situations. Other traumatizing experiences may include bullying and teasing (which may have not only occurred in childhood); childhood sexual or physical abuse, trauma, death or loss of friends, family members, or pets; and traumatic or abusive experiences with service providers or professionals. For those events subjectively experienced as traumatic, it is often difficult to ascertain the impact due to the tendency in this population to "get stuck" in feelings and the characteristic inflexible thinking, misunderstanding of social cues, and excellent (sometimes video-graphic) memory of past events. We have certainly seen the cumulative effect of combined traumatic events over time, which may require focused intervention by the therapist.

From a biopsychosocial perspective, it is important to identify potential triggers to dissociative phenomena in an individual's life and to alter his or her environment accordingly. Prior to completing a functional behavior analysis of challenging behavior, the clinician may observe that individuals with AS and PTSD present with challenging behavior arising "out of the blue." A detailed history should raise the threshold for including the possibility of PTSD in the diagnostic formulation. Commonly, individuals are reacting to unidentified environmental triggers originally paired with their physiological response to the initial trauma or series of traumatic events.

PSYCHOPHARMACOTHERAPY OF MENTAL HEALTH AND BEHAVIORAL CONCERNS

Although the provision of psychopharmacotherapy to children with autism has historically been a core treatment for medical and behavioral problems associated with this disorder, the psychopharmacotherapy of AS, particularly for adults, is a relatively new field of practice. Not surprisingly, therefore, adults with AS struggle to find a physician who feels competent to prescribe medications for the common comorbid psychiatric or behavioral problems present in AS. Physicians, whether they are psychiatrists, developmental pediatricians, or general practitioners, may have had experience with, and knowledge of, prescribing for children with ASDs and feel that this experience can be generalized to adults. In some cases it can be. However, due to a general inexperience in prescribing and reluctance of medical practitioners to engage in prescribing, we have found that pharmacological interventions are often not used when it could substantially improve an individual's quality of life.

On the other hand, when prescribing does occur, individuals may have negative experiences because it is not clear what symptom(s) the medication is intended to treat (in part, due to diagnostic over-shadowing), nor has a thorough discussion of the target behaviors or symptoms occurred. Sometimes, low doses are not used initially (Sloman, 2005) or medication is increased too quickly, giving rise to side effects to which individuals with AS may be more susceptible and find more difficult to tolerate (Towbin, 2003). Past experiences with medication use are especially important to explore with adults who have recently received a diagnosis of AS or who have been subjected to unsuccessful or inappropriate pharmacological treat-ments by an inexperienced clinician, or one who did not recognize that the patient had AS. Once these negative or unproductive expe-riences have occurred, it may be extremely difficult for the patient with AS to acknowledge the possible merits of psychopharmaco-therapy in the future. Finally, pharmacotherapy must be an inte-grated part of an overall treatment plan that may include psycho-therapy and other interventions; in the absence of integrated multidisciplinary community teams for adults with AS, creating such a comprehensive approach may be a difficult undertaking.

When psychopharmacology is combined with other treatments such as psychotherapy, the potential synergistic effects can be real-ized, to the patient's benefit. Often, team members or the individuals themselves have not articulated (1) *specific,* (2) *realistic,* or (3) *measur-able* goals that they expect to achieve by the introduction of medica-tion. A polypharmacological approach, which is indicated in some cases, further clouds possible treatment effects. Unfortunately, evi-dence-based information on the use of medication in adults with AS, which is accessible to the layperson is virtually nonexistent. Medica-tion compliance may also be a problem due to passive resistance or problems remembering to take medication at the prescribed time(s) and dose(s) (Stoddart, 2005, 2007b). Addressing the potential prob-lems of this population with self-reports in monitoring the effects of medications, Towbin (2003) notes:

Another hurdle is the shortcomings patients have in identifying their own internal mood states and emotions. As a result, the

221

clinician may be unable to gauge whether patients experience less subjective anxiety, sadness, or anger. The patient's psychological "comfort" may not be available to the clinician for rating improvement. To monitor progress, the clinician is compelled to draw on multiple observations, rely more or less exclusively on the patient's somatic experience, and to use highly concrete measures with patients. Treating adult patients who are living independently and are unwilling to allow others to participate in their treatment is particularly challenging. (p. 25)

The value of eliciting a family history of suspected comorbid mental health concerns and medication response or lack of response/adverse effects experienced by family members can assist the clinician in recommending specific medication from a particular class of medications indicated for that condition. In addition, a respectful inquiry into the individual's subjective experience of previously prescribed medication(s) often elicits an honest acknowledgment of nonadherence to recommended doses or duration of therapy, particularly in individuals with anxiety disorders who are hypervigilant to somatic changes and who may misattribute physical experiences to adverse medication effects. With sensitive guidance, these individuals may be willing to consider reviewing a cost–benefit analysis of a second trial with the same medication, beginning at a lower dose, and following a more conservative dose titration schedule, with the assurance that there may be strategies available to minimize the intensity of adverse effects if they are again experienced (e.g., using an antinausea medication to treat SSRI-time-limited induced nausea).

Reviewing documented "allergic responses" to previously prescribed medications sometimes reveals that the allergy was actually an adverse effect, and this information then opens the possibility of a second trial with the same medication, following the above principles, versus accepting that the drug is contraindicated due to an allergic reaction. These "allergic responses" are particularly common when extrapyramidal side effects (e.g., rigidity, tremor, drooling, and dsytonias) are experienced because of an atypical antipsychotic medication, particularly risperidone, initiated by an inexperienced physician at higher than optimal doses.

Review articles on the treatment of mental health concerns in individuals with ASDs have focused on target symptoms, particularly in the symptomatic treatment of behaviors of concern, recognizing that there is still no definitive approach to pharmacologically altering the core features of ASDs (Ghaziuddin, 2005; King, 2000; Kwok, 2003; Posey & McDougle, 2000; Sloman, 2005; Willemsen-Swinkels & Buitelaar, 2002). Attempts have been made to rationalize pharmacological treatment of symptomatic behaviors—such as emotional lability, overactivity, stereotypies, aggression, and self-injury—by best matches between our current understanding of the neuropathological and neurophysiological changes documented in ASDs and the presumed methods of action of various classes of psychotropic medications. Reviews have typically highlighted either the efficacy of drugs according to their proposed neurochemical method of action (dopaminergic, serotonergic, opioidergic, adrenergic, thymolytic, or glutaminergic) (Buitelaar & Willemsen-Swinkels, 2000) or by class (indirect serotonin agonists, typical antipsychotics, atypical antipsychotics, serotonin reuptake inhibitors, other antidepressants, opioid antagonists, and alpha-adrenergic agents).

Below, we briefly review some of the current literature on medication and ASDs. For each class of medication, a preliminary review of the action of the medication and examples of specific medications are given. An introduction to psychopharmacotherapy is beyond the scope of this book, and we would encourage the reader to consult general references with respect to general dosing, contraindications, and interactions, such as the excellent reference: *Clinical Handbook of Psychotropic Drugs* (Virani, Bezchlibnyk-Butler, & Jeffries, 2009). This handbook also contains useful patient information sheets. We feel that it is important for nonmedical clinicians to be familiar with psychopharmacotherapy, given the central role of medication use in this population, the task of psychoeducation about medications, and the lack of support adults with AS receive in the community with respect to this issue. We begin with a discussion of selective serotonin reuptake inhibitors.

Selective Serotonin Reuptake Inhibitors

Selective serotonin reuptake inhibitors (SSRIs) are one of the current primary treatments for depression and anxiety and other mental health disorders in the general population. Serotonin is a neurotransmitter which has been implicated as being involved in the etiology of depression, anxiety disorders, and other mental health disorders. The benefit of this class of drugs is that it is thought to be *selective*, acting primarily on serotonin receptors, and therefore has fewer adverse side effects than older classes of medications. SSRIs block serotonin reuptake sites, allowing serotonin to remain active in the synaptic cleft longer. Examples of SSRIs include fluoxetine (Prozac), fluvoxamine (Luvox), paroxetine (Paxil), sertraline (Zoloft), escitalopram (Cipralex) and citalopram (Celexa). SSRIs are the best studied of the antidepressants in the treatment of panic disorder, obsessive–compulsive disorder (OCD), social anxiety disorder, and major mood disorders.

Interest in this class of medications in our field has been prompted by studies of blood serotonin concentrations in individuals with ASDs dating back as far as 1961 (Burgess, Sweeten, McMahon, & Fujinami, 2006; Hranilovic et al., 2007; Kolevzon, Mathewson, & Hollander, 2006; Schain & Freedman, 1961). Approximately one-third of individuals with ASDs are thought to have hyperserotonemia; therefore, the potential role of SSRIs in the regulation of peripheral and central serotonin levels, and thus the symptoms associated with dysregulation (e.g., mood, anxiety, impulsivity, and aggression), is an important consideration (Kolevzon, Mathewson, & Hollander, 2006).

In reviewing data on the efficacy and tolerability of SSRIs in individuals with ASDs, Kolevzon and colleagues (2006) identified three randomized controlled trials (Buchsbaum et al., 2001; Hollander et al., 2004; McDougle et al., 1996). The first two studies investigated fluoxetine. The Hollander study was the first controlled study to demonstrate a reduction in repetitive behaviors in children and adolescents with ASDs using a liquid formulation of fluoxetine, which was well tolerated by trial participants. The Buchsbaum study demonstrated a reduction in anxiety in a small ($n = 6$) group of adults with ASDs. McDougle and colleagues included 30 adults with ASDs. Objective outcome measures demonstrated reduction in repetitive thoughts and behavior and in maladaptive behaviors and aggression in 8 of 15 subjects receiving fluvoxamine versus no improvement in 15 subjects receiving placebo.

Ten open-label or retrospective case reviews of SSRIs, including fluoxetine, sertraline, luvoxamine, citalopram, and escitalopram, were summarized in tabular form by Kolevzon and colleagues

(2006). Most of these studies showed improvement in global functioning and in signs and symptoms such as anxiety, aggression, and repetitive behavior. Although the various SSRIs were generally well tolerated, agitation (particularly in children) was severe enough to warrant discontinuation of the medication in a significant minority of subjects. These findings point to the need to begin with low doses, to titrate doses upward slowly, to use objective outcome measures, and to be vigilant to the possibility of SSRI-induced hypomania or mania. Kolevzon and colleagues conclude their review by noting: "SSRIs appear to demonstrate therapeutic benefit in the treatment of autism spectrum disorders" (p. 413).

Autism Speaks (2009) announced the results of an industry-sponsored double-blind placebo-controlled study evaluating the efficacy of fluoxetine in reducing repetitive behavior in children and adults with autism. The Study of Fluoxetine in Autism (SOFIA), conducted by the Autism Clinical Trials Network (ACTN), involved 19 medical centers and clinical sites in the United States, enrolling 158 participants between the ages of 5 and 17. A new low-dose form of fluoxetine, designed for use in a melt-in-the-mouth formulation, was assessed. Unfortunately and surprisingly, this study did not show that fluoxetine was more efficacious than placebo. This study hopefully does foreshadow the inclusion of children, youth, and adults with ASDs in more properly designed medication studies in the future.

Stimulants and Other Options

As a medication class, the stimulants are prescribed to address the symptoms of attention deficit hyperactivity disorder (ADHD) and target symptoms including hyperactivity, inattentiveness, and impulsivity. The most commonly prescribed stimulants are methylphenidate hydrochloride (Ritalin) and dextroamphetamine sulphate (Dexedrine). These medications are available in various formats that alter the length of time the medication is effective, and hence have different dosing schedules. Adderall is also available as a mixture of dextroamphetamine and racemic amphetamine salts. These medications act primarily by increasing the availability of norepinephrine and dopamine at the synaptic cleft (the space between cells or neurons in the brain).

Atomoxetine hydrochloride (Strattera) is the first nonstimulant medication to be approved for the treatment of ADHD in Canada. Strattera and Concerta (a long-acting methylphenidate) are recommended as drugs of first choice in the treatment of this disorder (Canadian ADHD Resource Alliance, 2006). As a selective norepinephrine reuptake inhibitor, atomoxetine increases the availability of the neurotransmitter norepinephrine. Atomoxetine may be particularly beneficial for individuals with a history of psychosis, Tourette syndrome, or substance abuse (as the stimulant class of medications may exacerbate these conditions). There have been reports that a small percentage of individuals prescribed atomoxetine may develop symptoms of depression and thoughts of self-harm.

Symptoms of impulsivity, inattentiveness, and overactivity are common in children with ASDs; some have suggested a prevalence of up to 60% (Tsai, 2000). Many adults whom we see in our practice have previously been appropriately diagnosed with ADHD, but this diagnosis does not explain the "gestalt" of their clinical presentation, which is better explained by the diagnosis of AS. Very little empirical information is available regarding these symptoms in *adults* with AS. Promising case descriptions of adults with AS and ADHD are beginning to emerge, however (Roy, Dillo, Bessling, Hinderk, & Ohlmeier, 2009). In comparison, a recent review found 41 studies of the pharmacological treatment of *children* with ASD and ADHD-like symptoms (Aman & Langworthy, 2000).

The literature regarding the use of these medications in individuals with ASDs has been mixed in terms of evaluations of efficacy. Early case reports and case series on the efficacy of the stimulants dextroamphetamine and methylphenidate were disappointing, leading to an early consensus that stimulants were contraindicated in ASDs (Aman, Van Bourgondien, Wolford, & Sarphare, 1995). Anecdotal reports continue to describe the exacerbation of irritability, insomnia, and aggression in this population's response to this class of medication (Posey & McDougle, 2000). Stigler and colleagues (Stigler, Desmond, Posey, Wiegand, & McDougle, 2004) found that individuals with AS were more likely to respond better to stimulants than individuals diagnosed with other subtypes of ASDs ($p < .01$); this has also been our clinical observation over the years. No known work has been completed in adults with AS on the use of Concerta, a controlled-release form of methylphenidate, or of Strattera (atomoxetine, a selective norepinephrine inhibitor); these are all drugs identified in recent practice guidelines as medications of first choice to treat ADHD (Canadian ADHD Resource Alliance, 2006).

With the support of the National Institute of Mental Health (NIMH), a network of pediatric psychopharmacological researchers at seven academic centers in the United States has established research units on pediatric psychopharmacology (RUPP). The RUPP Network has facilitated the establishment of multisite, high-enrollment studies to advance an improved understanding of pharmacological efficacy in this area. The RUPP Network demonstrated the superiority of methylphenidate over a placebo in 72 children with ASD (49% response), with adverse effects leading to discontinuation of study medication in 18% of subjects (RUPP Network, 2005). The RUPP Network has not completed trials involving adults with ASDs, to date.

Given the moderate efficacy of psychostimulants, additional options to address the behavioral problems of impulsivity, aggressiveness, and overactivity have been pursued. Clonidine (an alpha-adrenergic agonist), in both oral and transdermal forms, has been demonstrated to have a modest effect in one small double-blind study (Frankhauser, Karumanchi, German, Yates, & Karumanchi, 1992). Clonidine can be sedating and has modest tic-suppressing properties (Cohen, Riddle, & Leckman, 1992), making it a reasonable choice for individuals with the constellation of rage outbursts, sleep disturbances, and tics, typically with comorbid oppositional defiant disorder, an ASD, Tourette's syndrome, and ADHD-like features. Orthostatic hypotension, dry mouth, and oversedation are often dose-limiting factors or reasons for discontinuation of this medication.

Guanfacine, which has a similar mode of action and a longer half-life compared to clonidine, resulting in less sedation and orthostatic hypotension, has demonstrated some efficacy in open trials, but these trials have not included adults with AS (Jaselskis, Cook, & Fletcher, 1992). Others have assessed the response of children with ASD to guanfacine (Posey, Puntney, Sasher, Kem, & McDougle, 2004) and have reported that clinicians can expect a less robust treatment response to psychostimulants in children with ASD.

King et al. (2001) completed a double-blind, placebo-controlled study of amantadine as a treatment for ADHD in children with ASD. Amantadine is an excitatory amino acid with antagonistic activity at the N-methyl-d-aspartate (NMDA) subclass of glutaminergic receptors. In this study, patients did not report statistically significant behavioral change in response to amantadine. No known research of this nature has been completed involving adults with AS.

Antipsychotics

Antipsychotic medications are used to treat psychotic disorders such as schizophrenia. Traditional, or first-generation antipsychotics, include haloperidol (Haldol), chlorpromazine (Largactil or Thorazine), loxapine (Loxapac), trifluoperazine (Stelazine), perphenazine (Trilafon), fluphenazine (Fluanxol), and thioridazine (Mellaril), among others. These medications predominately treat the positive symptoms of schizophrenia (i.e., hallucinations, delusions, and disorganized behavior) and are less effective in treating the secondary symptoms of amotivation, blunted affect, anhedonia (a lack of enjoyment of previously pleasurable activities), and alogia (a reduction in spontaneous speech).

The second generation (or atypical antipsychotics) includes clozapine, risperidone (Risperdal), quetiapine (Seroquel), olanzapine (Zyprea), ziprasidone (Zeldox), and aripiprazole (Abilify). This class of medication acts through antagonism of serotonin and dopamine receptors. The drugs in this class have been demonstrated to be equally effective to the first-generation antipsychotics in treating the positive symptoms of schizophrenia (Lieberman et al., 2005). The atypical antipsychotics also appear to be more beneficial for the negative symptoms of schizophrenia, many of which resemble the core features of ASDs (Fisman & Steele, 1996).

The method of action of atypical antipsychotics is through the blockade (antagonism) of dopamine receptors. However, as there are a number of different dopamine-responsive systems in the brain, and since this class of medication also antagonizes serotonin, alpha-adrenergic, and cholinergic receptors, it can produce a number of adverse effects. These include acute neurological disorders (dystonias, dyskinesias, and akathesia) as well as tardive dyskinesia, a movement disorder. In addition, atypical antipsychotics have the potential to produce a possibly lethal condition called neuroleptic malignant syndrome (NMS), characterized by a fever, altered blood pressure and pulse, diaphoresis, alterations in level of consciousness, and extreme muscle rigidity. We have, unfortunately, seen NMS in a number of cases of adults with ASDs, but primarily those who have some cognitive disability and other medical issues. Despite having a decreased risk of tardive dyskinesia and NMS, the atypical antipsychotics carry a high risk of inducing a metabolic syndrome in the individuals to whom they are prescribed. This is characterized by weight gain, diabetes mellitus, and hyperlipidemias (i.e., an abnormally high level of lipids in the blood).

There is little information in the literature specifically addressing the impact of atypical antipsychotics on comorbid disorders in adults with ASDs. Barnard, Young, Pearson, Geddes, and O'Brien (2002) completed a systematic review of the use of atypical antipsychotics in individuals with autism, identifying 13 studies on risperidone, three using olanzapine, one using clozapine, one using amisulpride, and one using quetiapine. First, we turn our attention to the use of risperidone.

Risperidone

Anecdotally, in our practices we have seen remarkable progress in individuals with angry, explosive, or aggressive behavior on low doses of risperidone. On occasion, these doses have been used in combination with other classes of medications (e.g., SSRIs) and often in combination with psychotherapy and cognitive behavioral approaches. Typically, these doses have been low, in the 1–2 mg range, which has been suggested elsewhere (Sloman, 2005). In our clinical review of 100 adults with ASDs (most with some intellectual disability) it is noteworthy that risperidone was the most commonly prescribed antipsychotic in 16% of the cases; the mean dose was 2.2 mg (Stoddart, Burke, & Temple, 2002a). A case report did identify a significant calming effect in a 30-year-old individual with AS, presenting with a mixed anxious–depressive state, with a very small dose of risperidone (0.1 mg), after a period of nonadherence with a dose of 1 mg (Raheja, Libretto, & Singh, 2002). A 12-week double-blind placebo-controlled study of risperidone demonstrated a positive impact on repetitive behavior, aggression, anxiety, nervousness, and irritability (McDougle et al., 1998). Participants were diagnosed with autism or PDD, but not AS.

Promising research data have been discovered regarding the benefits of risperidone on challenging behavior and at least one of the core domains of ASD in children (McDougle et al., 2005). The initial study conducted by the RUPP Network, involving an 8-week double-blind, placebo-controlled comparison of risperidone in 101 children, showed a highly significant advantage favoring risperidone on the Irritability subscale of the Aberrant Behavior Checklist (ABC; 57% decrease vs. 14% decrease with placebo) and the Clinical Global Impressions scale (CGI; 75% improvement vs. 11% improvement; RUPP Network, 2002).

Recognizing that standardized scales may fail to reflect real change important to the individual family, a second study collected concerns of parents (tantrums, aggression, hyperactivity), rated these on a 9-point scale, and again demonstrated risperidone's superiority over a placebo, which proved colinear with CGI Improvement (CGI-I) and ABC Irritability subscales (Arnold, Vitiello, McDougle, Scahill, Shah, Gonzales, Chuang, et al., 2003). In addition, the scores for the Ritvo–Freeman Real Life Rating Scale (with subscales measuring social relationship to people and language) failed to demonstrate significant changes in the core ASD domains. However, changes were observed in restricted, repetitive, and stereotyped patterns of behavior using the Children's Yale–Brown Obsessive Compulsive Scale.

Finally, this landmark study reviewed observed weight gain in children in response to risperidone (citing a meta-analysis of 26 studies of risperidone-treated adults demonstrating a mean increase of 2.1 kg at 10 weeks; Allison et al., 1999). Despite a wide variation in changes in weight among individuals treated (from a loss of 4.0 kg to a gain of 15.3 kg), the study demonstrated that leptin levels (a hormone secreted by differentiated adipocytes in direct proportion to body fat stores) at 1 month did not predict weight gain at 6 months. Weight gain at 1 month did emerge as a potential indicator for significant weight gain at 6 months. Concern about weight gain with the use of risperidone is a major obstacle in practice to the treatment of individuals who might be genetically susceptible to weight gain or who are already obese.

Other Atypical Antipsychotics

Trials of the atypical antipsychotics olanzapine, quetiapine, ziprasidone, and aripiprazole in the treatment of ASDs, published between the years 1966 and 2007, have been reviewed (Stachnik & Nunn-Thompson, 2007). Clinical trial case reports in retrospective series were included. Published reports of the use of these four drugs were presented in tabular form. Nine reports involving olanzapine were identified. Only one double-blind placebo-controlled trial involving 11 children, including one with AS, was noted. Three of six children were identified as responding to olanzapine, based on a physician-rated CGI-I. Sedation and weight gain were identified as common adverse effects. We have clinically observed significant beneficial effects on intense interpersonal aggression, impulsivity, and rigidity of thinking in two male adults with AS in response to clozapine and in the absence of significant adverse effects.

A case report describing the use of aripiprazole in five children (only one with AS) was described by Stigler, Posey, and McDougle (2004). All children were reported to experience improvement in behavior. One adult with autism was included in a case series of five adults with intellectual disability. A reduction in aggression, facilitating the discontinuation of previously prescribed chlorpromazine and lorazepam, was noted (Shastri, Alla, & Sabaratnam, 2006).

McDougle, Kem, and Posey's (2002) case series of 12 individuals with autism taking ziprasidone demonstrated a 50% positive response. These authors also identified a retrospective review of ziprasidone in 10 adults with autism and profound intellectual disabilities. Seven of these individuals were judged to respond to ziprasidone. Of possibly greatest significance was the fact that eight of these individuals lost weight during treatment (Cohen, Fitzgerald, Khan, & Khan, 2004).

We identified four studies involving the use of quetiapine, but only one of these series included adults (Corson, Barkenbus, Posey, Stigler, & McDougle, 2004). Forty percent of individuals were judged to respond, whereas 50% experienced sedation, insomnia, pain, and weight gain. Anecdotally, I (R. K.) have had success utilizing quetiapine, primarily on a PRN basis (given its sedating properties) in doses of 25–150 mg every 2 hours, with a maximum of four doses in 24 hours, to address self-injurious behavior, aggression, and insomnia.

Open-label trials with olanzapine in children and adults with ASDs have demonstrated equivocal results (Kemner, Willemsen-Swinkels, de Jonge, Tuynman-Qua, & van Engeland, 2002; Stavrakaki, Antochi, & Emery, 2004). In a small open-label pilot study, Potenza, Holmes, Kanes, and McDougle (1999) demonstrated that olanzapine reduced hyperactivity and aggression and improved social functioning and language. The risks of significant negative metabolic consequences of olanzapine (obesity, diabetes, hypercholesterolemia, and hypertriglyceridemia) are concerns, however.

McDougle et al. (2002) presented a case series of 12 individuals (ages 8–20 years) with ASD (none with AS) who received open-label treatment with ziprasidone. Six of twelve patients were considered responders, in the absence of significant weight gain. As the fifth second-generation antipsychotic to be released in the United States and now in Canada, of available atypical antipsychotics, ziprasidone has the longest 5-HT2 (serotonin) to D2 (dopamine) binding ratio. It is unique in that it also possesses serotonin and norepinephrine uptake inhibiting properties (Tandon, Harrigan, & Zorn, 1997). McDougle et al. (2002) reviewed a study involving 12 subjects, ages 8–20 years. Although all subjects had ASDs, none was identified as having AS. Fifty percent of the subjects were considered responders. Acknowledging the small size of the study, the authors noted that subjects had infrequent dyskinesia and weight gain. A beneficial effect on the impaired social relatedness characteristics of ASD was observed.

The use of clozapine in children with ASDs is not well reported in the literature. The need for an initial 6-month period of weekly phlebotomies, given the risk of agranulocytosis and concern regarding adherence to this regime, leaves many clinicians hesitant to pursue this option. However, open-label reports of individuals with intellectual disability have demonstrated initial positive results (Cohen & Underwood, 1994; Thalayasingam, Alexander, & Singh, 2004). Published case reports have demonstrated improvements in aggression, self-injurious behavior, social functioning, and ability to participate in daily living in these individuals (Hammock, Levine, & Schroeder, 2001; Sajatovic, Ramirez, Kenny, & Meltzer, 1994).

Mood Stabilizers

Mood stabilizers are prescribed most commonly to decrease the intensity and frequency of the depressed, hypomanic, and manic phases experienced by individuals with bipolar disorders. They are defined as having no propensity to induce an episode of opposite polarity (e.g., inducing a switch from depression to mania) and have long-term prophylactic or maintenance value in decreasing the burden of this illness. The term *mood stabilizer* was first applied to the lithium salts: lithium carbonate and lithium citrate. These medications affect the neurotransmitters serotonin and norepinephrine, and have additional complex effects on intracellular messenger systems (Poindexter et al., 1998).

A number of anticonvulsant (antiseizure) medications have also been demonstrated to have mood-stabilizing properties. These include valproic acid (Depakene), carbamazapine (Tegretol), and lamotrigine (Lamictal). The anticonvulsants gabapentin (Neurontin) and topiramate (Topamax) have less support as mood stabilizers. The safe prescription of lithium carbonate, valproic acid, and carbamazapine is enhanced by the availability to measure their serum levels and individualize dosing according to these levels to minimize adverse effects. Recently, several atypical antipsychotics have also been demonstrated to have mood-stabilizing properties, both acutely and as maintenance medications. They can be used individually for this purpose or more commonly in combination with one or more of the above mood stabilizers, depending upon the severity of the individual's illness.

Lithium carbonate, divalproex, and the atypical antipsychotics olanzapine, risperidone, quetiapine, ariprazole, and ziprasidone are recommended drugs of first choice for the pharmacological treatment of acute bipolar mania (Yantham et al., 2005). The Canadian Network for Mood and Anxiety Treatments (CANMAT) guidelines stress the need for the completion of baseline laboratory investigations before the initiation of treatment for bipolar disorder (Yatham et al., 2005). Regular monitoring for weight changes, extrapyramidal side effects (in response to atypical antipsychotics), and polycystic ovarian syndrome in females is recommended. Monitoring of serum medication levels (particularly divalproex and lithium), renal function (lithium), hepatic function (all other mood stabilizers and second-generation antipsychotics), thyroid stimulating hormone (lithium), fasting blood sugars and lipid profiles (second-generation antipsychotics), and complete blood counts are also endorsed (American Psychiatric Association, 2002).

Beta-Blockers

Beta-adrenergic blocking medications compete with catecholamines at beta-adrenergic nerve receptor sites. Beta-blockers vary in their degree of lipid solubility, hence altering their ability to be transmitted across the blood–brain barrier. Propranolol, a nonselective beta-blocker (blocking B1 and B2 subtypes of catecholamine receptors), and metoprolol, a selective beta-blocker, are best studied for this purpose. Beta-blockers have been studied in the treatment of anxiety disorders, aggression, psychotic disorders, and akathesia (a syndrome of motor restlessness caused by traditional and, to a lesser extent, atypical antipsychotics). The outcomes of studies in individuals with developmental disabilities have been published in tabular form (Reiss & Aman, 1998). Guidelines for the use of beta-blockers have also been formulated (Fraser, Ruedrich, Kerr, & Levitas, 1998; Huggins, 1995; Ruedrich, Grush, & Wilson, 1990). We have seen a number of individuals in our practices who have historically engaged in high levels of aggression or rage and who have shown significant behavioral improvement with the use of beta-blockers. It should be noted that monitoring of blood pressure is important for those being treated for behavioral concerns with beta-blockers.

Benzodiazepines

The benzodiazepines are used to treat anxiety disorders and to induce sleep. They are also commonly used as one component of a continuum of supports included in a crisis prevention plan (a PRN protocol) to decrease the intensity and duration of an episode of challenging behavior. They act as central nervous system depressants through enhancing the neurotransmitter gamma-aminobutyric acid (GABA). Commonly prescribed benzodiazapines include lorazepam (Ativan), clonazapam (Rivotril), diazepam (Valium), oxazepam (Serax), and tenazapam (Restoril). They differ primarily in their pharmacokinetic properties, which alter their onset of action and the rate at which they are metabolized by the liver. This class of medication is generally recommended for short-term use only, given the potential risk of tolerance, physical dependency, and withdrawal symptoms if discontinued abruptly.

It is important to be cognizant of the increased risk of paradoxical disinhibiting responses to a benzodiazepine in individuals with

ASDs. Our experience with the use of benzodiazepines on a PRN basis is favorable, though utilization should be guided by the use of written PRN protocols to ensure safe and consistent utilization. In addition, it is very helpful to review their effectiveness using PRN efficacy charts that document (1) the antecedent or observed behavior prior to the administration of the benzodiazepine or atypical antipsychotic, (2) the time to observed response, (3) the nature of the observed response, and (4) a clinical judgment as to whether or not the response is favorable. Although the risk of tolerance and physical dependency, as well as a withdrawal syndrome, is theoretically possible with benzodiazepines, under the above cautious prescribing circumstances, we have observed these effects only rarely.

PRN Medications

The relative merits of PRN, or "as needed," medications as one component of a crisis plan have been debated. To some extent, concerns regarding the use of PRN medications have arisen in relation to historical contexts during which psychotropic medications were used as punishment, for staff convenience, as a substitute for meaningful psychosocial services, and in quantities that interfered with quality of life (Reiss & Aman, 1998). However, in recognition of the chronic, recurring nature of Axis I disorders, guidelines have been offered to incorporate PRN psychotropic medications into comprehensive biopsychosocial client-centered plans with success. In this paradigm, medications are allowed to work synergistically with other modalities of treatment and environmental manipulation to optimize quality of life (Kalachnik et al., 1995; King, Fay, & Croghan, 2000). Community-based education, emphasizing an understanding of the pharmacokinetics (i.e., the science describing an individual's response to a medication, including factors affecting the drug's absorption, distribution, metabolism, and excretion from the body) of available medication options, has been developed (King, Wilson, & Atchison, 2008).

The frequent use of PRN medication of any class should alert the interdisciplinary team to (1) consider increasing the dose of regularly prescribed medications (based on rational diagnostic formulation) to achieve optimally tolerated doses; (2) ensure that adequate time has been allowed (based on known pharmacokinetic properties of the prescribed drug) to avoid premature termination of a potentially positive drug trial; (3) consider alternative medications if optimal doses and durations of drug trials have been achieved, in the absence of a significantly objective positive response; and (4) reevaluate the choice of PRN medication or combination of PRN medications, the dose of the PRN medications prescribed, and the initially prescribed dosing interval, as well as the number of possible doses to be utilized in a 24-hour period.

Zelenski (2002) has presented a helpful psychiatric case management flowchart outlining algorithmic approaches to address both type 1 crises (acute and dangerous to self and others) and type 2 crises (disruptive, interfering with quality of life and social interaction, but short-lived and not necessarily dangerous). The utilization of benzodiazepines and traditional and atypical antipsychotics, alone or in combination, is endorsed in the algorithm addressing type 1 crises. The absence of the need for acute psychopharmacological interventions is stressed for type 2 crises. The antidepressant trazadone and antihistamines (including hydroxyzine or diphenhydramine) are cited as possible pharmacological options. Based on our experience, we do not necessarily support the use of the latter recommendations, given the potential for significant adverse effects (including oversedation, dry mouth, blurred vision, and dizziness) and the accumulating clinical evidence supporting the use of the medications recommended in the type 1 crisis algorithm.

Table 6.2 lists potential advantages and disadvantages of choosing a medication in the benzodiazepine, traditional, or atypical antipsychotic class. In extreme situations, combinations of a drug from each of these classes may be indicated. Given their favorable bioavailability profile when given intramuscularly, lorazepam, a benzodiazepine, and olanzapine, an atypical antipsychotic, are popular options (King et al., 2000).

COMBINED PSYCHOPHARMACOLOGY AND PSYCHOTHERAPY

Often, psychopharmacology and psychotherapy are used in combination to treat some of the comorbid mental health or behavioral symptoms present in adults with AS. Treatment effects vary widely in response to pharmacological or other types of intervention in this clinical group. The task of assessing and monitoring the mental health symptoms is often left to the nonmedical Asperger specialist who might have a more intimate and long-term perspective of the waxing and waning of mental health symptoms; general (consulting) psychiatrists or busy family physicians may defer to nonmedical specialists in assessing a patient's response to a pharmacological intervention. This deference is largely due to the lack of mental health expertise in ASDs, the limited number of psychiatrists available for following a patient, and the role of the general medical practitioner in overseeing patients with mental health problems in the absence of specialist practitioners. The psychotherapist has a unique opportunity to collect information over a course of long-term involvement from the adult with AS, his or her family members, or other members of the support team, such as special needs counselors at postsecondary institutions.

Since many individuals express concern about side effects and the long-term implications of medication use, a psychoeducational task is to discuss the use of medication in the treatment of mental health symptoms. Although some of the information may have been given verbally by the prescribing physician, it may be overwhelming for individuals to integrate and retain all the information that they are provided in appointments, so review by informed nonmedical clinicians is helpful. One of the most common concerns relates to the literal interpretation of the list of possible side effects that most pharmacies now provide with prescriptions. The individual with AS may feel that many or all of the side effects listed on the information sheet are likely to occur, rather than realizing that the side effects listed occurred with varying frequencies in the medication trial. Some clients may have conferred with others or obtained information on the Internet about adverse reactions. Towbin (2003) notes:

> Building a relationship and gaining the patient's trust can be hard to accomplish; patients often feel forced to take medication and commonly recoil from the idea of medication treatment. Understandably, many patients are so frightened of the effects of medications that they cannot put those fears aside enough to try one. The amount of anxiety that makes it ap-

TABLE 6.2. ADVANTAGES AND DISADVANTAGES OF BENZODIAZEPINES, TRADITIONAL ANTIPSYCHOTICS, AND ATYPICAL ANTIPSYCHOTICS

BENZODIAZEPINES[a]		TRADITIONAL ANTIPSYCHOTICS[b]		ATYPICAL ANTIPSYCHOTICS[c]	
ADVANTAGES	DISADVANTAGES	ADVANTAGES	DISADVANTAGES	ADVANTAGES	DISADVANTAGES
Familiarity to individuals and caregivers	The existence of multiple drugs within this class results in varying prescribing practices among physicians	The ideal antipsychotic should have: • A rapid onset of action • An initial sedative affect • Few neurological adverse affects • A longer duration of action to minimize administration frequency • Good local tolerability if given intramuscularly or intravenously	A risk of paradoxical response secondary to oversedation and akathisia	A decreased propensity for adverse extrapyramidal effects and tardive dyskinesia	A risk of agranulocytosis, particularly in the first six months of treatment with clozapine
General efficacy (although a risk of paradoxical disinhibition exists)	These drugs differ in their rate and route of elimination as well as the presence or absence or active metabolites		Acute neurological adverse affects (including dystonia, spasmodic torticollis, oculogyric crisis), each with a potentially negative impact on subsequent compliance	Decreased risk of hyperprolactinemia (except risperidone)	A theoretical risk of respiratory depression with combined use of lorazepam and clozapine
Rapid oral absorption	Intramuscular absorption is variable in this class and inconsistent, with the exception of lorazepam and midazolam		Exacerbation of seizure disorder	Improved impact on the negative symptoms of schizophrenia	Dose-related risk of seizures with cloazapine
Potential to raise or at least not lessen seizure thresholds				Interaction with both dopaminergic and serotonergic systems	Significant weight gain

(Continued)

TABLE 6.2. (CONTINUED)

BENZODIAZEPINES[a]		TRADITIONAL ANTIPSYCHOTICS[b]		ATYPICAL ANTIPSYCHOTICS[c]	
ADVANTAGES	DISADVANTAGES	ADVANTAGES	DISADVANTAGES	ADVANTAGES	DISADVANTAGES
	Significant intraindividual differences with respect to response and adverse affects		Adverse sedative and anticholinergic affects that may produce delirium		
	Rapid oral absorption		Exacerbation in PTSD of dissociative phenomena		

Note: PTSD = posttraumatic stress disorder.

[a]Benzodiazepines include lorazepam, clonazepam, diazepam, oxazepam and tenazapam.

[b]Traditional antipsychotics include haloperidol, chlorpromazine, loxapine, trifluoperazine, perphenazine, fluphenazine and thioridazine.

[c]Atypical antipsychotics include risperidone, clozapine, olanzapine and quetiapine.

propriate to consider medication for a patient can also interfere
with him or her adhering to a prescription. (p. 24)

The therapist might also review with clients what impact the
medication and psychotherapy will have and how they might see
that impact exhibited in their day-to-day life. This symptom-focused
treatment discussion can replace commonly held misperceptions
that the medication (or psychotherapy) will "change them." Some of
our adult patients have reported that the medication has resulted in
less creativity or slowed thinking, and this complaint needs to be
sensitively explored. Another common concern is that a physician
who has prescribed "antipsychotic" medication has deemed the individual to be "psychotic." Finally, all individuals need to understand
that prescription of medication for mental health problems is an
"inexact science" and that there may be a need for trials of a number
of medications and dosages within a class of medications (e.g.,
SSRIs) before the optimal effect is achieved.

CONCLUSION

For clinicians who have or are developing clinical practices that focus
on ameliorating the major psychosocial sequela of AS in adults, the
challenges can be both rewarding and frustrating. Treatment specialists who can act as mentors to novice clinicians are few, and there is
sparse psychotherapeutic and psychopharmacotherapeutic practice
literature and research to guide assessment and interventions—an
issue that we address in the final chapter. On the whole, adult clients
who have lived with AS are keen teachers and responsive patients,
when psychotherapy and psychopharmacotherapy are guided by
patient-centered, respectful practice and the best available evidence.
When psychotherapists and medical professionals work collaboratively, we have seen the best outcomes. In the next chapter, we review other interventions that compliment these two core treatments
in adult AS. Both the complexity and the uncertainly of this practice
area will continue to attract new clinicians trained in medicine and
psychotherapy to work in this emerging field.

Chapter 7

COMPLEMENTARY INTERVENTIONS AND EVIDENCE-INFORMED PRACTICE IN ADULT ASPERGER SYNDROME

This final chapter underscores our findings throughout this book: Although we have gained a vast knowledge base about the range of clinical presentations of AS, we have just begun the journey of understanding the breadth of helpful clinical practices in this field, especially as they relate to AS in adults. In order to meet this need, knowledge dissemination and translation between various service, policy, research and medical sectors requires continued attention. In this chapter, we reinforce the need for a clinical approach that is multidisciplinary, multifaceted, and collaborative in nature to most efficiently support adults with AS and ameliorate the symptoms with which they struggle.

ADJUNCTIVE INTERVENTIONS

With this goal as our guide, we review 10 key adjunctive interventions: (1) psychoeducation, (2) family therapy, (3) couple and parenting therapy, (4) occupational therapy, (5) behavioral therapy and coaching, (6) case management, (7) employment counseling,

(8) groups, (9) academic advising, and (10) inpatient treatment. There is yet little empirical evidence of the efficacy of some of these interventions. We nevertheless offer them because of the significant positive and synergistic effect that they have had in our clients' lives after diagnosis. This chapter thereby suggests a research agenda that has yet to be explored. We end with a brief discussion of evidence-based practice and present an example of the contextual and resource challenges that confront research efforts in the psychotherapeutic treatment of adults with ASDs.

Psychoeducation

Education about ASD and related symptoms is central to many interventions in our field, and has long been recognized as important (Bristol & Schopler, 1984; Edwards & Bristol, 1991; Gaus, 2007; Konstantareas, 1990; Singer, Ethridge, & Aldana, 2007). With this clinical group, after a diagnostic assessment, further exploration of an individual's own presentation of AS is important. When a diagnosis is communicated verbally by the diagnostician, either at the assessment meeting or at a feedback appointment, the client's uptake of the information may be limited by their ability to process a verbal presentation, or if she is (emotionally) overwhelmed by the content.

It is often helpful if another person, such as a parent, spouse, sibling, or close friend, attends the feedback appointment. As this supporting person may not be knowledgeable about ASDs, it is important that general information about disorders on the spectrum be provided. It is necessary that individuals have access to printed copies of their assessment report, or a summary of the report, in which the findings and diagnosis are explained. Sometimes a second appointment is required after the individual has had time to read and think about the information and identify questions he or she may have. As well, the treating clinician often helps the individual with AS fully understand the findings and discuss the implications for his or her support and treatment.

Considering the fragmentation of most services for adult ASD in North America, other professionals actively treating the individual should have access to this diagnostic information as well. (Occasionally, we have seen that those providing the diagnosis are also involved in providing ongoing services, but this is the exception in Canada.) Treating clinicians will see that the in-depth assessment, as described in Chapter 2, was not offered casually (as is sometimes the case) and fully comprehend why the diagnosis was provided. As well, they will gain insight into other comorbid issues that may be a focus of treatment or affect treatment outcome. Throughout the course of treatment, issues may arise related to learning, attention, mental health, sensory problems, or activities of daily living (ADLs), and these issues should lead both the treating clinician and client back to the initial assessment report. If new issues are revealed throughout the process of clinical intervention, aspects of the individual's presentation may warrant a reevaluation or suggest a new problem for evaluation. Ideally, recommendations from the existing assessment report form the beginning of a collaboratively negotiated treatment plan, if a course of treatment is pursued.

Considering that many individuals with AS will have a poor understanding of emotional expression and regulation (and may have a positive finding of alexithymia), education about emotions is a central task of therapeutic involvement, especially when mental health problems are part of the presenting clinical picture. Individuals with AS may need to receive reassurance that their experience of moods is common. For example, a young man who experienced a range of feelings and beliefs about the sudden death of his mother was comforted to know there was no "right way to grieve" and that his range of emotions was symptomatic of a significant loss. This process of grief psychoeducation in the context of psychotherapy may have been a protective factor when he was faced with the sudden death of his father, a few years later (Stoddart & McDonnell, 1999). Education about mental health problems and interventions is central to ameliorating poor mental health in this client group, and is a component of many cognitive–behavioral programs addressing mood and anxiety problems (Antony & Swinson, 2008; Greenberger & Padesky, 1995; Leahy & Holland, 2000). The information that is contained in these cognitive–behavioral protocols can either be used as presented or adapted to individual needs.

Education about available services preceding or following a diagnosis is another important area for discussion. The clinician may draw the client's attention to listings of local resources on the Internet or help the client locate services. Although the range of organizations available to adults with AS is limited, it is helpful for the clinician to develop a resource list of existing services. Because many

243

adults with AS have had previous negative experiences with service providers, it is essential for the referring clinician to be knowledgeable about the services' familiarity with AS and their success of past work with adults who have mild ASDs. Some individuals may not qualify for services without a diagnosis of an ASD, and this is important for patients to know. If the organization provides services to adults with a range of developmental disabilities or mental health disorders, it is useful to know the degree to which the other clients of the program are affected by these clinical issues. It is not appropriate that people with AS participate in programming with those who have a moderate or severe intellectual disability, for example.

Discussion of self-advocacy skills when applying for those services is also needed. If, for example, clients emphasize only their strengths in an initial phone call, those services that provide support to persons with developmental delays may reject them, perceiving that there is no potential role for them. Ideally, adults with AS with multiple needs should have access to case management services (which we discuss below); however, patients often become their own advocate and case coordinator while accessing multiple services and supports. These services might include those discussed later in this chapter, such as groups or employment programs.

Bibliotherapy is the provision of therapeutic information through books and other written formats. It has been used as an adjunctive therapy for various psychological concerns, including psychiatric problems (Katz & Watt, 1992). An example is the use of self-help books or manuals. A meta-analysis on the effectiveness of bibliotherapy for a range of issues found favourable results when compared to traditional types of therapy (Marrs, 1995), as did a recent systematic review for the use of bibliotherapy for mental health problems (Fanner & Urquhart, 2008).

There is now an abundance of books on AS that can be used to promote therapeutic change. For example, autobiographical accounts include those by Grandin (1995, 2008), Grandin and Duffy (2008), O'Neill (1999), Schneider (1999), and Willey (1999). Other sources of autobiographical information are the numerous Internet sites and blogs hosted by individuals with ASDs. These are valuable sources for ensuring that core symptoms of AS, as well as symptoms of related disorders, are understood and normalized. They are affirming of the individual's experience. However, we caution our clients that some of the information on the Internet can be mislead-ing, lack research evidence, or present a narrow view of adult ASDs. The naïveté of individuals with AS can make them especially vulner-able to those who promote costly, untested, and even dangerous interventions. We always counsel our clients to discuss the use of materials or substances with a credible professional (e.g., physician, therapist, occupational therapist).

Literature on AS and related issues may also provide a useful start-ing point for discussion in individual, couple, and family therapy contexts. The literature on marriage and sexuality specific to AS, for example (Bentley, 2007; Hendrickx & Newton, 2007; Slater-Walker & Slater-Walker, 2002), provides a common understanding for the com-mencement of couple therapy. Other books that provide helpful intro-ductions to AS include Attwood's first very popular book and most recent volume (Attwood, 1998, 2007). A common frustration for the individuals with whom we have worked is that much of the published literature is focused on children; however, this trend is changing as more adults with ASDs are writing about their own experiences, and clinicians are becoming interested in the adult population.

Family Therapy

Meta-analyses of the efficacy of marital and family therapy (MFT) demonstrate its effectiveness for a wide range of presenting issues (Pinsof & Wynne, 1995). Shadish and colleagues reviewed 163 ran-domized clinical trials (RCTs) and concluded that MFT is effective, as demonstrated by an effect size that is considerably larger than those seen in many medical RCTs ($d = .51$). The odds of a client doing bet-ter in MFT than receiving no treatment are roughly two out of three (Shadish, Ragsdale, Glaser, & Montgomery, 1995).

MFT has been shown to be efficacious in the treatment of major mental illness, including affective disorders and schizophrenia. As an adjunct to pharmacological intervention in our population, family therapy may involve a strong psychoeducational component that serves to (1) engage the family in early treatment, (2) create a "no-fault" environment, (3) educate the family about symptoms and treat-ments, and (4) provide coping strategies, communication training, problem-solving training, and crisis management. With this interven-tion, relapse rates for psychiatric patients have shown significant re-ductions when compared to controls (Goldstein & Miklowitz, 1995).

245

Unfortunately, marital and family therapists are not adequately familiar with the signs and symptoms of AS. A recent study demonstrated on that only one-fifth of American Association of Marriage and Family Therapy (AAMFT) members accurately identified a child with AS using a case vignette methodology (Carlson, McGeorge, & Halvorson, 2007). It is encouraging, however, that an increasing number of referrals to our center come from marriage and family therapists when there is suspected AS. There has been a surprising dearth of academic literature on family intervention in the ASD population, with some exceptions (e.g., Carlson et al., 2007; Fidell, 2000; Munro, 2010; Konstantareas, 1990; Sofronoff & Farbotko, 2002; Sofronoff, Leslie, & Brown, 2004; Stoddart, 1998, 1999).

We believe that the family has a vital role to play in supporting the effective assessment (see Chapter 2) and treatment of adults with AS. Unfortunately, the parental role is often overlooked or disregarded by clinicians because the individual appears capable, may be insightful, and is an adult. Given the potential system-level resource of the family during the assessment process and throughout intervention, it is important that we address the needs of the entire family system, including those of parents and siblings.

Exploration of significant family tensions may be an integral piece of the individual psychotherapeutic encounter with affected adults. Although we believe that effective family therapy can be carried out by the identified client's individual therapist, at times it is more productive to refer a family to another therapist for family treatment. This is especially true in cases where there is extreme family conflict, and preservation of the therapeutic alliance with the identified patient is a priority.

Given the prevalence of late diagnosis in many individuals, family members may have misunderstood the behaviors and abilities of the affected individual. Negative character attributions such as "lazy" or "rude" by family members, in the absence of a correct diagnostic opinion, should be carefully deconstructed in the context of therapy. Family members may not be candidates for therapeutic involvement with the individual because of lack of desire, their age, illness, or because they live at a distance. In many centers, involvement of siblings or parents in ongoing treatment is rare for adult patients. In our experience, even one or two appointments with family members can be very helpful in dispelling previously held negative beliefs about their family member with AS, and in providing an important perspective and information for inclusion in ongoing clinical work. Such a family appointment is also beneficial in helping family members understand, particularly if they were involved in the initial referral, that just because a reason for problematic behaviors has been identified, it does not mean that the affected individual will have the desire or ability to change the behaviors which others find troublesome. Whether they are realistic or unrealistic, expectations of family members about what the individual with AS can accomplish might also be explored.

As with many psychological issues, AS traits may be seen across generations of families, as discussed in Chapters 1 and 2. Gillberg (1991) noted the presence of both mental health issues and Asperger traits/syndrome in one of the first cross-generational case series that was published. Others have empirically examined traits that are suggestive of a broader autism phenotype (BAP; Bailey, Palferman, Heavey, & Le Couteur, 1998; Baron-Cohen & Hammer, 1997; Bolton et al., 1994; Dorris, Espie, Knott, & Salt, 2004; Fombonne, Bolton, Prior, Jordan, & Rutter, 1997). The implication of this finding for the front-line clinician is that a number of family members may struggle with their own AS traits or related neurological issues and mental health problems. The influence of these factors in parenting the client with AS requires consideration and assessment.

We have found that the cross-generational effects of these untreated psychological and ASD traits can be profound. Themes of feelings of abandonment, perceived or actual abuse, lack of engagement with the child and disinterest in parenting are common. We have seen fathers of young adults with AS who have their own AS traits, and they have been parented by men who also have/had strong AS traits. Discussion of these occurrences is common in both the assessment process and postdiagnosis. Although the cross-generational effects of unrecognized AS can be tragic, the newfound realization that these may be genetically borne traits can promote understanding, normalization, and acceptance.

We have previously discussed the fact that parents may need support in a number of areas: moderating their degree of influence or guidance, addressing their feelings of guilt and disillusionment with professionals after a late diagnosis, preparing for the future needs of their adult child, obtaining information on available sources of support and services, and addressing their own needs at their life stage (Stoddart, 2005c). Especially in cases of a late diagnosis, parents and other family members may need guidance and education from professionals as to the influence of AS on their young adult's life. As noted in Chapter 2, overinvolvement of family members can be diagnostic. Tensions around degree of parental involvement often reflect the patient's self-awareness that he or she is not developmentally typical, and that family members' anxieties are warranted because of previously unsuccessful experiences in the individual's attempts to transition to independence. Families and the identified patient become entrenched in a "power struggle" without the benefit of a neutral and informed mediator. Future planning for their AS child is often a concern for parents, as is the potential stress and burden on siblings in years to come. In some cases, parents report they are "burned out" and feel that they can no longer help their adult child. It is important to clarify the therapeutic role in these cases to ensure that the family does not have unrealistic expectations of what the clinician can accomplish.

The most effective support that we can sometimes provide is enabling parents to speak with other parents of affected adults. Despite our clinical experience, we can never replace the comfort and support that a parent of a person with AS can provide another. This may also come in the form of reading parent accounts (Quint, 2005), although accounts from parents of adults are the exception. It is remarkable how many families we see in our practices have suffered for years without support, services, or an appropriate diagnostic opinion, despite their valiant attempts to seek these for their family member. Many parents of individuals we see are still advocating for their adult children well into their 60s, 70s, and even their 80s. Their commitment to their adult children, even as they may be struggling with their own health issues and other family stressors, is remarkable.

Fidell (2000) has noted that the reason for referral to family therapy may often not be the issue that a family identifies, and that the process of "being heard" in itself has important therapeutic value for many families:

> . . . a psychiatrist referred a family whose 20-year-old son had recently been diagnosed as having Asperger's syndrome. His opinion was that the family needed help in coming to terms

with this diagnosis. However, the family was much more concerned with the son's aggressive behaviour. We used this as a basis for discussion and, in the process, the family developed a more helpful understanding of the syndrome. During the course of therapy the family's dissatisfaction with both social and educational services emerged. Our evaluation indicated how pleased family members were with the service they had currently received however, because they felt that their concerns were listened to. (p. 313)

Family therapy may also be offered without the "identified patient" present (Stoddart, 1999). This may be the only option available to families who are seeking assistance for their adult child who is not amenable to being assessed for AS when it is suspected by family members. In our experience, this refusal of assessment often occurs in situations where there is chronic substance abuse or when the relationship between parents and the adult child has deteriorated over many years and there are irreconcilable differences. In cases where there is "enabling" of inappropriate behavior involving drugs or alcohol, these families may need specialized family intervention or treatment from an addictions center, and the specialist in AS may be able to refer them to family supports such as Al-Anon. Although not ideal, it is important to recognize that significant systemic changes can be made for both the individual and the family even in these difficult situations, without the cooperation of the identified client. It is advisable to also engage the resource of siblings or other family members who may have a better relationship with the identified client in these high-conflict situations.

Couple and Parenting Therapy

Clinicians are increasingly being asked to intervene in couple and parenting relationships when one or both partners have AS. They are facing this challenge with few established best practices and almost no research. The intersection of intimate relationships and AS is now being given attention in both the media (Moore, 2008) and in published literature (Aston, 2001, 2003, 2009; Bentley, 2007; Jacobs, 2003; Thompson, 2008). Insightful books are also being written by affected adults who are in relationships (Newport & Newport, 2002; Slater-Walker & Slater-Walker, 2002).

Although formal professional supports were not found to be predictive of individual or marital adaptation by Renty and Roeyers (2007), the authors note that this finding reflects the lack of such supports for married individuals. When professional sources of support do exist, efforts should be made by these professionals to strengthen and educate the informal support network of individuals with AS (Renty & Roeyers, 2007). For example, partners of individuals with AS can benefit from inclusion in individual counseling; psychoeducational and support groups; workshops; and from phone, personal, or e-mail communication with other partners. It is imperative that the spouse of a partner on the spectrum has a solid knowledge of the characteristics of ASD and how they influence his or her relationship. A therapist working with such a couple should have knowledge of the unique needs of an individual with AS (or ASD) and be able to adapt counseling techniques to meet the needs of both partners (Aston, 2001). This understanding, along with provision of specific strategies in addressing challenges, can be helpful for these partners in negotiating the struggles inherent in relationships.

Jean Shinoda Bolen (1989) has provided a profile of the "Cassandra woman" modeled after the relationship between Apollo and Cassandra in Greek Mythology. Cassandra was seen as hysterical and not believed by others. This situation parallels the experience of many wives when they report to friends, family members, and professionals that their husband is demonstrating characteristics that suggest AS. Sometimes wives do not have knowledge of the label of AS, but they describe their husband as aloof, as exhibiting strong (even obsessive) interests, as neglecting issues of family management, excluding important activities of daily living, and/or as having anger and social problems. Other traits thought to exist of the Cassandra woman are low self-esteem; feelings of confusion, anger, and guilt; depression; and loss of self. The Apollo archetype is illustrative of the man with AS: "The Apollo archetype favors thinking over feeling, distance over closeness, objective assessment over subjective intuition" (Shinoda Bolen, 1989, p. 135).

Cassandra symptoms have been described by Aston (2008) as relating to women who have married men with AS or ASDs. This paradigm is seen by some members of the AS community as excessively pathologizing and blaming of the individual with AS, and we think, can lead the "neurotypical" partner to take little or no responsibility for the state of the relationship. A linear causal theory posits that the man with AS is "the cause" of all the relationship problems; this view is not necessarily helpful or correct in our experience. Instead, we espouse a circular etiology of marital dysfunction in which both partners are able to understand their contributions to their difficulties, take responsibility for them, and actively address them. It is noteworthy that many of the women we see clinically are understandably depressed, anxious, and troubled because of the state of their marriage, but they may also have had longstanding mental health conditions that preceded the marriage. Many of these women are naturally nurturing individuals and may be employed in caring professions such as nursing, social services, or teaching. One woman with an older husband with AS noted that she "just overtook a mother role" (Bolte & Bosch, 2004, p. 12).

Interestingly, in our experience, women we see with AS reflect a similar level of hyperanxiety over not having their symptoms recognized by their spouse (or other family members or friends) similar to woman whose husband has AS and is not believed. We have found that women with AS tend to present as more outgoing, without necessarily feeling the comfort they project. They also tend to exhibit obsessive and compulsive traits that suggest they are organized, but the application of these traits may be specific to one area and lead the person to feel ineffectual in other areas. These features often imply skills that are not present, and the woman experiences internal pain and a response from others that suggest she is exaggerating her situation. We have seen some of these women cope via rage outbursts or incidents involving self-harm; others internalize and become agoraphobic and depressed.

Many times, a child with an ASD further complicates stressful marital situations. Discussion of relationship problems may be intertwined with the management of behavior problems in the affected child, and approaches to his or her intervention. Sometimes parental differences start with the child's assessment and diagnostic process. Fathers often report "He is just like me when I was his age!" and feel that there is little to be concerned about. Mothers, on the other hand, view social and behavioral concerns as more troublesome. When one of the parents also has an ASD, specific traits of that person, such as rigidity around scheduling, household disorganization, and lack of emotional responsiveness, will complicate the issue. A lack of trust and respect in the marital relationship often undermines parenting approaches, and vice versa. This combination of issues requires a dual role for the therapist as both marital therapist and parenting consultant.

As discussed in Chapter 5, there are typically various couple-related issues that present as clinical problems to be addressed in counseling when one of the partners is affected by AS. Figure 7.1 illustrates the interactional pattern that we observe between partners, when one individual has AS. On a consistent basis, we observe this cyclical interaction between unaffected partners and their affected spouses, in which conflict and emotional distance are fueled by misunderstanding and false attributions for distancing and aloof behavior. This cycle is perpetuated by the unaffected spouse, more often

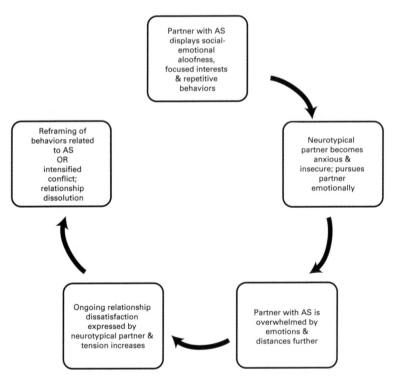

FIGURE 7.1. A COMMON INTERACTIONAL CYCLE BETWEEN PARTNERS WHEN ONE HAS ASPERGER SYNDROME.

the woman, by not having her emotional or even instrumental needs met while recognizing the many admirable qualities in her spouse.

The parent with AS faces some challenges beyond the usual parenting challenges. Some of these depend on whether the person is a single parent or part of a couple; others tend to be gender-specific. If a parent is single and has few natural supports, it is useful to connect him or her with parenting resources or develop some form of support circle. Parents who have AS may have difficulties with scheduling their own activities, planning for future events, and organizing materials. Therefore, when it comes to developing a routine for a child, ensuring that school materials are prepared or planning for weekend activities, the problem is compounded. If there is a spouse, he or she frequently ends up being the person to plan family vacations, make doctor appointments, go to school meetings, and take children to out-of-home events. If the person with AS does do the scheduling, he or she may be overly rigid. For example, he or she may develop a schedule that says that everyone in the house must be in bed at a certain time, and no flexibility is provided for either the spouse or the teenage child. Obsessive and compulsive behaviors may become an expectation for the child; the parent with AS may insist that the child line up cans of food alphabetically, organize the clothes in his or her closet by color, or engage in similar habits.

We have had parents with AS ask us how to play with their child. Because parents with AS may have been focused on one or two special interests during their childhood, they haven't developed the breadth of play and are unsure how to engage in it. Some parents with AS are also unable to engage in imaginary activities. When the child is young, we have encouraged action songs and games, as these provide cues. Blocks and similar building activities tend to be a preference for those with AS. We also encourage the parent to take the child to play groups, story hours, or some form of preschool so that the child can engage socially and have play models other than the parent. The inability of a father with AS to engage with his children was exhibited in a family assessment when both the therapist and mother were on the floor in the clinic playing with the two young children. The father seated on a chair, overlooking the playful chaos on the floor, soon became bored, and eventually opened his briefcase and began shuffling through and reading work papers. Other fathers we work with constantly check their BlackBerrys or other electronic devices and inappropriately text to colleagues during family therapy sessions.

Parents who have AS sometimes abide by specific diets that may not be nutritious. This again becomes problematic as they want their child to be healthy, but may be unable to tolerate the tastes, smells, and textures of foods that are healthier. Such a parent needs guidance in putting together a menu for the family that can blend the needs of everyone and allow that parent to prepare, if not eat, a healthy diet.

Empathy is an issue that becomes more problematic as the child goes to the parent for support, particularly on social issues, and the parent cannot understand the child's needs. In a two-parent family, the child will typically be able to receive support from one parent. In a one-parent family, an extended family member, close friend, or participant in a support circle may become a surrogate around such issues. As the above issues highlight, parenting for an individual with AS can cause specific challenges that may require not only family therapy or individual therapy, but some practical interventions, such as are discussed in the behavioral therapy and coaching section, below.

Occupational Therapy

The activities and mandate of the profession of occupational therapy is sometimes misunderstood. "Occupational therapy is the art and science of enabling engagement in everyday living, through occupation; of enabling people to perform the occupations that foster health and well-being; and of enabling a just and inclusive society so that all people may participate to their potential in the daily occupations of life" (Townsend & Polatajko, 2007, p. 372). Further, the Canadian Association of Occupational Therapists notes: "Occupational therapists define an *occupation* as much more than a chosen career. *Occupation* refers to everything that people do during the course of everyday life" (CAOT; 2010). Many occupational therapists who work in the field of ASDs are trained to assess and treat those with sensory integration dysfunctions (SID).

Individuals who have complex or extreme sensory-processing or movement-planning difficulties can experience serious discomfort and impairment in their daily functioning. We have found that for these individuals, a specialized occupational therapy consultation from somebody well versed in the problems of SID and treatment has been beneficial. Occupational therapists who specialize in SID develop protocols to aid the person with an ASD or to overcome the impact of this disorder. This is referred to as sensory integration therapy (SIT). It is noteworthy that there has been some debate in the behavioral literature about the efficacy of SIT, as it has not been adequately researched. When studies have been carried out, effectiveness has not been demonstrated (Gresham, Beebe-Frankenburger, & MacMillan, 1999; Herbert, Sharp, & Gaudiano, 2002). Attempts are being made to increase research in this area. One example of a successful outcome was a single-subject study of a child showing improvements in behavior with the use of SIT (Roberts, King-Thomas, & Boccia, 2007).

For those who are not affected excessively, or who have symptoms in a specific sensory domain, remediation may simply involve recognizing and addressing the specific difficulties they have. For example, those with aversion to certain textures or tactile sensations, dealing practically with the issue may suffice (e.g., cutting the labels out of clothing or not buying aversive clothing textures). Some individuals who crave the sensation of pressure or snugness around them tell us that they sleep against the wall, in a sleeping bag, or use a body pillow. Others wrap themselves in shawls or wear tight clothing. Some individuals are extremely sensitive to light and may see halos around lights or develop tics in response to certain lighting. These individuals may benefit from specially prepared tinted lenses, from adjusting the lighting in certain rooms, or even by using sunglasses in settings where light is overwhelming. Simple environmental accommodations may also be appropriate in educational or employment settings, such as taking exams in a private room or implementing a no-perfume policy in the workplace.

Behavioral and Life Skill Coaching Approaches

Although most individuals with AS with whom we work are able to engage successfully in traditional forms of individual psychotherapy, there are others who need more concrete approaches. This is the case when the symptoms of AS are very intense or when the individual has a coexisting learning or clinical disorder. At our center, many adults with AS have comorbid issues regarding mood, attention, executive functions, and anxiety and may require a more "hands-on" or practical approach. One woman with severe social anxiety requires a case manager to help her coordinate services. Another with executive functioning difficulties has asked for assistance in planning her daily routine and accomplishing tasks at home. A man who has AS and ADHD has befitted from using an organizational coach at home to keep him organized and his living environment less cluttered.

Use of coaching techniques assists the individual with AS in practical day-to-day tasks, and may feel less stigmatizing than traditional forms of psychotherapy. These activities may be performed by an occupational therapist, a behavioral therapist, a support worker who visits the home, a family member or a case manager. Problems and goals should be clearly stated and defined in terms of behaviors to be promoted or reduced, and steps to accomplishing the goals should be explicitly articulated and monitored. Our clients require assistance in developing strategies, working out solutions to problems, and in applying new techniques. Often, we integrate this approach into traditional forms of psychotherapy.

Other methods of support may include role-playing social interactions and monitoring behavior in natural environments; using scripts or social stories (Gray, 1998) to address issues such as high anxiety, topics appropriate for conversation, hygiene, or to overcome problematic behaviors; recording and developing means to reduce obsessive or self-harming behaviors; developing and practicing methods of relaxation; partializing, scheduling, and completing tasks, including leisure and adaptive activities; and developing means of self-cuing. These may be seen as "soft" behavioral methods, as opposed to the more structured and comprehensive methods utilized in applied behavior analysis (ABA), or other intense methods of reducing problematic behaviors and teaching new skills that are employed for children who have autism (Myers & Johnson, 2007). The individuals with whom we work who have AS are more often living independently or semi-independently, and so their interventions (outside of the therapeutic setting) are self-administered.

Cognitive–behavioral modification (Quinn, Swaggart, & Myles, 1994) is a structured approach that leads to self-management of behavior acquired through modeling, practice, self-monitoring, and self-reinforcement. Reviews of the literature suggest that this and other forms of self-management have been implemented with those who function on the higher end of the spectrum and are found to be effective (Huang & Wheeler, 2006). There are some extreme situations for those who have AS and comorbid disorders in which self-management techniques are not possible, and where traditional behavioral approaches may be required. For example, we have worked with individuals who require support through more rigorous approaches, developed by a trained behavioral therapist or psychologist in the community, or through admission to mental health facilities or specialized group homes. Although this scenario is more likely to be necessary for adults with autism, we do find that in a small number of cases, this also applies to those with AS. In these situations, our approach would include a functional analysis to determine what is causing or maintaining the behavior of concern, the development of a structured and consistently administered program focused on reducing the problematic behavior and increasing more adaptive behaviors, and the use of positive reinforcement to increase and maintain the desirable behaviors (Burke & Baker, 2010).

Case Management

Although case management is often viewed as the purview of social workers (Stoddart, 1998; Stoddart et al., 2005), we propose that all professionals, despite their professional training, must be aware of and sensitive to the need for case management because services for this clinical group are fragmented and decentralized. Primary to case management is the requirement of regular and effective communication about (1) each professional's assessment of the presenting complaints, (2) his or her specific role in ameliorating those issues, (3) the progress of the individual in treatment, (4) the measure of success, and (5) the introduction of new interventions or problems to be targeted.

As previously noted, families of adults with AS, and the individuals with AS themselves, have struggled for years with the task of coordinating service and ensuring communication among professionals. Many have told their stories multiple times, and it is not uncommon for families and individuals to lose all hope in "the system." Therefore, they are often relieved to have good case coordination facilitated by a professional. The resulting synergy and effectiveness of professionals, who have a similar understanding of client and family needs, working respectfully together in a collaborative manner, can be remarkable. Mohr and colleagues have suggested that the key elements of a collaborative model are (1) a shared model and understanding of different models; (2) effective communication; (3) respect for and willingness to learn from each other; (4) multi-disciplinary input; (5) ability to solve dynamic tensions; and (6) adequate resources (Mohr, Curran, Coutts, & Dennis, 2002).

A recent situation of a young man with high-functioning autism and severe addictions illustrates this need. Although there were many professionals involved with the case, including a general practitioner, counselor, educators, and community psychiatrist, as well as the family, effective treatment would have been facilitated if there were effective case coordination and if the local autism specialist center was involved as a resource, educating the team of community professionals about autism. Often, cases such as these build new connections for further collaboration across service systems. The most complex of cases involving adults with AS may involve multiple service providers with discipline-specific perspectives, from fiscally divided service sectors. These service providers might include: medical practitioners, vocational counsellors, autism service providers, (individual, family or couples) psychotherapists, academic advisors, residential service providers, occupational or behavioral therapists, mental health or addictions specialists, and case coordinators or managers.

Others have advocated that a "systemic approach to service planning and delivery promotes an integrated service system for individuals with dual diagnoses and in turn, provides a range of comprehensive supports involving a number of service providers and sectors. The goal is to build a network based on a continuum of integrated services and supports" (Dart, Gapen, & Morris, 2002, p. 284). Dart et al. describe an ideal continuum of care as consisting of three components: (1) prevention and early intervention, (2) intervention and treatment, and (3) long-term care and support. Regardless of the model one subscribes to, it is important that roles of the professionals are clearly defined and understood by the individual with AS and their family, as well as by the other professionals involved.

Employment Counseling

In Chapter 5, we discussed some of the problems that might be encountered by individuals with AS regarding employment. We see three groups of individuals in practice that are affected by employment issues: young adults who have not been successful in navigating the transition from post-secondary education or high school to employment, those who have had many short-term jobs, and those who have been employed successfully but experience a mid-career failure or "crisis." Work is therefore a key theme in therapy for those who have difficulty finding or keeping employment.

Psychological themes that might be addressed in therapy related to employment are significant for this group because of an overrepresentation of males and the psychological importance of employment for some males in terms of self-esteem and self-worth. Unemployment or underemployment might be especially difficult for our clients who come from highly accomplished families. While their brothers and sisters are going into professional programs in university in pursuit of challenging careers, adults with AS are struggling to find and keep the most basic employment. Individuals with AS are often coached by others, and there is counsel in the literature by affected individuals to pursue employment in their areas of interest (e.g., Grandin & Duffy, 2008). Although this focus can result in a successful work experience, it can also lead to disappointment and even feelings of grief and loss. One young man, who took an animation program in college because of his interest in cartooning and computer games, was devastated to discover that his artistic skills were not "market-ready." Another who graduated with a degree in physics was unable to find employment in his field of interest because of the lack of local demand for undergraduates with science degrees. These disappointments need to be processed carefully; often, signs of depression can be closely related to these seeming employment "failures."

We have seen many individuals who pursued a career based on a superficial understanding of what it involved and then ended up completing college or university programs for careers they ultimately dislike or for which they find themselves poorly suited. A number of individuals we have seen have several degrees or diplomas, yet ultimately work in a position that is totally unrelated to any of them. We also find that those with AS often expect to like all aspects of their job and do not want to do it if there is some portion of the job that is less satisfying. They are often surprised to hear that most of us engage in aspects of our work that is less satisfying, but it is the balance of more positive aspects than negative that keep us working in our chosen profession.

Mid-career individuals may find themselves in managerial jobs with which they are not able to cope due to organizational, sensory, or social deficits. Despite advanced knowledge in their area of employment, they are unable to move beyond a "glass ceiling" due to a lack of "soft skills." Sometimes, aware of social difficulties, a person may refuse a promotion that requires more interpersonal interactions, and this refusal ultimately puts the existing position in jeopardy. Many of the mid-career adults we see in practice have gone without a diagnosis, and their problems at work compel them or their employer to seek psychological assistance or assessment. An important role for the employment counselor is to mediate between client and the employer as to what reasonable changes can be made in the workplace because of the diagnosis, and what accommodations might optimize the individual's work performance. In such cases, union officials may also be involved, and it is important to work closely with them in order to ensure that the worker's rights under the union agreement are respected.

In some cities, supported employment is available and can be instrumental in helping individuals on the autism spectrum gain entry to the workforce. Howlin, Alcock, and Burkin (2005) reviewed a supported employment service for individuals with high-functioning ASDs. Sixty-eight percent of the supported individuals found employment, and most of it was permanent. Other research has shown that individuals in supported programs had higher job levels, were employed longer, and received higher wages than individuals who were not in a supported program (Mawhood & Howlin, 1999). A determinant of employment success is a close liaison with employers to explore fitting job opportunities and match individuals' skills and abilities to jobs (Mawhood & Howlin, 1999). In cities where there is no specific employment agency that specializes in supporting adults with ASDs, other services for individuals with disabilities might be helpful. In all cases, however, it is essential that personnel involved in employment supports have a working knowledge of the typical strengths and areas of need for adults on the spectrum and available measures with which to address them positively and proactively. Again, an agency's involvement with clients who have more severe mental health problems or developmental disabilities requires careful consideration, when using employment supports for adults with AS.

Groups

Unfortunately, there is scarce literature on the use of groups for adults who are on the mild end of the autism spectrum. Until now, much of the published literature has focused on child groups, and is on social skills development (Coucouvanis, 2005; Krasny, Williams, Provencal, & Ozonoff, 2003; Marriage, Gordon, & Brand, 1995; Mishna & Muskat, 1998). These group reports suffer from a lack of empirical evidence of effectiveness for the main variables of interest, usually relating to social skills. Many reports are not able to demonstrate that even if the social skills are learned in the groups, they generalize to naturalistic environments.

For adults with milder forms ASDs, groups can be powerful means by which to educate and provide mutual support and a forum for discussion of common concerns about the participants' life situations. Howlin and Yeates (1999) note that considering the fact that groups are neither time intensive nor expensive to run, they may help to fill the lack of community services for this population. After a review of their adult social skills group at the Maudsley Hospital, they proposed we need (1) more information on the most effective ways of organizing such groups, (2) strategies for combining clinical practice with appropriate research methodology, and (3) effective means of ensuring that skills acquired can be maintained and generalized (Howlin & Yeates, 1999).

A byproduct of the increasing use of electronic social media, list serves, and Internet blogs is that individuals with ASDs have an opportunity to meet others in "virtual groups." These are, for some, less threatening than conventional means of socializing and highly advantageous to many because they no longer feel isolated. But, as previously discussed with respect to intimate relationships, these individuals may also gain a false impression of how significant the online relationships are. Locally, we have seen many of our clients gravitate to activity-based groups such as those that are organized through "meet-ups." This way of meeting others capitalizes on parallel engagement in interests (i.e., "parallel play") versus intimidating means of meeting others such going to night clubs or bars. Many individuals with AS report that when they are focused less on the social interaction, their anxiety is decreased and they are able to find common topics of conversation.

The first author (K. P. S.) has had the opportunity to work with three types of groups involving adults with AS. In the first instance, a clinic-based group was developed for mutual therapeutic support and education. The goals of the group were (1) to reduce isolation and provide mutual support about common concerns; (2) to educate group members about their diagnosis and treatment and explore coping strategies; (3) to allow the therapist an opportunity to observe social interaction of each of the group members with peers and provide direct feedback in their individual sessions; (4) to enact specific behavioral goals in the context of the group that had been decided upon in their previous individual sessions; and (5) to encourage social contact with group members outside the group meetings.

Potential members for the group were screened before group involvement during their individual therapy sessions. The group planned to meet every other week for ten 1-hour sessions. The format of the group was loosely structured, as it was believed that since most of the participants had engaged in a course of individual therapy, they would be aware of those issues that they would benefit from discussing in the group. The only structure that was provided was at the beginning of each session when a "check-in" occurred. The role of the therapist was to facilitate the group process with the aim of playing a less active role as the group progressed, and to enable to group members to enter into a greater level of disclosure with the other members. In the first few group sessions, the leader suggested topics for discussion (e.g., family relationships, living situation) when the members were unable to raise their own issues.

A second type of group with which we have had experience is the community-based recreational group. These types of groups are becoming increasingly common throughout North America and the United Kingdom. The community group organized in Toronto, Canada, continues to operate as a program of the Asperger Society of Ontario a decade later. It meets in various locations around the city; activities have included playing billiards; going bowling; attending amusement parks, plays, and musicals; and having dinner at members' houses. There continues to be a great need for groups of this nature; however, some individuals with AS are concerned about appearing in public with "disabled" individuals, do not want to associate with others with ASDs, and would rather be included in an integrated social situation. In terms of the management of the group, we found that it took considerable organization and effort to ensure that all the group members arrived at the correct location in the city at the right time and made it home on time and safely. We also had to deal with members in the group behaving inappropriately, getting lost or intoxicated at the social outing. There was ongoing concern about the homogeneity of individuals in the group, as we now know that adults with the diagnosis of AS can vary widely in their social skills, behavior, ability to problem-solve, and knowledge of community norms. As well, we feel that the label of AS is often applied mistakenly, based on their appearance in a structured clinical setting, whereas the individual is much more impaired in common social situations. One young man attending this group, when confronted with a dark restaurant and a menu, went out on the street to read his menu under the light of the streetlamp!

We have also had the opportunity to run groups with adults with a focus on mood and anxiety disorders (Stoddart & Duhaime, 2011). Not only do these types of groups provide an opportunity to meet others who are similarly affected, but time to share coping strategies and experiences. This far, we have found it helpful to separate participants into groups based on age range and gender, so that group members are somewhat homogeneous in their life experiences and current struggles. Others have also provided a case series using a standard published CBT protocol (Weiss & Lunsky, 2010).

Academic Advising

Academic advisors in postsecondary institutions may take on various roles that include providing referrals and advice, acting as a tutor, facilitating accommodations, acting as group facilitator for students with ASDs, or helping with time management (Manett, 2007). Manett, in his capacity as disability advisor at the University of Toronto, identified 13 students diagnosed with an ASD from his caseload of 250 students. Of these, all the students needed extra time to complete tests and assignments (ranging from 1.25 to 2.25 times), 10 requested private or semiprivate space in which to complete tests,

10 required some breaks (from 10 minutes to an hour, as needed). Others requested one exam per day, a dictionary, an aid sheet, distraction music, or a scribe (Manett, 2007). Specialized tutoring, a modified curriculum, peer supports, supportive counseling, and regularly scheduled meetings with the disability adviser may be required. Other colleges and universities have noted additional accommodations including housing, flexibility with classroom attendance, ability to leave class when symptoms occur, environmental alterations for exams (e.g., lighting and acoustics), priority enrollment, and alternatives to group work and projects (Smith, 2007). Advocating for the student within the postsecondary setting is the overarching role of the academic advisor.

Those students who do not take advantage of disability services and supports may find their education stressful, especially when preexisting symptoms are not addressed properly, making coursework difficult or impossible to complete. Others may excel, even without ongoing academic supports. In our experience, if there are questions about whether the student with AS requires support at the postsecondary level, it is best to arrange the support at the beginning of his or her enrollment and then monitor the person's use of the supports and their effect on academic performance. At least, the services of the disability office can be presented as a "transitional support" to aid the student in adjusting to a new level of academic independence. Certainly, the needs that arise because of the many transitions in young adulthood are well documented (Adreon & Durocher, 2007; Stoddart, 2005c). If these supports are not required and the student adjusts well, involvement can be faded, reduced, or removed altogether. However, if the service is not established early, the student may fall further behind and be less able to seek out supports once the path of isolation and/or failure has begun. Figure 7.2 presents an example of a letter of introduction that was provided to a professor, coauthored by the student and her disability counselor.

Hospitalization and Inpatient Addiction Programs

At times, full or partial hospitalization in either general or psychiatric facilities is necessary for adults with AS. We resort to hospitalization as a last option for instances where there is chronic and extreme aggressive behavior, when an individual is at risk of significant

Dear Professor Jones,

Jennifer is a student in your humanities class. She has a mild form of autism called Asperger syndrome. This letter is an introduction to some of her strengths, which can be used in class, and some of her challenges, for which she will need some accommodations and your understanding.

Strengths

When Jennifer is interested in a subject, she is an eager, fully engaged student who will not only immerse herself in the subject but is more than willing to help struggling classmates get through the material. Jennifer is an independent learner and will go out of her way to understand the material. For her, words become pictures, and the pictures become interconnected patterns of ideas. Because of this, she is able to make intellectual leaps and draw otherwise unobserved connections, all of which are an asset to theoretical analysis and critical thought. So far, she has maintained an A average in her classes, organized several political events, organized and taught several study groups, produced large research papers, and presented her findings at various universities. When it comes to school, Jennifer works very hard.

Challenges

1. **Scheduling:** Jennifer needs to know well ahead of time if there are any changes to the course outline. Further, the course outline must include full details of each assignment throughout the year as well as the nature of the examinations. If this is not clear in the syllabus, please provide that information as soon as possible.

2. **Learning:** When Jennifer is keenly interested in a subject, she is a fast learner and requires a lot of information to keep her intellectually stimulated. In this case, providing additional readings would be helpful to her. Sometimes, however, only one aspect of a subject will be of interest to her, leaving her unable to enjoy an enriched learning environment. Jennifer may have relevant information to contribute, but during oral exchanges, have difficulty formulating this into words without some additional time to prepare. If the essay assignments are not based on the area in which she is interested, it becomes difficult for her to understand the directions or to engage in the assignment. In this case, she may wish to negotiate the assignment with you, so that she can continue to enjoy the course.

FIGURE 7.2. EXAMPLE OF A LETTER OF INTRODUCTION FOR A STUDENT IN POSTSECONDARY EDUCATION

---

3. Communicating and Social Interaction: Please do not single Jennifer out during question-and-answer period unless she initiates the conversation. Knowing when to speak is difficult for her. Social interaction and eye contact may be problematic for her in class. Small-group interactions like tutorials may not be possible for her. She may also not understand metaphors or humor in class. Although she tries her best to be polite and follow the rules for social conduct, this is an area that she has had to learn artificially, and she may sometimes be unable to perform the appropriate mannerisms.

Possible Accommodations

If necessary, accommodations can be negotiated with her accessibility adviser (name). Suggestions include:

1. Provide optional work that she can do for the same mark that other students get for attendance and/or participation.

2. It would be helpful if all assignments were made available at the beginning of the term. This includes details such as structure and content of assignments, length, and any specific components that must be used. The content of some assignments may need to be negotiated.

3. Any changes in room or in the readings need to be announced ahead of time.

4. Group projects will need to be negotiated with her.

5. Jennifer will be writing all tests/exams through the Accessibility Center.

6. Jennifer will require a consistent seating location in the lecture hall/classroom.

FIGURE 7.2. CONTINUED

self-harm, in cases of severe addictions, or when pharmacological management needs to be closely monitored or altered. Partial hospitalization has been defined as "an ambulatory treatment program that includes the major diagnostic, medical, psychiatric, psychosocial and pre-vocational treatment modalities designed for patients with serious mental disorders who require coordinated, intensive, comprehensive and multidisciplinary treatment not provided in an outpatient setting" (West, Casarino, Dibella, & Gross, 1980, p. 47).

Unfortunately, multiple organizational, structural, and process problems have complicated attempts to successfully utilize inpatient psychiatric facilities to provide comprehensive psychosocial assessments and treatments for adults with AS and other ASDs. These include (1) a lack of adequate training among mental health practitioners regarding the primary needs of individuals with ASDs; (2) the unpredictability of externalizing behaviors of other patients; (3) the high risk of exposure to unknown sensory hypo- and hypersensitivities and a lack of awareness of these; (4) difficulties communicating and implementing previous positive community support approaches in the context of an under resourced milieu; (5) fiscal restraints and resource demands, creating obstructions to providing adequate periods of time available for comprehensive assessments; (6) differences in cultural values between community-based programs and medically oriented inpatient units; (7) challenges performing a functional behavioral analysis in inpatient units when these behaviors are often correlated with in vivo (community-specific) antecedents; (8) trouble generalizing skill development gains made in the hospital to community-based settings; and (9) reluctance of this patient group to engage in inpatient (group) treatment programs. For these reasons, less intrusive treatment measures need to be utilized first. It has been our experience that when inpatient treatment has been required, those who have an ASD but have not yet been diagnosed have been admitted to general psychiatric units. However, those who have received an ASD diagnosis may be streamed into mental health and behavioral inpatient units for those with developmental disorders, although admission is sometimes restricted to those with an IQ of less than 70.

Findings of a report that focused on the prevalence of dual diagnosis (i.e., the presence of a mental health problem and a developmental disability) in the specialty hospital system in Ontario, Canada, indicated that these individuals had more severe symptoms, fewer resources, and required a higher level of care than other patients served by this system (Lunsky & Puddicombe, 2005). Subsequent roundtable discussions in this report highlighted (1) the severe limitations of intensive community-based resources; (2) inadequate interministry collaboration; (3) a shortage of appropriate housing on being discharged from hospital; (4) lack of knowledge, expertise, and human resources; and (5) a focus on management rather than on

267

attempts to understand and reduce aggression in hospital (Lunsky & Puddicombe, 2005).

This report also details numerous recommendations to improve quality of care. These include the enhancement of professional expertise in both the mental health and developmental sectors; enhanced training through agency partnerships; the use of teleconferencing; training support workers in specialty hospitals; cross-sector secondments (i.e., a temporary transfer to another job or post within the same organization) and secondments between hospital and community; enhanced interministerial partnerships; increased linkages, partnerships, and collaboration throughout hospital stays through joint care management; and improved linkages between professionals and families. We suspect that the findings of this report are not specific to Ontario. In fact, systemic inadequacies are often magnified when the complex needs of adults with ASDs are involved.

Attempts have been made to assist personnel in specific disciplines, such as nursing, to optimize their understanding of the needs of individuals with ASD, although these attempts remain challenging to implement in busy emergency rooms of general hospitals and offices of family physicians, with few specific practice guidelines. Primary health care providers (i.e., family physicians, pediatricians, nurses, and emergency room physicians) are often "the first point of contact" in the health care system for many individuals with developmental disabilities and are often are faced with making significant decisions which can promote (or perpetuate) physical or mental health conditions (Hennen, 2007; Sullivan et al., 2006).

Sullivan et al. (2006) have published Canadian "Consensus Guidelines for Primary Health Care of Adults with Developmental Disabilities," also applicable to adults with ASDs. These authors identified the complexity of health issues in individuals with all developmental disabilities (DD), stressing the need to provide adequate health care to identify these issues and to prevent morbidity and premature death. They also draw attention to ethical issues such as informed consent and avoidance of harm, advocating that DD are not grounds for care providers to withhold or withdraw medically indicated interventions, and that interventions should be based on patients' best interests. These ethical issues have been discussed by Heng and Sullivan (2003), and the issue of informed consent, applicable to treatment of adults with AS in both community and hospital-based settings, has been addressed by Rush and Frances (2000, 2002).

There is a lack of literature regarding the future of optimal hospital-based mental health facilities for adults with ASD and mental health concerns. START (Systemic Therapeutic Assessment Respite and Treatment), a community-based system designed to assist individuals with mental illness, behavioral disorders, or DD in the northeastern Massachusetts, has been described by Beasley and Kroll (1994). The authors identified four factors complicating the treatment of adults with DD in acute care settings: (1) Mental illness often presents in a nonspecific way, usually with maladaptive behavior; (2) inpatient staff cannot rely on patient self-reports for diagnosing mental illness; (3) objective behavioral data are often necessary to make a valid diagnosis; and (4) outpatient treatment (particularly medication) may mask diagnostically relevant symptomatology.

Beasley and Kroll (1994) enumerated six functions that define quality of care for psychiatric inpatient units serving persons with DD: (1) The unit is able to monitor clinical course and treatment efficacy using objective measures of change 24 hours per day; (2) the unit is able to use nonpharmacological intervention to manage out-of-control behavior; (3) the unit creates psychiatric formulations that take into account developmental and social factors; (4) the unit psychiatrists prescribe psychotropic medication only when there is a clear formulation based on a syndrome or symptom cluster model; (5) the unit provides meaningful activities; and (6) family members, community care providers, and patient advocates are included in the clinical decision making (p. 4). These functions continue to be valid today in designing optimal acute care settings for adults with AS and mental health concerns.

Burge and colleagues (2002) described the characteristics of individuals with DD and their admissions to psychiatric wards in two acute care hospitals in Kingston, Ontario. Length of stay of this group was compared to the comparison group of inpatient admissions involving individuals without DD. The main length of stay, in contrast to concerns expressed above, of individuals with DD was not greater than the comparison sample. Gender (males had longer stays than females), referral source, and diagnosis (individuals with mood disorders and schizophrenia had greater lengths of stay) were identified as variables significantly associated with length of stay in individuals with DD. Consistent with prevalence studies documented in this chapter, these authors noted that individuals with DD accounted for 2.5% of all acute psychiatric admissions during the study, despite only representing 1% of the general population (Burge et al., 2002).

In attempting to address challenges frequently encountered in accessing effective mental health services for individuals living with DD in community settings, Luiselli et al. (Luiselli, Benner, Stoddard, Weiss, & Liscuwski, 2001) reviewed the efficacy of partial hospitalization services for a group of 38 adults with mild DD and psychiatric disorders. The Aberrant Behavior Checklist was used to evaluate outcomes from this service. Outcome data indicated that 39.4% (15/18) patients demonstrated uniform improvement, 60.5% (23/30) had mixed outcomes, and 0% (0/30) had no improvement. The authors concluded that partial hospitalization services can be an efficacious therapeutic option for individuals with DD living in the community. This study does not indicate whether any of the subjects reviewed also had AS (Luiselli et al., 2001).

King and colleagues (2009) reported a retrospective review of a variety of demographic, diagnostic, and treatment utilization characteristics of a group of adults with DD and ASD (three individuals had ASD) supported by an assertive community treatment (ACT) team in Brockville, Ontario. A total of 43 clients, supported by the team, were reviewed. King et al. conclude with a description of a variation to ACT standards to address the specific needs of adults with DD and ASD and mental health concerns. These modifications include (1) the need for flexible admission criteria to the team; (2) the need to partner with other agencies in both the mental health and developmental sectors, rather than maintaining a "can-do-all approach"; (3) the need to encourage subspecialty areas of expertise among team members; (4) the need to educate hospital-based support teams regarding the needs of individuals supported by the team and to provide a seamless continuum of care from community to hospital and back; and (5) the need to be aware of the high incidence of abuse and a diagnosis of PTSD in individuals supported by the team, and the need to develop specialized team facilitative resources to address these.

On occasion, we have also referred our clients to inpatient addictions programs. Although some addiction treatment programs are reluctant to engage in treatment with an adult on the autism spectrum, others have had increasing experience with these individuals and are comfortable admitting them. The task of the ongoing clinician therefore becomes one of consultant or collaborator with the addiction program, thereby forging a working relationship between the program and the client. These are useful and fitting roles. For the case manager who has as an adult with AS as a client, the addiction program may request information about the client and how AS affects the client. As well, recommendations might be made about how the individual would receive the most benefit from the treatment program. For specific patients, a determination needs to be made as to the pros and cons of outpatient versus inpatient treatment. When considering inpatient treatment, experiences of feeling overwhelmed and further stigmatized by entering a large mental health or addictions treatment facility may need to be explored.

In devising a possible inpatient plan for treatment of addictions in an adult with AS, the following questions should be raised with the addiction treatment service either by members of the client's professional team, the individual him- or herself, or family members:

- What degree of social interaction will be required during the program?
- Will participation in group treatment be required?
- Will passive involvement in groups be viewed as resistance to treatment?
- How will involvement with other patients in the program be monitored?
- Will the individual have regularly scheduled programs and appointments?
- Will the patient share a room with others or will a private room be provided?
- What is the program's understanding of and experience with AS?
- How will information about the program be communicated to the patient?
- Will information be sought from and conveyed to spouses and family members?
- Do "no contact" rules exist in the program?
- Is there support for ADLs (e.g., completing laundry) in the program?

- Are there sensory issues in the facility that need to be addressed?
- How are food likes and dislikes managed in the program?
- What is the program's response to "noncompliance"?
- How will behavior issues common in individuals with AS be addressed?
- Will a psychiatric/medication consultation be available in the program?

EVIDENCE-BASED PRACTICE IN ASDS

Evidence-based medicine has been defined as

> . . . the conscientious, explicit, and judicious use of current best evidence in making decisions about the care of individual patients. The practice of evidence based medicine means integrating individual clinical expertise with the best available external clinical evidence from systematic research. By individual clinical expertise we mean the proficiency and judgment that individual clinicians acquire through clinical experience and clinical practice. (Sackett, Rosenberg, Gray, Haynes, & Richardson, 1996, p. 71)

Further refinement of this model has suggested that clinical expertise is the combination of three areas: research evidence, patients' preferences and actions, and clinical state and circumstances (Haynes, Devereaux, & Guyatt, 2002).

Other professions such as psychology and social work have emphasised evidence-based practices in addition to medicine. In keeping with social work's attention to contextual and systemic issues, Regehr and colleagues note: "We would add that organizational mission, mandate, and context also should be included to include consideration of environmental strengths and barriers that exist outside the individual" (Regehr, Stern, & Shlonsky, 2007, p. 410). Gibbs (2003) has suggested that there are six steps to becoming an evidence-based practitioner: (1) convert information need into an answerable question; (2) find current best evidence; (3) critically appraise the evidence; (4) integrate critical appraisal with practice experience and client's strengths, values, and circumstances; (5)

evaluate effectiveness and efficiency in exercising steps 1–4 and seek ways to improve them; and (6) teach others to follow the same process.

In many practice areas in the field of ASDs, dissemination of knowledge regarding the requirements of evidence-based practices is a concern. Increasingly, websites, books, conferences and papers are providing guidance on the extent of empirical evidence for a treatment or intervention, in an attempt to refute effectiveness claims for unsubstantiated treatments and promote the uptake of evidence-based information for those interventions with a body of research evidence (Freeman, 2007; McClure & Le Couteur, 2007; Perry & Condillac, 2003; Rhoades, Scarpa, & Salley, 2007; Stahmer & Aarons, 2009; Stoddart, 2007c; Vismara, Young, Stahmer, Griffith, & Rogers, 2009). Much of this concern is focused on early intervention and on treatment for children and adolescents. Understandably, some parents choose "alternative" treatments in this context, refusing to wait for evidence-based data to support proposed interventions. This trend has resulted in persistent anecdotal claims of efficacy for multiple alternative modes of therapy.

Sadly, the evidence in adult ASDs and AS is lacking to an even greater extent. We espouse the use of available published peer-reviewed intervention approaches to address the clinical issues that are core to AS, as well as those that have been identified as comorbidities. For those situations where there is no prior clinical evidence, treatments that have been used successfully for other related disorders (e.g., social anxiety) might be attempted, possibly with modifications. Ultimately, we agree that the process of applying evidence-based interventions is contextually informed (Regehr et al., 2007).

The Case of Psychotherapeutic Interventions

One of the major interventions for this population—individual, couple, and group psychotherapy—lacks evidence at the present time. There are several reasons for this. The first is likely the lack of trained psychotherapists or counselors who have practiced in the field of ASDs and developmental disabilities. We have practiced in both of these fields and found the scarcity of therapists who can work confidently with these populations is alarming—and we were located in or near major metropolitan centers. Although those who provide psychotherapy to children and youth are few, professionals experienced in addressing issues of adults with ASDs and developmental disabilities are even more scarce.

Many psychotherapeutic interventions for the general population prove difficult to evaluate, and approaches can vary widely even within a common therapeutic paradigm. Heterogeneity among individuals in our clinical population of interest also presents challenges to methodological rigor. Issues such as ensuring treatment fidelity and identifying common outcomes across a diverse range of presenting problems remain significant methodological obstacles that outcome-based research in this field will continue to face.

In service settings, by definition, research and evaluation of interventions are generally considered secondary to clinical programming, instead of a core component of those programs. Funded settings tend to be under resourced, and even when there is recognition that evaluation of services is important, clinical activities take precedence, and too often, program evaluation is ignored. Clinicians–researchers–evaluators in our field are rare, and some (more experienced) clinicians have moved into private practices that involve a physical move away from funded research opportunities, academic research centers, or research colleagues. Research in ASDs is strongly biomedical, behavioral, and child-oriented, and funding bodies are just beginning to recognize the need for outcome research that addresses the psychosocial needs of this adult group. Potential partnerships that can be forged between academic, research, and service organizations are promising. In one instance, a local autism organization asked a mental health organization to vet applications for research using their in-house research expertise while the autism organization raised the funds.

Concerns have been voiced about the lack of training in professions such as psychiatry (Bradley & Lunsky, 2001; Lunsky & Puddicombe, 2005) and social work (Burge, Druick, Caron, & Ouellette-Kuntz, 1998; Burge, Druick, Caron, Ouellette-Kuntz, & Paquette, 1999) and about the lack of undergraduate and graduate education received in North America and abroad in developmental disabilities and dual diagnosis. The first author (K. P. S.) routinely hears that his hour-and-a-half lecture on AS and ASDs is the first that graduate students have heard on the topic in 5 or 6 years of undergraduate and graduate education combined. Work with individuals with ASDs or developmental disabilities may be seen by clinicians as unchallenging and thus an unattractive field in which to practice; students also lack clinical training and exposure to these groups in clinical and research internships.

Finally, with limited financial resources and limited evidence for efficacy, governments and policy makers are inclined to support brief and directed interventions that are yoked to evidence of their efficacy and effectiveness (Stoddart et al., 2001). Although the last decade has seen substantial contributions to the literature on individual, brief, and group interventions indicating the efficacy in this population, we are just beginning to see proper funding channeled to this clinical population and the services that they need.

CONCLUSION

This chapter has highlighted 10 adjunctive interventions in the field of adult AS. Continued work is required to pull seemingly disparate views and paradigms into comprehensive and collaborative assessment and treatment approaches for this population. Due to the increased recognition of ASDs generally, and AS in adults specifically, the need for evidence-based interventions for this clinical group will continue to mount. This need can only be addressed as policy and treatment systems across divided sectors work together to respectfully learn from these consumers, their families, and the service systems that are struggling to support them.

REFERENCES

Abell, F., & Hare, D. J. (2005). An experimental investigation of the phenomenology of delusional beliefs in people with Asperger syndrome. *Autism: International Journal of Research and Practice, 9*(5), 515–531.

Abrahamson, S. (2007). Did Janet Frame have high-functioning autism? *New Zealand Medical Journal, 120*(1263), 63–67.

Adler, L. A., Kessler, R. C., & Spencer, T. (2003). Adult ADHD Self-Report Scale-v1.1 (ASRS-v1.1) Symptom Checklist. New York, NY: World Health Organization.

Adreon, D., & Durocher, J. S. (2007). Evaluating the college transition needs of individuals with high-functioning autism spectrum disorders. *Intervention in School and Clinic, 42*(5), 271–279.

AIDS Committee of Toronto. (2008). Aids Committeee of Toronto Services. Retreived on January 24, 2010 from http://www.actoronto. org

Allison, D. B., Mentore, J. L., Heo, M., Chandler, L. P., Cappelleri, J. C., Infante, M. C., & Weiden, P. J. (1999). Antipsychotic-induced weight gain: A comprehensive research synthesis. *American Journal of Psychiatry, 156*(11), 1686–1696.

Al-Mahmood, R., McLean, P., Powell, E., & Ryan, J. (1998). Towards success in tertiary study with Asperger's syndrome and other autism spectrum disorders. Melbourne, Australia: Victorian Cooperative Projects Higher Education Students with a Disability Committee, University of Melbourne.

Aman, M. G., & Langworthy, K. S. (2000). Pharmacotherapy for hyperactivity in children with autism and other pervasive developmental disorders. *Journal of Autism and Developmental Disorders, 30*(5), 451–459.

Aman, M. G., Van Bourgondien, M. E., Wolford, P. L., & Sarphare, G. (1995). Psychotropic and anticonvulsant drugs in subjects with autism: Prevalence and patterns of use. *Journal of the American Academy of Child and Adolescent Psychiatry, 34*(12), 1672–1681.

American Psychiatric Association. (1952). *Diagnostic and statistical manual of mental disorders.* Washington, DC: Author.

American Psychiatric Association. (1968). *Diagnostic and statistical manual of mental disorders (2nd ed.).* Washington, DC: Author.

American Psychiatric Association. (1980). *Diagnostic and statistical manual of mental disorders (3rd ed.).* Washington, DC: Author.

American Psychiatric Association. (1987). *Diagnostic and statistical manual of mental disorders (3rd ed., rev.).* Washington, DC: Author.

American Psychiatric Association. (1994). *Diagnostic and statistical manual of mental disorders (4th ed.).* Washington, DC: Author.

American Psychiatric Association. (2000). *Diagnostic and statistical manual of mental disorders (4th ed., text rev.).* Washington, DC: Author.

American Psychiatric Association. (2002). *Practice guidelines for the treatment of patients with bipolar disorder (Rev. ed.).* Arlington, VA: American Psychiatric Association.

American Psychiatric Association. (2010). DSM-5 development. Available at www.dsm5.org.

American Speech–Language–Hearing Association (1996). Central auditory processing: Current status of research and implications for clinical practice. Task force on central auditory processing consensus development. *American Journal of Audiology, 5,* 41–54.

Anderson, S., & Morris, J. (2006). Cognitive behaviour therapy for people with Asperger syndrome. *Behavioural and Cognitive Psychotherapy, 34,* 293–303.

Andreasen, N. C., & Olsen, S. (1982). Negative v positive schizophrenia: Definition and validation. *Archives of General Psychiatry, 39*(7), 789–794.

Annas, G. J., & Elias, S. (1999). Thalidomide and the Titanic: Reconstructing the technology tragedies of the twentieth century. *American Journal of Public Health, 89*(1), 98–101.

Antony, M. M., & Swinson, R. P. (2008). The shyness and social anxiety workbook (2nd ed.). Oakland, CA: New Harbinger.

Aquilla, P., Yack, E., & Sutton, S. (2005). Sensory and motor differences for individuals with Asperger syndrome: Occupational therapy assessment and intervention. In K. P. Stoddart (Ed.), Children, youth and adults with Asperger syndrome: Integrating multiple perspectives (pp. 197–210). London: Jessica Kingsley.

Arnold, L. E., Vitiello, B., McDougle, C., Scahill, L., Shah, B., Gonzales, N. M., et al. (2003). Parent-defined target symptoms respond to risperidone in RUPP autism study: Customer approach to clinical trials. *Journal of American Academy of Child and Adolescent Psychiatry, 42*(12), 1443–1450.

Arshad, M., & Fitzgerald, M. (2004). Did Michelangelo (1475–1564) have high-functioning autism? *Journal of Medical Biography, 12*(2), 115–120.

Asperger, H. (1944). Die "autistischen psychopathen" im kindeslater ["Autistic psychopathy" in childhood]. *Archive fur Psychiatrie un Nervenkrankheiten, 117,* 76–136.

Asperger, H. (1991). "Autistic psychopathy" in childhood. In U. Frith (Ed.), Autism and Asperger syndrome (pp. 37–92). Cambridge: Cambridge University Press.

Asperger Society of Ontario. (2006). Report of the adult housing and supports committee. Toronto, ON: Author.

Aston, M. C. (2001). The other half of Asperger syndrome: A guide to living in an intimate relationship with a partner who has Asperger syndrome. London: National Autistic Society.

Aston, M. C. (2003). Aspergers in love: Couple relationships and family affairs. London: Jessica Kingsley.

Aston, M. C. (2005). Growing up in an Asperger family. *Counselling Children and Young People, Summer,* 200–209.

Aston, M. C. (2008). Website of Maxine Aston. Retrieved November 17, 2008 from www.maxineaston.co.uk/cassandra/healing.shtml.

Aston, M. C. (2009). The Asperger couple's workbook: Practical advice and activities for couples and counsellors. London: Jessica Kingsley.

Attwood, T. (1998). Asperger's syndrome: A guide for parents and professionals. London: Jessica Kingsley.

Attwood, T. (1999a). The pattern of abilities and development of girls with Asperger's syndrome. Available at www.aspergerfoundation. org.uk.

Attwood, T. (1999b, March 22). Practical strategies to help partners of people with Asperger syndrome. Workshop hosted by the National Autistic Society, London.

Attwood, T. (2004). Exploring feelings: Cognitive behavior therapy to manage anger. Arlington, TX: Future Horizons.

Attwood, T. (2007). The complete guide to Asperger's syndrome. London: Jessica Kingsley.

Autism Society Canada. (2007). Report of the Advisory Committee of Adults on the Spectrum. Ottawa, ON: Author.

Autism Speaks (2009, February 19). Autism: Fluoxetine Not Effective In Reducing Repetitive Behaviors, Study Shows. *Science Daily.*

Ayres, J. (1979). Sensory integration and the child. Los Angeles, CA: Western Psychological Services.

Bagby, R. M., Parker, J. D. A., & Taylor, G. J. (1994). The twenty-item Toronto Alexithymia Scale–1: Item selection and cross-validation of the factor structure. *Journal of Psychosomatic Research, 38*(1), 23–32.

Bailey, A., Le Couteur, A., Gottesman, I., Bolton, P., Simonoff, E., Yuzda, E., et al. (1995). Autism as a strongly genetic disorder: Evidence from a British twin study. *Psychological Medicine, 25*(1), 63–77.

Bailey, A., Palferman, S., Heavey, L., & Le Couteur, A. (1998). Autism: The phenotype in relatives. *Journal of Autism and Developmental Disorders, 28*(5), 369–392.

Baird, G., Simonoff, E., Pickles, A., Chandler, S., Loucas, T., Meldrum, D., et al. (2006). Prevalence of disorders of the autism spectrum in a population cohort of children in South Thames: The Special Needs and Autism Project (SNAP). *Lancet, 368,* 210–215.

Bandler, R., Grinder, J., & Satir, V. (1976). Changing with families: A book about further education for being human. Palo Alto, CA: Science and Behavior Books.

Bargary, G., & Mitchell, K. J. (2008). Synaesthesia and cortical connectivity. *Trends in Neurosciences, 31*(7), 335–342.

Barnard, A. L., Young, A. H., Pearson, A. D. J., Geddes, J., & O'Brien, G. (2002). A systematic review of the use of atypical antipsychotics in autism. *Journal of Psychopharmacology, 16*(1), 93–101.

Barnard, J., Harvey, V., Potter, D., & Prior, A. (2001). Ignored or ineligible? The reality for adults with autistic spectrum disorders. London: National Autistic Society.

Barnhill, G. P. (2007). Outcomes in adults with Asperger syndrome. *Focus on Autism and Other Developmental Disabilities, 22*(2), 116–126.

Barnhill, G. P., Hagiwara, T., Myles, B.S., & Simpson, R.L. (2000). Asperger syndrome: A study of the cognitive profiles of 37 children and adolescents. *Focus on Autism and Other Developmental Disabilities, 15*(3), 146–153.

Baron-Cohen, S. (1988). An assessment of violence in a young man with Asperger's syndrome. *Journal of Child Psychology and Psychiatry, 29*(3), 351–360.

Baron-Cohen, S. (1991). The development of a theory of mind in autism: Deviance and delay? *Psychiatric Clinics of North America, 14*(1), 33–51.

Baron-Cohen, S. (1995). Mindblindness: An essay on autism and theory of mind. Cambridge, MA: MIT Press.

Baron-Cohen, S. (2003). The essential difference: Men, women and the extreme male brain. London: Allen Lane.

Baron-Cohen, S. (2008). Autism, hypersystemizing and truth. *Quarterly Journal of Experimental Psychology, 61*(1), 64–75.

Baron-Cohen, S. (2009). Autism: The empathizing systemizing (E-S) theory. *Annals of the New York Academy of Sciences, 1156,* 68–80.

Baron-Cohen, S., Bor, D., Billington, J., Asher, J., Wheelwright, S., & Ashwin, C. (2007). Savant memory in a man with colour–number synaesthesia and Asperger syndrome. *Journal of Consciousness Studies, 14*(9–10), 114–129.

Baron-Cohen, S., & Hammer, J. (1997). Parents of children with Asperger syndrome: What is the cognitive phenotype? *Journal of Cognitive Neuroscience, 9*(4), 548–554.

Baron-Cohen, S., Hoekstra, R. A., Knickmeyer, R., & Wheelwright, S. (2006). The Autism-Spectrum Quotient (AQ) Adolescent Version. *Journal of Autism and Developmental Disorders, 36*(3), 343–350.

Baron-Cohen, S., Jolliffe, T., Mortimore, C., & Robertson, M. (1997). Another advanced test of theory of mind: Evidence from very high functioning adults with autism or Asperger syndrome. *Journal of Child Psychology and Psychiatry, 38*(7), 813–822.

Baron-Cohen, S., Knickmeyer, R. C., & Belmonte, M. K. (2005). Sex differences in the brain: Implications for explaining autism. *Science, 310*(5749), 819–823.

Baron-Cohen, S., Mortimore, C., Moriarty, J., Izaguirre, J., & Robertson, M. (1999). The prevalence of Gilles de la Tourette's syndrome in children and adolescents with autism. *Journal of Child Psychology and Psychiatry and Allied Disciplines, 40*(2), 213–218.

Baron-Cohen, S., Richler, J., Bisarya, D., Gurunathan, N., & Wheelwright, S. (2003). The systemizing quotient: An investigation of adults with Asperger syndrome or high-functioning autism, and normal sex differences. *Philosophical Transactions of the Royal Society B: Biological Sciences, 358*(1430), 361–374.

Baron-Cohen, S., & Wheelwright, S. (2004). The empathy quotient: An investigation of adults with Asperger syndrome or high functioning autism, and normal sex differences. *Journal of Autism and Developmental Disorders, 34*(2), 163–175.

Baron-Cohen, S., Wheelwright, S., Robinson, J. & Woodbury-Smith, M. (2005). The Adult Asperger Assessment (AAA): A diagnostic method. *Journal of Autism and Developmental Disorders, 35*(6), 807–819.

Barry-Walsh, J. B., & Mullen, P. E. (2004). Forensic aspects of Asperger's syndrome. *Journal of Forensic Psychiatry and Psychology, 15*(1), 96–104.

Bartak, L., & Rutter, M. (1976). Differences between mentally retarded and normally intelligent autistic children. *Journal of Autism and Childhood Schizophrenia, 6*, 109–120.

Bartz, J. A., & Hollander, E. (2008). Oxytocin and experimental therapeutics in autism spectrum disorders. In I. D. Neumann & R. Landgraf (Eds.), Advances in vasopressin and oxytocin: From genes to behaviour to disease (pp. 451–462). Amsterdam: Elsevier.

Bauman, M., & Kemper, T. L. (1985). Histoanatomic observation of the brain in early infantile autism. *Neurology, 35*(6), 866–874.

Beasley, J. B., & Kroll, J. (1994). The Start Comprehensive Psychiatric Evaluation (SCOPE): Preliminary considerations and diagnostic protocol. *NADD Newsletter, 11*(6), 1–5.

Beaumont, R., & Newcombe, P. (2006). Theory of mind and central coherence in adults with high-functioning autism or Asperger syndrome. *Autism: International Journal of Research and Practice, 10*(4), 365–382.

Beck, A. T., & Steer, R. A. (1990). Beck Anxiety Inventory manual. San Antonio, TX: Psychological Corporation.

Beck, A. T., Steer, R. A. & Brown, G. K. (1996). Beck Depression Inventory–II. San Antonio, TX: The Psychological Corporation.

Bentley, K. (2007). Alone together: Making an Asperger marriage work. London: Jessica Kingsley.

Berney, T. (2004). Asperger syndrome from childhood into adulthood. *Advances in Psychiatric Treatment, 10*(5), 341–351.

Berthier, M. L., Santamaria, J., Encabo, H., & Tolosa, E. S. (1992). Recurrent hypersomnia in two adolescent males with Asperger's syndrome. *Journal of the American Academy of Child and Adolescent Psychiatry, 31*(4), 735–738.

Bertrand, J., Mars, A., Boyle, C., Bove, F., Yeargin-Allsopp, M., & Decoufle, P. (2001). Prevalence of autism in a United States population: The Brick Township, New Jersey, investigation. *Pediatrics, 108*(5), 1155–1161.

Bettelheim, B. (1967). The empty fortress: Infantile autism and the birth of the self. New York: Free Press.

Biddle, B. J. (1979). Role theory: Expectations, identities and behaviors. New York: Academic Press.

Bird, G., Silani, G., Brindley, R., White, S., Frith, U., & Singer, T. (2010). Empathic brain responses in insula are modulated by levels of alexithymia but are not autism. *Brain, 133*(5), 1515–1525.

Bishop, D. V. M. (1989). Autism, Asperger's syndrome and semantic–pragmatic disorder: Where are the boundaries? *British Journal of Disorders of Communication, 24*(2), 107–121.

Bishop, D. V. M. (2000). Pragmatic language impairment: A correlate of SLI, a distinct subgroup, or part of the autistic continuum? In D. V. M. Bishop & L. B. Leonard (Eds.), Speech and language impairments in children: Causes, characteristics, intervention and outcome (pp. 99–113). Hove, UK: Psychology Press.

Bissonnette, B. (2009). Workplace disclosure: Strategies for individuals with Asperger's syndrome and NLD. Available at www.forwardmotion.info.

Blackshaw, A. J., Kinderman, P., Hare, D. J., & Hatton, C. (2001). Theory of mind, causal attribution and paranoia in Asperger syndrome. *Autism: International Journal of Research and Practice, 5*(2), 147–163.

Bodfish, J. W. (2004). Treating the core features of autism: Are we there yet? *Mental Retardation and Developmental Disabilities Research Review, 10*(4), 318–326.

Bolte, S., & Bosch, G. (2004). Bosch's cases: A forty year follow up of patients with infantile autism and Asperger's syndrome. *German Journal of Psychiatry, 7,* 10–13.

Bolte, S., Ozkara, N., & Poustka, F. (2002). Autism spectrum disorders and low body weight: Is there really a systematic association? *International Journal of Eating Disorders, 31*(3), 349–351.

Bolte, S., & Poustka, F. (2004). Comparing the intelligence profiles of savant and nonsavant individuals with autistic disorder. *Intelligence, 32*(2), 121–131.

Bolton, P., Macdonald, H., Pickles, A., Rios, P., Goode, S., Crowson, M., et al. (1994). A case-control family history study of autism. *Journal of Child Psychology and Psychiatry, 35*(5), 877–900.

Bolton, P. F., Park, R. J., Higgins, J. N. P., Griffiths, P.D., & Pickles, A. (2002). Neuro-epileptic determinants of autism spectrum disorders in tuberous sclerosis complex. *Brain, 125*(6), 1247–1255.

Bonfardin, B., Zimmerman, A.W., & Gaus, V. (2007). Pervasive developmental disorders. In R. Fletcher, E. Loschen, C. Stavrakaki, & M. First (Eds.), Diagnostic manual—intellectual disability: A textbook of diagnosis of mental disorders in persons with intellectual disability (pp. 107–125). Kingston, NY: NADD Press.

Bradley, E., & Bryson, S. (1998). Psychiatric illness in mentally handicapped adolescents (and young adults) with autistic disability. Toronto, ON: Surrey Place Centre.

Bradley, E., & Burke, L. (2002). The mental health needs of persons with developmental disabilities. In D. M. Griffiths, C. Stavrakaki, & J. Summers (Eds.), Dual diagnosis: An introduction to the mental health needs of persons with developmental disabilities (pp. 45–79). Sudbury, ON: Habilitative Mental Health Resource Network.

Bradley, E., & Lunsky, Y. J. (2001). Developmental disability training in Canadian psychiatry residency programs. *Canadian Journal of Psychiatry, 46*(2), 138–143.

Brasic, J. R., & Gianutsos, J. G. (2000). Neuromotor assessment and autistic disorder. *Autism: International Journal of Research and Practice, 4*(3), 287–298.

Bristol, M. M., & Schopler, E. (1984). Stress and coping in families of autistic adolescents. In E. Schopler & G. B. Mesibov (Eds.), The effects of autism on the family (pp. 251–278). New York: Plenum Press.

Brown, T. E. (1996). Brown ADD Scales. San Antonio, TX: The Psychological Corporation.

Brown, C., & Dunn, W. (2002). Adolescent/Adult Sensory Profile User's Manual. San Antonio, TX: Psychological Corporation.

Buchsbaum, M. S., Hollander, E., Haznedar, M. M., Tang, C., Spiegel-Cohen, J., Wei, T. C., et al. (2001). Effect of fluoxetine on regional cerebral metabolism in autistic spectrum disorders: A pilot study. *International Journal of Neuropsychopharmacology, 4*(2), 119–125.

Buitelaar, J. K., & Willemsen-Swinkels, S. H. (2000). Medication treatment in subjects with autistic spectrum disorders. *European Child and Adolescent Psychiatry, 9*(Suppl. 1), 185–197.

Burd, L., Fisher, W., & Kerbeshian J. (1987). A prevalence study of pervasive developmental disorders in North Dakota. *Journal of the American Academy of Child and Adolescent Psychiatry, 26*(5), 700–703.

Burge, P., Druick, D., Caron, M. C., & Ouellette-Kuntz, H. (1998). Fieldwork: Are students prepared to work with persons with developmental disabilities? *Social Worker, 66*(3), 15–27.

Burge, P., Druick, D., Caron, M. C., Ouellette-Kuntz, H., & Paquette, D. (1999). Coursework on developmental disabilities: A national survey of Canadian schools of social work. *Canadian Social Work Review, 16*(1), 49–64.

Burge, P., Ouelette-Kuntz, H., Saeed, H., McCreary, B., Paquette, D., & Sim, F. (2002). Acute psychiatric inpatient care for people with a dual diagnosis: Patient profiles and lengths of stay. *Canadian Journal of Psychiatry, 47*(3), 243–249.

Burger-Veltmeijer, A. (2007). Gifted or autistic? The 'Grey Zone'. In K. Tirri & M. Ubani (Eds.) Policies and programs in gifted education (pp. 115–124). University of Helsinki: Department of Applied Sciences of Education.

Burgess, N., Sweeten, T., McMahon, W., & Fujinami, R. (2006). Hyperserotoninemia and altered immunity in autism. *Journal of Autism and Developmental Disorders, 36*(5), 697–704.

Burgoine, E., & Wing, L. (1983). Identical triplets with Asperger's syndrome. *British Journal of Psychiatry, 143*, 261–265.

Burke, L. (2005). Psychological assessment of more able adults with autism spectrum disorders. In K. P. Stoddart (Ed.), Children, youth and adults with Asperger syndrome: Integrating multiple perspectives (pp. 211–225). London: Jessica Kingsley.

Burke, L. (2007, November). Screening and diagnosis in teens and adults with autism spectrum disorders: The need goes on. National Autism Research Symposium, Sponsored by Canadian Institutes of Health Research, Toronto, ON.

Burke, L. & Baker, K. (2010, April). Act five: Has the script changed? Paper presented at the Human Rights for Persons with Intellectual Disabilities Conference, Niagara Falls, ON.

Burnette, C. P., Mundy, P. C., Meyer, J. A., Sutton, S. K., Vaughan, A. E., & Charak, D. (2005). Weak central coherence and its relations to theory of mind and anxiety in autism. *Journal of Autism and Developmental Disorders, 35*(1), 63–73.

Butcher, J. N., Graham, J. R., Ben-Porath, Y. S., Tellegen, A., Dahlstrom, W. G. & Kraemer, B. (2001). Minnesota Multiphasic Personality Inventory-2 (MMPI-2): Manual for administration, scoring, and interpretation (Rev. Ed.). Minneapolis: University of Minnesota Press.

Butzer, B., & Konstantareas, M. (2003). Depression, temperment and their relationship to other characteristics in children with Asperger's disorder. *Journal on Developmental Disabilities, 10*(1), 67–72.

Centers for Disease Control (2010). Retrieved from http://www.cdc.gov/ncbddd/autism/

Campbell, J. (2005). Diagnostic assessment of Asperger's disorder: A review of five third-party rating scales. *Journal of Autism and Developmental Disorders, 35*(1), 25–35.

Canadian ADHD Resource Alliance. (2006). Canadian ADHD practice guidelines. Toronto, ON: Author.

Canadian Association of Occupational Therapists. (2010). Occupational therapy: Definition. Available online at http://www.caot.ca.

Cardaciotto, L. A., & Herbert, J. D. (2004). Cognitive behavior therapy for social anxiety disorder in the context of Asperger's syndrome: A single-subject report. *Cognitive and Behavioral Practice, 11*(1), 75–81.

Carlson, T. S., McGeorge, C. R., & Halvorson, S. (2007). Marriage and family therapists' ability to diagnose Asperger's syndrome: A vignette study. *Contemporary Family Therapy, 29*(1–2), 25–37.

Carter, A. E., & McGoldrick, M. (Eds.). (1980). The family life cycle: A framework for family therapy. New York: Guardian.

Cederlund, M., & Gillberg, C. (2004). One hundred males with Asperger syndrome: A clinical study of background and associated factors. *Developmental Medicine and Child Neurology, 46*(10), 652–660.

Chaing, H.-M., & Lin, Y.H. (2007). Reading comprehension instruction for students with autism spectrum disorders: A review of the literature. *Focus on Autism and Other Developmental Disabilities, 22*(4), 259–267.

Chamberlain, E. (2003). Behavioural Assessment of the Dysexecutive Syndrome (BADS). *Journal of Occupational Psychology, Employment and Disability, 5*(2), 33–37.

Channon, S. (2004). Frontal lobe dysfunction and everyday problem-solving: Social and non-social contributions. *Acta Psychologica, 115* (2–3), 235–254.

Channon, S., Charman, T., Heap, J., Crawford, S., & Rios, P. (2001). Real-life-type problem-solving in Asperger's syndrome. *Journal of Autism and Developmental Disorders, 31*(5), 461–469.

Charlot, L. R., Doucette, A. C., & Mezzacappa, E. (1993). Affective symptoms of institutionalized adults with mental retardation. *American Journal of Mental Retardation, 98*(3), 408–416.

Charman, T. (2002). The prevalence of autism spectrum disorders: Recent evidence and future challenges. *European Child and Adolescent Psychiatry, 11*(6), 249–256.

Chen, P. S., Chen, S. J., Yang, Y. K., Yeh, T. L., Chen, C. C., & Lo, H. Y. (2003). Asperger's disorder: A case report of repeated stealing and the collecting behaviours of an adolescent patient. *Acta Psychiatrica Scandinavica, 107*(1), 73–75.

Chick, J., Waterhouse, L., & Wolff, S. (1979). Psychological construing in schizoid children grown up. *British Journal of Psychiatry, 135,* 425–430.

Chow, S. L., Leung, G. M., Ng, C., & Yu, E. (2009). A screen for identifying maladaptive internet use. *International Journal of Mental Health and Addiction, 7*(2), 324–332.

Chudley, A. E., Conry, J., Cook, J. L., Loock, C., Rosales, T., & LeBlanc, N. (2005). Fetal alcohol spectrum disorder: Canadian guidelines for diagnosis. *Canadian Medical Association Journal, 175*(5 Suppl.), S1–S21.

Clark, D. A. (2005). Lumping versus splitting: A commentary on subtyping in OCD. *Behavior Therapy, 36*(4), 401–404.

Clark, D., & Beck, A. T. (2002). Clark–Beck Obsessive-Compulsive Inventory Manual. San Antonio, TX: Psychological Corporation.

Cohen, D. J., Riddle, M. A., & Leckman, J. F. (1992). Pharmacotherapy of Tourette's syndrome and associated disorders. *Psychiatric Clinics of North America, 15*(1), 109–129.

Cohen, S. A., Fitzgerald, B. J., Khan, S. R., & Khan, A. (2004). The effect of a switch to ziprasidone in an adult population with autistic disorder: Chart review of naturalistic, open-label treatment. *Journal of Clinical Psychiatry, 65*(1), 110–113.

Cohen, S. A., & Underwood, M. T. (1994). The use of clozapine in a mentally retarded and aggressive population. *Journal of Clinical Psychiatry, 55*(10), 440–444.

Conners, C. K., Erhardt, D., & Sparrow, E. (1999). Conners' Adult ADHD Rating Scales. New York: Multi-Health Systems.

Cook, E. H., & Scherer, S. W. (2008). Copy-number variations associated with neuropsychiatric conditions. *Nature, 455*(7215), 919–923.

Corson, A., Barkenbus, J., Posey, D., Stigler, K. & McDougle, C. (2004). A retrospective analysis of quetiapine in the treatment of pervasive developmental disorders. *Journal of Clinical Psychiatry, 65*(11), 1531–1536.

Coucouvanis, J. (2005). Super skills: A social skills group program for children with Asperger syndrome, high-functioning autism, and related challenges. Shawnee Mission, KS: Autism Asperger Publishing.

Craig, J. S., Hatton, C., Craig, F. B., & Bentall, R. P. (2004). Persecutory beliefs, attributions, and theory of mind: Comparison of patients with paranoid delusions, Asperger's syndrome, and healthy controls. *Schizophrenia Research, 69*(1), 29–33.

Croen, L. A., Grether, J. K., Hoogstrate, J., & Selvin, S. (2002). The changing prevalence of autism in California. *Journal of Autism and Developmental Disorders, 32*(3), 207.

Crosland, K. A., Zarcone, J. R., Lindauer, S. E., Valdovinos, M. G., Zarcone, T. J., Hellings, J. A., et al. (2003). Use of functional analysis methodology in the evaluation of medication effects. *Journal of Autism and Developmental Disorders, 33*(3), 271–279.

Dakin, C. (2005). Life on the outside: A personal perspective on Asperger syndrome. In K. P. Stoddart (Ed.), Children, youth and adults with Asperger syndrome: Integrating multiple perspectives (pp. 352–361). London: Jessica Kingsley.

Dart, L., Gapen, W., & Morris, S. (2002). Building responsive service systems. In D. Griffiths, C. Stravakaki, & J. Summers (Eds.), Dual diagnosis: An introduction to the mental health needs of persons with developmental disabilities (pp. 283–323). Sudbury, ON: Habilitative Mental Health Resource Network.

Dawson, G., Webb, S., Schellenberg, G. D., Dager, S., Friedman, S., Aylward, E., & et al. (2002). Defining the broader phenotype of autism: Genetic, brain, and behavioural perspectives. *Development and Psychopathology, 14*(3), 581–611.

Delis, D. C., Kaplan, E., & Kramer, J. H. (2001). Delis-Kaplan Executive Function System. San Antonio, TX: The Psychological Corporation.

DeLong, G. R., & Dwyer, J. T. (1988). Correlation of family history with specific autistic subgroups: Asperger's syndrome and bipolar affective disease. *Journal of Autism and Developmental Disorders, 18*(4), 593–600.

DeLong, R. (1994). Children with autistic spectrum disorder and a family history of affective disorder. *Developmental Medicine and Child Neurology, 36*, 674–687.

Denmark, J. L. (2002). The relationship between autism and fragile X syndrome: A review of the research. *Journal on Developmental Disabilities, 9*(2), 29–43.

Department of Justice Canada (April, 1993). News release: Amendments to the criminal code respecting family violence against women. Ottawa, ON: Government of Canada.

Despert, J. L. (1951). Some considerations relating to the genesis of autistic behavior in children. *American Journal of Orthopsychiatry, 21*(2), 335–350.

Dewey, M. (1991). Living with Asperger's syndrome. In U. Frith (Ed.), Autism and Asperger syndrome (pp. 184–206). Cambridge, UK: Cambridge University Press.

DiCicco-Bloom, E., Lord, C., Zwaigenbaum, L., Courchesne, E., Dager, S. R., Schmitz, C., et al. (2006). The developmental neurobiology of autism spectrum disorder. *Journal of Neuroscience, 26*(26), 6897–6906.

Dillon, M. R. (2007). Creating supports for college students with Asperger syndrome through collaboration. *College Student Journal, 41*(2), 499–504.

Dodd, S. (2005). Understanding Autism. Marrickville, N.S.W.: Elsevier Australia.

Dominick, K. C., Davis, N. O., Lainhart, J., Tager-Flusberg, H., & Folstein, S. (2007). Atypical behaviors in children with autism and children with a history of language impairment. *Research in Developmental Disabilities, 28*(2), 145–162.

Donoghue, K., Stallard, P., & Kucia, J. (2011). The clinical practice of Cognitive Behavioural Therapy for children and young people with a diagnosis of Asperger's Syndrome. *Clinical Child Psychology and Psychiatry, 16*(1), 89–102

Dorris, L., Espie, C. A., Knott, F., & Salt, J. (2004). Mind-reading difficulties in the siblings of people with Asperger's syndrome: Evidence for a genetic influence in the abnormal development of a specific cognitive domain. *Journal of Child Psychology and Psychiatry, 45*(2), 412–418.

Dubin, N. (2007). Asperger syndrome and bullying: Strategies and solutions. London: Jessica Kingsley.

Duchaine, B., & Nakayama, K. (2005). Dissociations of face and object recognition in developmental prosopagnosia. *Journal of Cognitive Neuroscience, 17*(2), 249–261.

Dunn, W., Saiter, J., & Rinner, L. (2002). Asperger syndrome and sensory processing: A conceptual model and guidance for intervention planning. *Focus on Autism and Other Developmental Disabilities, 17*(3), 172–185.

Dykens, E., Volkmar, F., & Glick, M. (1991). Thought disorder in high-functioning autistic adults. *Journal of Autism and Developmental Disorders, 21*(3), 291–301.

Dziuk, M. A., Gidley Larson, J. C., Apostu, A., Mahone, E. M., Denckla, M. B., & Mostofsky, S. H. (2007). Dyspraxia in autism: Association with motor, social and communicative deficits. *Developmental Medicine and Child Neurology, 49*(1), 734–739.

D'Zurilla, T. J., Nezu, A. M., & Maydeu-Olivares, A. (2002). Social Problem-Solving Inventory—Revised. North Tonawanda, NY: Multi-Health Systems.

Edwards, D. R., & Bristol, M. M. (1991). Autism: Early identification and management in family practice. *American Family Physician, 44*(5), 1755–1764.

Eisenberg, L. (1957). The fathers of autistic children. *American Journal of Orthopsychiatry, 27*(4), 715–724.

Eisenberg, L., & Kanner, L. (1956). Early infantile autism 1943–1955. *American Journal of Orthopsychiatry, 26*(3), 556–566.

Egerton, R. B., Bollinger, M., & Herr, B. (1984). The Cloak of Competence: After two decades. *American Journal of Mental Deficiency, 88*(4), 345–351.

Ellis, H. D., Ellis, D. M., Fraser, W., & Deb, S. (1994). A preliminary study of right hemisphere cognitive deficits and impaired social judgments among young people with Asperger syndrome. *European Child and Adolescent Psychiatry, 3*(4), 255–266.

Engström, I., Ekström, L., & Emilsson, B. (2003). Psychosocial functioning in a group of Swedish adults with Asperger syndrome or high-functioning autism. *Autism: International Journal of Research and Practice, 7*(1), 99–110.

Epstein, T., & Salzman-Benaiah, J. (2005). Tourette syndrome and Asperger syndrome: Overlapping symptoms and treatment implications. In K. P. Stoddart (Ed.), Children, youth and adults with Asperger syndrome: Integrating multiple perspectives (pp. 72–83). London: Jessica Kingsley.

Erickson, C. A., Stigler, K. A., Corkins, M. R., Posey, D. J., Fitzgerald, J. F., & McDougle, C. J. (2005). Gastrointestinal factors in autistic disorder: A critical review. *Journal of Autism and Developmental Disorders, 35*(6), 713–727.

Eveloff, H. H. (1960). The autistic child. *Archives of General Psychiatry, 3*(1), 66-81.

Evenhuis, H., Henderson, C. M., Beange, H., Lennox, N. & Chicoine, B. (2000). *Healthy aging in adults with intellectual disabilities: Physical health issues.* Geneva, Switzerland: WHO.

Fanner, D., & Urquhart, C. (2008). Bibliotherapy for mental health service users Part 1: A systematic review. *Health Information and Libraries Journal, 25*(4), 237–252.

Farrell, E. F. (2004). Asperger's confounds colleges. *Chronicle of Higher Education, 57*(7), A35.

Fenigstein, A., & Vanable, P. A. (1992). Paranoia and self-consciousness. *Journal of Personality and Social Psychology, 62,* 129–138.

Fennell, M. (1998). Depression. In K. Hawton, P. M. Salkovskis, J. Kirk, & D. M. Clark (Eds.), Cognitive behaviour therapy for psychiatric problems: A practical guide (pp. 169–234). Oxford: Oxford Medical.

Fidell, B. (2000). Exploring the use of family therapy with adults with a learning disability. *Journal of Family Therapy, 22*(3), 308–323.

Figueira, I., & Jacques, R. (2002). Social anxiety disorder: Assessment and pharmacological management. *German Journal of Psychiatry, 5*(2) 40–48.

Fine, J., Bartolucci, G., Ginsberg, G., & Szatmari, P. (1991). The use of intonation to communicate in pervasive developmental disorders. *Journal of Child Psychology and Psychiatry, 32*(5), 771–782.

First, M. B., Spitzer, R. L., Gibbon, M., & William, J. B. W. (1996). Structured Clinical Interview for DSM-IV Axis 1 Disorders—Patient Edition (SCID-I/P, Version 2.0). New York: New York State Psychiatric Institute, Biometrics Research Department.

Fisman, S., & Steele, M. (1996). Use of risperidone in pervasive developmental disorders: A case series. *Journal of Child and Adolescent Psychopharmacology, 6*(3), 177–190.

Fitzgerald, M. (2000). Did Ludwig Wittgenstein have Asperger's syndrome? *European Child Adolescent Psychiatry, 9*(1), 61–65.

Fitzgerald, M. (2002). Did Ramanujan have Asperger's disorder or Asperger's syndrome? *Journal of Medical Biography, 10*(3), 167–169.

Fitzgerald, M. (2007). Editorial: Suicide and Asperger's syndrome. *Crisis, 28*(1), 1–3.

Fitzgerald, M., & Corvin, A. (2001). Diagnosis and differential diagnosis of Asperger syndrome. *Advances in Psychiatric Treatment, 7*(4), 310–318.

Fombonne, E. (2001). What is the prevalence of Asperger disorder? *Journal of Autism and Developmental Disorders, 31*(3), 363–364.

Fombonne, E. (2003). Epidemiological surveys of autism and other pervasive developmental disorders. *Journal of Autism and Developmental Disorders, 33*(4), 365–382.

Fombonne, E., & Cook, E. (2003). MMR and autism: Consistent epidemiological failure to support the putative association. *Molecular Psychiatry, 8*, 133–134.

Fombonne, E., Bolton, P., Prior, J., Jordan, H., & Rutter, M. (1997). A family study of autism: Cognitive patterns and levels in parents and siblings. *Journal of Child Psychology and Psychiatry, 38*(6), 667–683.

Fombonne, E., Simmons, H., Ford, T., Meltzer, H., & Goodman, R. (2001). Prevalence of pervasive developmental disorders in the British nationwide survey of child mental health. *Journal of the American Academy of Child and Adolescent Psychiatry, 40*(7), 820–827.

Fombonne, E., & Tidmarsh, L. (2003). Epidemiologic data on Asperger disorder. *Child and Adolescent Psychiatric Clinics of North America, 12*(1), 15–21.

Frankhauser, M. P., Karumanchi, V. C., German, M. L., Yates, A., & Karumanchi, S. D. (1992). A double-blind, placebo-controlled study of the efficacy of transdermal clonidine in autism. *Journal of Clinical Psychiatry, 53*(3), 77–82.

Fraser, W. I., Ruedrich, S., Kerr, M., & Levitas, A. (1998). Beta-adrenergic blockers. In S. Reiss & M. G. Aman (Eds.), Psychotropic medication and developmental disabilities: The international consensus handbook (pp. 271–289). Columbus, OH: Ohio State University, Nisonger Center.

Frazier, J. A., Doyle, R., Chiu, S., & Coyle, J. T. (2002). Treating a child with Asperger's disorder and comorbid bipolar disorder. *American Journal of Psychiatry, 159*(1), 13–21.

Freeman, R. D., Fast, D. K., Burd, L., Kerbeshian, J., Robertson, M. M., & Sandor, P. (2000). An international perspective on Tourette syndrome: Selected findings from 3500 individuals in 22 countries. *Developmental Medicine and Child Neurology, 42*(7), 436–447.

Freeman, S. K. (2007). The complete guide to autism treatments—a parent's handbook: Make sure your child gets what works! Lynden, WA: SKF Books.

Frith, U. (1989). Autism: explaining the enigma. Oxford: Blackwell.

Frith, U. (Ed.). (1991). Autism and Asperger syndrome. Cambridge: Cambridge University Press.

Frith, U. (2004). Emmanuel Miller lecture: Confusions and controversies about Asperger syndrome. *Journal of Child Psychology and Psychiatry, 45*(4), 672–686.

Furusho, J., Matsuzaki, K., Ichihashi, I., Satoh, H., Yamaguchi, E., & Kumagai, K. (2001). Alleviation of sleep disturbance and repetitive behaviour by a selective serotonin reuptake inhibitor in a boy with Asperger's syndrome. *Brain and Development, 23*(2), 135–137.

Gallagher, S. A. & Gallagher, J. J. (2002). Giftedness and Asperger's syndrome: A new agenda for education. *Understanding Our Gifted, 14*(2), 7–12.

Gallucci, G., Hackerman, F. & Schmidt, C. W. (2005). Gender Identity Disorder in an adult male with Asperger's Syndrome. *Sexuality and Disability, 23*(1), 35–40.

Garber, K.B., Visootsak, J., & Warren, S.T. (2008). Fragile X syndrome. *European Journal of Human Genetics, 16*(6) 666–672.

Garland, T. (2005). Test review: WASI. *Journal of Occupational Psychology, Employment, and Disability, 7*(2), 130–135.

Garnett, M.S., & Attwood, T. (1998). Australian Scale for Asperger's Syndrome. In T. Attwood, Asperger's syndrome: A guide for parents and professionals (pp. 17–20). London: Jessica Kingsley.

Gaus, V. L. (2007). Cognitive–behavioral therapy for adult Asperger syndrome. New York: Guilford Press.

Gaus, V. (2011). Adult Asperger syndrome and the utility of Cognitive-Behavioral Therapy. *Journal of Contemporary Psychotherapy, 41*(1), 47–56.

Ghaziuddin, M. (2005). Mental health aspects of autism and Asperger syndrome. London: Jessica Kingsley.

Ghaziuddin, M., Butler, E., Tsai, L., & Ghazuiddin, N. (1994). Is clumsiness a marker for Asperger syndrome? *Journal of Intellectual Disability Research, 38*, 519–527.

Ghaziuddin, M., & Gerstein, L. (1996). Pedantic speaking style differentiates Asperger syndrome from high-functioning autism. *Journal of Autism and Developmental Disorders, 26*(6), 585–595.

Ghaziuddin, M., Tsai, L. Y., & Ghaziuddin, N. (1991). Brief report: Violence in Asperger syndrome: A critique. *Journal of Autism and Developmental Disorders, 21*(3), 349–354.

Ghaziuddin, M., Tsai, L. Y., & Ghaziuddin, N. (1992a). A comparison of the diagnostic criteria for Asperger syndrome. *Journal of Autism and Developmental Disorders, 22*(4), 643–649.

Ghaziuddin, M., Tsai, L. Y., & Ghaziuddin, N. (1992b). A reappraisal of clumsiness as a diagnostic feature of Asperger syndrome. *Journal of Autism and Developmental Disorders, 22*(4), 651–656.

Ghaziuddin, M., Weidmer-Mikhail, E., & Ghaziuddin, N. (1998). Comorbidity of Asperger syndrome: A preliminary report. *Journal of Intellectual Disability Research, 42*(4), 279–283.

Gibbs, L. E. (2003). Evidence-based practice for the helping professions: A practical guide with integrated multimedia. Pacific Grove, CA: Thompson Brooks/Cole.

Gilbert, P. (2002). Understanding the biopsychosocial approach: Conceptualisation. *Clinical Psychology, 14*, 13–17.

Gilchrist, A., Green, J., Cox, A., Burton, D., Rutter, M., & Le Couteur, A. (2001). Development and current functioning in adolescents with Asperger syndrome: A comparative study. *Journal of Child Psychology and Psychiatry, 42*(2), 227–240.

Gillberg, C. (1983). Identical triplets with infantile autism and the fragile-X syndrome. *British Journal of Psychiatry, 143*, 256–260.

Gillberg, C. (1989). Asperger syndrome in 23 Swedish children. *Developmental Medicine and Child Neurology, 31*(4), 520–531.

Gillberg, C. (1991). Clinical and neurobiological aspects of Asperger syndrome in six family studies. In U. Frith (Ed.), Autism and Asperger syndrome. Cambridge, UK: Cambridge University Press.

Gillberg, C. (1992). Subgroups in autism: Are there behavioural phenotypes typical of underlying medical conditions? *Journal of Intellectual Disability Research, 36*(3), 201–214.

Gillberg, C. (1995). Clinical Child Neuropsychiatry. Cambridge, UK: Cambridge University Press.

Gillberg, C. (1998). Asperger syndrome and high-functioning autism. *British Journal of Psychiatry, 172*, 200–209.

Gillberg, C. (2002a). [Charles XII seems to have fulfilled all the criteria of Asperger syndrome]. *Lakartidningen, 99*(48), 4837–4838.

Gillberg, C. (2002b). A guide to Asperger Syndrome. Cambridge: Cambridge University Press.

Gillberg, C., & Billstedt, E. (2000). Autism and Asperger syndrome: Co-existence with other clinical disorders. *Acta Psychiatrica Scandanavica, 102*(5), 321–330.

Gillberg, C., & Ehlers, S. (1998). High-functioning people with autism and Asperger syndrome: A review of the literature. In E. Schopler, G. B. Mesibov, & L. J. Kunce (Eds.), Asperger syndrome or high-functioning autism? (pp. 79–106). New York: Plenum Press.

Gillberg, C., Gillberg, C., Rastam, M., & Wentz, E. (2001). The Asperger Syndrome (and high-functioning autism) Diagnostic Interview (ASDI): A preliminary study of a new structured clinical interview. *Autism: International Journal of Research and Practice, 5*(1), 57–66.

Gilliam, J. E. (2002). Gilliam Asperger's Disorder Scale: Examiner's Manual (GADS). Austin, TX: PRO-ED.

Gilliam, J. E. (2006). Gilliam Autism Rating Scale—Second Edition: Examiner's Manual (GARS-2). Austin, TX: PRO-ED.

Glessner, J. T., Wang, K., Cai, G., Korvatska, O., Kim, C. E., Wood, S., et al. (2009). Autism genome-wide copy number variation reveals ubiquitin and neuronal genes. *Nature, 459*(7246), 569–573.

Gold, N., & Whelan, M. (1992). Elderly people with autism: Defining a social work agenda for research and practice. In F. J. Turner (Ed.), Mental health and the elderly: A social work perspective. New York: Free Press.

Goldstein, G., Johnson, C., & Minshew, N. (2001). Attentional processes in autism. *Journal of Autism and Developmental Disorders, 31*(4), 433–440.

Goldstein, M. J., & Miklowitz, D. J. (1995). The effectiveness of psycho-educational family therapy in the treatment of schizophrenic disorders. *Journal of Marital and Family Therapy, 21*(4), 361–376.

Goodman, W. K., Price, L. H., Rasmussen, S. A., Mazure, C., Flieschmann, R. L., Hill, C. L., et al. (1989). The Yale–Brown Obsessive Compulsive Scale: I. Development and reliability. *Archives of General Psychiatry, 46*(1), 1006–1011.

Gordon, C. T., State, R. C., Nelson, J. E., Hamburger, S. D., & Rapoport, J. L. (1993). A double-blind comparison of clomipramine, desipramine, and placebo in the treatment of autistic disorder. *Archives of General Psychiatry, 50*(6), 441–447.

Gordon, H., & Grubin, D. (2004). Psychiatric aspects of the assessment and treatment of sex offenders. *Advances in Psychiatric Treatment, 10,* 73–80.

Gordon, S. (2011, January 17). Video game 'addiction' tied to depression, anxiety in kids. *U.S. News and World Report,* 1.

Grandin, T. (1992). An inside view of autism. In E. Schopler & G. B. Mesibov (Eds.), High-functioning individuals with autism (pp. 105–126). New York: Plenum Press.

Grandin, T. (1995). Thinking in pictures and other reports from my life with autism. New York: Vintage Books.

Grandin, T., & Barron, S. (2005). Unwritten rules of social relationships: Decoding social mysteries through the unique perspectives of autism. Arlington, TX: Future Horizons.

Grandin, T., & Duffy, K. (2008). Developing talents: Careers for individuals with Asperger syndrome and high-functioning autism (2nd ed.). Shawnee Mission, KS: Autism Asperger Publishing.

Grant, D. A., & Berg, E. A. (1948). A behavioral analysis of degree of reinforcement and ease of shifting to new responses in Weigl-type card sorting problems. *Journal of Experimental Psychology, 38*(4), 404–411.

Gray, C. A. (1998). Social stories and comic strip conversations with students with Asperger syndrome and high-functioning autism. In E. Schopler, G. B. Mesibov, & L. J. Kunce (Eds.), Asperger's syndrome or high-functioning autism? (pp. 167–198). New York: Plenum Press.

Greenberger, D., & Padesky, C. A. (1995). Mind over mood: Change the way you feel by changing the way you think. New York: Guilford Press.

Gresham, F. M., Beebe-Frankenburger, M. E., & MacMillan, D. L. (1999). A selective review of treatments for children with autism: Description and methodological considerations. *School Psychology Review, 28*(1), 559–576.

Griffiths, D. M. & Gardner, W. I. (2002). The integrated biopsychosocial approach to challenging behaviours. In T. Cheetham, J. Summers, C. Stavrakaki & D. Griffiths (Eds.), Dual Diagnosis: An introduction to the mental health needs of persons with developmental disabilities (pp. 81–114). Sudbury, ON: The Habilitative Mental Health Resource Network.

Gunter, H. L., Ghaziuddin, M. & Ellis, H. D. (2002). Asperger's syndrome: Tests of right hemisphere functioning and interhemispheric communication. *Journal of Autism and Developmental Disorders, 32*(4), 263–281

Gurney, J. G., Fritz, M. S., Ness, K. K., Sievers, P., Newschaffer, C. J., & Shapiro, E. G. (2003). Analysis of prevalence trends of autism spectrum disorder in Minnesota. *Archives of Pediatric and Adolescent Medicine, 157*(7), 622–627.

Gutkovich, Z. A., Carlson, G. A., Carlson, H. E., Coffey, B., & Wieland, N. (2007). Asperger's disorder and comorbid bipolar disorder: Diagnostic and treatment challenges. *Journal of Child and Adolescent Psychopharmacology, 17*(2), 247–255.

Hamilton, M. (1960). A rating scale for depression. *Journal of Neurology, Neurosurgery, and Psychiatry, 23*, 56–62.

Hamilton, M. (1967). Development of a rating scale for primary depressive illness. *British Journal of Social and Clinical Psychology, 6*(4), 278–296.

Hammock, R., Levine, W. R., & Schroeder, S. R. (2001). Brief report: Effects of clozapine on self-injurious behavior of two risperidone nonresponders with mental retardation. *Journal of Autism and Developmental Disorders, 31*(1), 109–113.

Hancock, L. (2008). Asperger Mentorship Program at York University. *Autism Matters: A Publication of Autism Ontario, 5*(4), 13–14.

Happé, F., Briskman, J., & Frith, U. (2001). Exploring the cognitive phenotype of autism: Weak "central coherence" in parents and siblings of children with autism: I. Experimental tests. *Journal of Child Psychology and Psychiatry, 42*(3), 299–307.

Hare, D. J. (1997). The use of cognitive–behavioural therapy with people with Asperger syndrome. *Autism: International Journal of Research and Practice, 1*(2), 215–225.

Hare, D. J., & Paine, C. (1997). Developing cognitive behavioural treatments for people with Asperger's Syndrome. *Clinical Psychology Forum, 110*, 5–8.

Harnadek, M. C. S., & Rourke, B. P. (1994). Principal identifying features of the syndrome of nonverbal learning disabilities in children. *Journal of Learning Disabilities, 27*(3), 144–154.

Harrison, P. L., & Oakland, T. (2003). Adaptive Behavior Assessment System Second Edition (ABAS–II) Manual. San Antonio, TX: Psychological Corporation.

Harrison, V. (1996). ColorCards. Bichester, UK: Speechmark Publishing.

Haskins, B. G., & Silva, J. A. (2006). Asperger's disorder and criminal behavior: Forensic–psychiatric considerations. *Journal of the American Academy of Psychiatry and the Law, 34*(3), 374–384.

Haynes, R. B., Devereaux, P. J., & Guyatt, G. H. (2002). Physicians' and patients' choices in evidence based practice. *British Medical Journal, 324*(7350), p. 1350.

Heaton, R. K., Chelune, G. J., Tally, J., Kay, G. G., & Curtiss, G. (1993). Wisconsin Card Sorting Test Manual—Revised and Expanded. Odessa, FL: Psychological Assessment Resources.

Heimberg, R. G., & Becket, R. E. (2002). Cognitive–behavioral treatment for social phobia: Basic mechanisms and clinical strategies. New York: Guilford Press.

Heinrichs, R. (2003). Perfect targets: Asperger syndrome and bullying. Shawnee Mission, KS: Autism Asperger Publishing.

Hellings, J. (1999). Psychopharmacology of mood disorders in persons with mental retardation and autism. *Mental Retardation and Developmental Disabilities Research Reviews, 5*, 270–278.

Hénault, I. (2005). Sexuality and Asperger syndrome: The need for so-cio-sexual education. In K. P. Stoddart (Ed.), Children, youth and adults with Asperger syndrome: Integrating multiple perspectives (pp. 110–122). London: Jessica Kingsley.

Hénault, I. (2006). Asperger's syndrome and sexuality: From adolescence through adulthood. London: Jessica Kingsley.

Hendrickx, S., & Newton, K. (2007). Asperger syndrome: A love story. London: Jessica Kingsley.

Hendriksen, J. G. M., & Vles, J. S. H. (2008). Neuropsychiatric disorders in males with Duchenne muscular dystrophy: Frequency rate of at-tention-deficit hyperactivity disorder (ADHD), autism spectrum dis-order, and obsessive–compulsive disorder. *Journal of Child Neurology, 23*(5), 477–481.

Heng, J., & Sullivan, W. F. (2003). Ethical issues relating to consent in providing treatment and care. In I. Brown & M. Percy (Eds.), Developmental Disabilities in Ontario (pp. 725–735). Toronto, ON: Ontario Association on Developmental Disabilities.

Hennen, B. K. E. (2007). Priorities for persons with developmental dis-abilities and their families in 2006: A three part series. *Clinical Bulletin of the Developmental Disabilities Division, 18*(1), 1–11.

Herbert, J. D., Rheingold, A. A., & Goldstein, S. G. (2002). Brief cogni-tive behavioral group therapy for social anxiety disorder. *Cognitive and Behavioral Practice, 9*, 1–8.

Herbert, J. D., Sharp, I. R., & Gaudiano, B. A. (2002). Separating fact from fiction in the etiology and treatment of autism. *Scientific Review of Mental Health Practice, 1*(1), 23–43.

Herbert, M. R. (2010). Contributions of the environment and environ-mentally vulnerable physiology to autism spectrum disorders. *Current Opinion in Neurology, 23*(2), 103–110.

Hill, E. L., & Bird, C. M. (2006). Executive processes in Asperger syn-drome: Patterns of performance in a multiple case series. *Neuro-psychologia, 44*(14), 2822–2835.

Hingsburger, D. (1995). Hand made love: A guide for teaching about male masturbation through understanding and video. Eastman, PQ: Diverse City Press.

Hingsburger, D. (1996). Under cover dick: A guide for teaching about condom use through video and understanding. Eastman, PQ: Diverse City Press.

Hingsburger, D., & Haar, S. (2000). Finger tips: Teaching women with disabilities about masturbation through understanding and video. Eastman, PQ: Diverse City Press.

Hirsch, A. (2009). Gary McKinnon should be extradited, court rules. Retrieved July 31, 2009 from www.guardian.co.uk.

Hodges, S. (2003). Borderline personality disorder and posttraumatic stress disorder: Time for integration? *Journal of Counseling and Development, 81*(4), 409–417.

Hofvander, B., Delorme, R., Chaste, P., Nyden, A., Wentz, E., Stahlberg, O., et al. (2009). Psychiatric and psychosocial problems in adults with normal-intelligence autism spectrum disorders. BMC Psychiatry, 9, 35.

Holden, J. J. A., & Liu, X. (2005). The genetics of autism spectrum disorders. In K. P. Stoddart (Ed.), Children, youth and adults with Asperger syndrome: Integrating multiple perspectives (pp. 268–281). London: Jessica Kingsley.

Hollander, E., Bartz, J., Chaplin, W., Phillips, A., Sumner, J., Soorya, L., et al. (2007). Oxytocin increases retention of social cognition in autism. *Biological Psychiatry, 61*(4), 498–503.

Hollander, E., Novotny, S., Hanratty, M., Yaffe, R., DeCaria, C. M., Aronowitz, B. R., et al. (2003). Oxytocin infusion reduces repetitive behaviors in adults with autistic and Asperger's disorders. *Neuropsychopharmacology, 28*(1), 193–198.

Hollander, E., Phillips, A., Chaplin, W., Zagursky, K., Novotny, S., Wasserman, S., et al. (2004). A placebo controlled crossover trial of liquid fluoxetine on repetitive behaviors in childhood and adolescent autism. *Neuropsychopharmacology, 30*(3), 582–589.

Honda, H., Shimizu , Y., Imai, M., & Nitto, Y. (2005). Cumulative incidence of childhood autism: A total population study of better accuracy and precision. *Developmental Medicine and Child Neurology, 47*(1), 10–18.

Honda, H., Shimizu, Y., & Rutter, M. (2005). No effect of MMR withdrawal on the incidence of autism: A total population study. *Journal of Child Psychology and Psychiatry and Allied Disciplines, 46*(6), 572–579.

Horvath, K., Papadimitriou, J. C., Rabsztyn, A., Drachenberg, C., & Tildon, J.T. (1999). Gastrointestinal abnormalities in children with autistic disorder. *Journal of Pediatrics, 135*(5), 559–563.

Howlin, P. (2000a). Assessment instruments for Asperger syndrome. *Child Psychology and Psychiatry Review, 5*(3), 120–129.

Howlin, P. (2000b). Outcome in adult life for more able individuals with autism or Asperger syndrome. *Autism: International Journal of Research and Practice, 4*(1), 63–83.

Howlin, P., Alcock, J., & Burkin, C. (2005). An 8 year follow-up of a specialist supported employment service for high-ability adults with autism or Asperger syndrome. *Autism: International Journal of Research and Practice, 9*(5), 533–549.

Howlin, P., & Yeates, P. (1999). The potential effectiveness of social skills groups for adults with autism. *Autism: International Journal of Research and Practice, 3*(3), 299–307.

Hranilovic, D., Bujas-Petkovic, Z., Vragovic, R., Vuk, T., Hock, K., & Jernej, B. (2007). Hyperserotonemia in Adults with Autistic

Disorder. *Journal of Autism and Developmental Disorders, 37*(10), 1934–1940.

Huang, A. X., & Wheeler, J. J. (2006). Effective interventions for individuals with high-functional autism. *International Journal of Special Education, 21*(3), 165–175.

Huband, N., McMurran, M., Evans, C. & Duggan, C. (2007). Social problem–solving plus psychoeducation for adults with personality disorder. *British Journal of Psychiatry, 190*(4), 307–313.

Huggins, J. (1995). Diagnostic and Treatment Model Version 16—Revised, Universal PDD/ADHD/DD Models & D & TM–IV. Toronto ON: Bitemarks.

Hughes, J. R. (2009). Update on autism: A review of 1,300 reports published in 2008. *Epilepsy and Behavior, 16*(4), 569–589.

Humphrey, N., & Lewis, S. (2008). "Make me normal": The views and experiences of pupils on the autistic spectrum in mainstream secondary schools. *Autism: International Journal of Research and Practice, 12*(1), 23–46.

Irlen, H. (1991). Reading by the colors. New York: Avery.

Isaev, D. N., & Kagan, V. E. (1974). Autistic syndromes in children and adolescents. *Acta Paedopsychiatrica, 40*(5), 182–190.

Jacobs, B. (2003). Loving Mr. Spock: Understanding an aloof lover. Arlington, TX: Future Horizons.

James, I. A., Mukaetova-Ladinska, E., Reichelt, F. K., Briel, R., & Scully, A. (2006). Diagnosing Aspergers syndrome in the elderly: A series of case presentations. *International Journal of Geriatric Psychiatry, 21*(10), 951–960.

Jansen, P. (2005) Asperger syndrome: Perceiving normality. In K. P. Stoddart (Ed.), Children, youth and adults with Asperger syndrome: Integrating multiple perspectives (pp. 313–322). London: Jessica Kingsley.

Järbrink, K., McCrone, P., Fombonne, E., Zandén, H., & Knapp, M. (2007). Cost–impact of young adults with high-functioning autistic spectrum disorder. *Research in Developmental Disabilities, 28*(1), 94–104.

Jaselskis, C. A., Cook, E. H., Jr., & Fletcher, K. E. (1992). Clonidine treatment of hyperactive and impulsive children with autistic disorder. *Journal of Clinical Psychopharmacology, 12*(5), 322–327.

Jobe, L. E., & White, S. W. (2007). Loneliness, social relationships, and a broader autism phenotype in college students. *Personality and Individual Differences, 42*(8), 1479–1489.

Johnson, C. P., & Myers, S. M. (2007). Identification and evaluation of children with autism spectrum disorders. *Pediatrics, 120*(5), 1183–1215.

Jolliffe, T., & Baron-Cohen, S. (1997). Are people with autism and Asperger syndrome faster than normal on the Embedded Figures Test? *Journal of Child Psychology and Psychiatry, 38*(5), 527–534.

Jolliffe, T., & Baron-Cohen, S. (2001). A test of central coherence theory: Can adults with high-functioning autism or Asperger syndrome integrate fragments of an object? *Cognitive Neuropsychiatry, 6*(3), 193–216.

Jones, P. B. & Kerwin, R. W. (1990). Left temporal lobe damage in Asperger's syndrome. *British Journal of Psychiatry, 156*(4), 570–572.

Kadesjö, B., Gillberg, C., & Hagberg, B. (1999). Brief Report: Autism and Asperger Syndrome in seven-year-old children: A total population study. *Journal of Autism and Developmental Disorders, 29*(4), 327–331.

Kalachnik, J. E., Leventhal, B. L., James, D. H., Sovner, R., Kastner, T. A., Walsh, K., et al. (1995). Guidelines for the use of psychotropic medication. Columbus, OH: Ohio State University Nisonger Center.

Kalyva, E. (2009). Comparison of eating attitudes between adolescent girls with and without Asperger syndrome: Daughters' and mothers' reports. *Journal of Autism and Developmental Disorders, 39*(3), 480–486.

Kanner, L. (1943). Autistic disturbances of affective contact. *Nervous Child, 2*(3), 217–250.

Kaplan, H. I., & Sadock, B. J. (1985). Comprehensive textbook of psychiatry—IV (Vol. 1). Baltimore, MD: Williams & Wilkins.

Katz, G., & Watt, J. (1992). Bibliotherapy: The use of books in psychiatric treatment. *Canadian Journal of Psychiatry, 37*(3), 173–178.

Katz, J., & Tillery, K. (2003). Central auditory processing. In L. Verhoeven & H. van Balkom (Eds.), classification of developmental language disorders: Theoretical issues and clinical implications (pp. 191–208). Mahwah, NJ: Erlbaum.

Kay, S. R., Fiszbein, A., & Opler, L. A. (1987). The Positive and Negative Syndrome Scale (PANSS) for schizophrenia. *Schizophrenia Bulletin, 13*(2), 261–276.

Kay, S. R., Opler, L. A., & Lindenmayer, J. (1988). Reliability and validity of the Positive and Negative Syndrome Scale for schizophrenia. *Psychiatry Research, 23*(1), 99–110.

Kemner, C., Willemsen-Swinkels, S. H. N., de Jonge, M., Tuynman-Qua, H., & van Engeland, H. (2002). Open-label study of olanzapine in children with pervasive developmental disorder. *Journal of Clinical Psychopharmacology, 22*(5), 455–460.

Kennerknect, I., Grueter, T., Welling, B., Wentzek, S., Horst, J., Edwards, S., et al. (2006). First report of prevalence of non-syndromic hereditary prosopagnosia (HPA). *American Journal of Medical Genetics, 140A*(15), 1617–1622.

Kerbeshian, J., Burd, L., & Fisher, W. (1987). Lithium carbonate in the treatment of two patients with infantile autism and atypical bipolar symptomatology. *Journal of Clinical Psychopharmacology, 7*(6), 401–405.

Kerbeshian, J., & Burd, L. (1996). Case study: Comorbidity among Tourette syndrome, autistic disorder, and bipolar disorder. *Journal of the American Academy of Child and Adolescent Psychiatry, 35*(5), 681–685.

Kerbeshian, J., Burd, L., Randall, T., Martsolf, J., & Jalal, S. (1990). Autism, profound mental retardation and atypical bipolar disorder in a 33-year-old female with a deletion of 15q12. *Journal of Mental Deficiency Research, 34*(2), 205–210.

King, B. H. (2000). Pharmacological treatment of mood disturbances, aggression, and self-injury in persons with pervasive developmental disorders. *Journal of Autism and Developmental Disorders, 30*(5), 439–445.

King, B. H., Wright, D. M., Handen, B. J., Sikich, L., Zimmerman, A. W., McMahon, W., et al. (2001). Double-blind, placebo-controlled study of amantadine hydrochloride in the treatment of children with autistic disorder. *Journal of the American Academy of Child and Adolescent Psychiatry, 40*(6), 658–665.

King, D., Delfabbro, P., & Griffiths, M. (2009). The psychological study of video game players: Methodological challenges and practical advice. *International Journal of Mental Health and Addiction, 7*(4), 555–562.

King, R. (2005). In support of psychotherapy for people who have mental retardation. *Mental Retardation, 43*(6), 448–450.

King, R. (2006). Charting for a purpose—Phase II: Optimal treatment of bipolar disorder in individuals with developmental disabilities. *Mental Health Aspects of Developmental Disabilities, 9*(2), 54–68.

King, R., Fay, G., & Croghan, P. (2000). Pre re nata: Optimal use of psychotropic PRN medication. *Mental Health Aspects of Developmental Disabilities, 3*(1), 1–9.

King, R., Fay, G., Prescott, H., Turcotte, P., & Preston, M. (2004). Selecting treatments for repetitive behaviors in pervasive developmental disorders. *Psychiatric Annals, 34*(3), 221–228.

King, R., Fay, G., Turcotte, P., Weildon, H., & Preston, M. (2002). Repetitive behaviors in pervasive developmental disorders: Distinguishing core features from compulsions. *Mental Health Aspects of Developmental Disabilities, 5*(4), 109–117.

King, R., Jordan, A., Mazurek, E., Earle, K., Earle, E., & Runham, A. (2009). Assertive community treatment—dually diagnosed: The hyphen was the easy part. *Mental Health Aspects of Developmental Disabilities, 12*(1), 1–7.

King, R., & McCartney, J. (1999). Charting for a purpose: Optimal treatment of bipolar disorder in individuals with developmental disabilities. *Mental Health Aspects of Developmental Disabilities, 2*(2), 50–58.

King, R., Wilson, J., & Atchison, J. A. (2008). PRN protocols: Applying pharmacokinetic principles to practice; supporting individuals with developmental disabilities and mental health concerns in community settings. *Mental Health Aspects of Developmental Disabilities, 11*(3), 79–84.

Kirby, A. (2002). What happens to children with D.C.D. when they grow up? *Dyspraxia Foundation Professional Journal, 1,* 3–9.

Klauck, S. M. (2006). Genetics of autism spectrum disorder. *European Journal of Human Genetics, 14*(6), 714–720.

Klin, A. (1994). Asperger syndrome. *Child and Adolescent Psychiatric Clinics of North America, 3,* 131–148.

Klin, A., Pauls, D., Schultz, R., & Volkmar, F.R. (2005). Three diagnostic approaches to Asperger syndrome: Implications for research. *Journal of Autism and Developmental Disorders, 35*(2), 221–234.

Klin, A., Volkmar, F. R., Sparrow, S. S., Cicchetti, D.V., & Rourke, B.P. (1995). Validity and neuropsychological characterization of Asperger syndrome: Convergence with nonverbal learning disabilities syndrome. *Journal of Child Psychology and Psychiatry and Allied Disciplines, 36*(7), 1127–1140.

Kohn, Y., Fahum, T., Ratzoni, G., & Apter, A. (1998). Aggression and sexual offense in Asperger's syndrome. *Israel Journal of Psychiatry and Related Sciences, 35*(4), 293–299.

Kolevzon, A., Mathewson, K. A., & Hollander, E. (2006). Selective serotonin reuptake inhibitors in autism: A review of efficacy and tolerability. *Journal of Clinical Psychiatry, 67*(3), 407–414.

Konstantareas, M. M. (1990). A psychoeducational model for working with families of autistic children. *Journal of Marital and Family Therapy, 16*(1), 59–70.

Konstantareas, M. M. (2005). Anxiety and depression in children and adolescents with Asperger syndrome. In K. P. Stoddart (Ed.), *Children, youth and adults with Asperger syndrome: Integrating multiple perspectives* (pp. 47–59). London: Jessica Kingsley.

Kraemer, B., Delsignore, A., Gundelfinger, R., Schnyder, U., & Hepp, U. (2005). Comorbidity of Asperger syndrome and gender identity disorder. *European Child and Adolescent Psychiatry, 14*(5), 292–296.

Krasny, L., Williams, B. J., Provencal, S., & Ozonoff, S. (2003). Social skills interventions for the autism spectrum: Essential ingredients and a model curriculum. *Child and Adolescent Psychiatric Clinics of North America, 12*(1), 107–122.

Krigsman, A., Boris, M., Goldblatt, A. & Stott, C. (2010). Clinical presentation and histologic findings at ileocolonoscopy in children with autism spectrum disorder and chronic gastrointestinal symptoms. *Autism Insights, 2,* 1–11.

Kristiansen C. M., Felton, K. A., Hovdestad, W. E. & Allard, C. B. (1996, January) The Ottawa Survivor's Study: A summary of the findings. Paper presented at the Barbara Schlifer Commemorative Clinic, Toronto, ON.

Krug, D., & Arick, J. (2003). Krug Asperger's Disorder Index. Austin, TX: PRO-ED.

Kulka, R. A., Schlenger, W. E., Fairbank, J. A., Hough, R. L., Jordan, B. K., Marmar, C. R., et al. (1990). Trauma and the Vietnam war generation: Report of findings from the national Vietnam veterans readjustment study. New York: Brunner/Mazel.

Kwok, H. (2003). Psychopharmacology in autism spectrum disorders. *Current Opinion in Psychiatry, 16*(5), 529–534.

Kwon, S., Kim, J., Choe, B., Ko, C., & Park, S. (2007). Electrophysiologic assessment of central auditory processing by auditory brainstem responses in children with autism spectrum disorders. *Journal of Korean Medical Science, 22*(4), 656–659.

Landrigan, P. J. (2008). Environmental toxicants and neurodevelopment. Workshop proceedings from "Autism and the Environment: Challenges and Opportunities for Research", Forum on Neuroscience and Nervous System Disorders Board on Health Sciences Policy. Washington, DC: Institute of Medicine of the National Academies.

Landrigan, P. J. (2010). What causes autism? Exploring the environmental contribution. *Current Opinion in Pediatrics, 22*(2), 219–225.

Lauritsen, M. B., Pedersen, C. B., & Mortensen, P. B. (2004). The incidence and prevalence of pervasive developmental disorders: A Danish population-based study. *Psychological Medicine, 34*(7), 1339–1346.

Lawton, S. C., & Reichenberg-Ullman, J. (2007). Asperger syndrome: Natural steps toward a better life. Santa Barbara, CA: Greenwood Publishing Group.

Leahy, R. L., & Holland, S. J. (2000). Treatment plans and interventions for depression and anxiety disorders. New York: Guilford Press.

Leask, S. J., Done, D. J., & Crow, T. J. (2003). Authors' reply to A. Ambelas: Children, neurological soft signs, and schizophrenia. *British Journal of Psychiatry, 182*, 362–363.

Ledgin, N. M. (2002). Asperger's and self-esteem: Insight and hope through famous role models. Arlington, TX: Future Horizons.

LeCouteur, A., Lord, C., & Rutter, M. (2003). Autism Diagnostic Interview—Revised (ADI-R). Los Angeles: Western Psychological Services.

Leighton, J., Bird, G., Charman, T., & Heyes, C. (2008). Weak imitative performance is not due to a functional "mirroring" deficit in adults with autism spectrum disorders. *Neuropsychologia, 46*(4), 1041–1049.

Lerner, M. D., Spies, J. R., Jordan, B. L., & Mikami, A. Y. (2009, May). Critical self-referent attributions potentiate social skills intervention response in adolescents with Asperger syndrome and high-functioning autism. Paper presented at the Eighth Annual International Meeting for Autism Research, Chicago, Il.

Lesch, K. P. (2004). Gene–environment interaction and the genetics of depression. *Journal of Psychiatry and Neuroscience, 29*(3), 174–184.

Levy, S., & Parkin, C. M (2003). Are we yet able to hear the signal through the noise? A comprehensive review of central auditory processing disorders—issues of research and practice. *Canadian Journal of School Psychology, 18*(1–2), 153–182.

Lewis, M., Bodfish, J. W., Powell, S. B., Parker, D. E., & Golden, R. N. (1996). Clomipramine treatment for self-injurious behavior of individuals with mental retardation: A double-blind comparison with placebo. *American Journal on Mental Retardation, 100*(6), 654–665.

Lieberman, J. A., Stroup, T. S., McEvoy, J. P., Swartz, M. S., Rosenheck, R. A. et al., (2005) Effectiveness of antipsychotic drugs in patients with chronic schizophrenia. *New England Journal of Medicine, 353*(12), 1209–122.

Limoges, E., Mottron, L., Bolduc, C., Berthiaume, C., & Godbout, R. (2005). Atypical sleep architecture and the autism phenotype. *Brain, 128*(5), 1049–1061.

Lindblad, T. (2005). Communication and Asperger syndrome: The speech–language pathologist's role. In K. P. Stoddart (Ed.), Children, youth and adults with Asperger syndrome: Integrating multiple perspectives (pp. 125–139). London: Jessica Kingsley.

Little, C. (2002). What is it? Asperger's syndrome or giftedness: Defining the differences. *Gifted Child Today, 25*(1), 58–63.

Little, L. (2002). Middle-class mothers' perceptions of peer and sibling victimization among children with Asperger's syndrome and nonverbal learning disorders. *Issues in Comprehensive Pediatric Nursing, 25*(1), 43–57.

Liu, M., & Peng, W. (2009). Cognitive and psychological predictors of the negative outcomes associated with playing MMOGs (massively multiplayer online games). *Computers in Human Behavior, 25*(6), 1306–1311.

Loeb, P. A. (1996). Independent Living Scales. San Antonio, TX: Psychological Corporation.

Lopata, C., Thomeer, M. L., Volker, M. A., & Nida, R. E. (2006). Effectiveness of a cognitive–behavioral treatment on the social behaviors of children with Asperger disorder. *Focus on Autism and Other Developmental Disabilities, 21*(4), 237–244.

Lord, C., Rutter, M., DiLavore, P., & Risi, S. (2001). Autism Diagnostic Observation Schedule (ADOS) Manual. Los Angeles, CA: Western Psychological Services.

LoVullo, S. V. & Matson, J. L. (2009). Comorbid psychopathology in adults with Autism Spectrum Disorders and intellectual disabilities. *Research in Developmental Disabilities, 30*(6), 1288–1296.

Lowry, M. A. (1997). Unmasking mood disorders: Recognizing and measuring symptomatic behaviors. *Habilitative Mental Healthcare Newsletter, 16*, 1–6.

Lowry, M. A., & Sovner, R. (1992). Severe behavior problems associated with rapid-cycling bipolar disorder in two adults with profound mental retardation. *Journal of Intellectual Disability Research, 36*(3), 269–281.

Ludlow, A. K., Wilkins, A. J., & Heaton, P. (2006). The effect of colored overlays on reading ability in children with autism. *Journal of Autism and Developmental Disorders, 36*(4), 507–516.

Ludlow, A. K., Wilkins, A. J., & Heaton, P. (2007). Colored overlays enhance visual perceptual performance in children with autism spectrum disorders. *Research in Autism Spectrum Disorders, 2*(3), 498–515.

Luiselli, J. K., Benner, S., Stoddard, T., Weiss, R., & Liscuwski, K. (2001). Evaluating the efficacy of partial hospitalization services for adults with mental retardation and psychiatric disorders: A pilot study using the Aberrant Behavior Checklist (ABC). *Mental Health Aspects of Developmental Disabilities, 4*(2), 61–67.

Lunsky, Y. J., & Puddicombe, J. (2005). Dual diagnosis on Ontario's speciality (psychiatric) hospitals: Qualitative findings and recommendations. Toronto, ON: Centre for Addiction and Mental Health.

Lynch, M. E. (2004). A report of the parent-initiated use of dietary interventions and nutritional supplements as a treatment for individuals with an autism spectrum disorder. *International Journal of Disability, Community and Rehabilitation, 3*(4), 1–17.

Lyon, G. R., Fletcher, J. M., Shaywitz, S. E., Shaywitz, B. A., Torgesen, J. K., Wood, F.B., et al. (2001). Rethinking learning disabilities. In C. E. Finn, A. J. Rotherham, & C. R. Hokanson (Eds.), Rethinking special education for a new century (pp. 259–287). Washington, DC: Thomas B. Fordham Foundation and the Progressive Policy Institute.

Mace, F. C., & Mauk, J. E. (1995). Bio-behavioral diagnosis and treatment of self-injury. *Mental Retardation and Developmental Disabilities Research Reviews, 1*(2), 104–110.

Macintosh, K. E., & Dissanayake, C. (2004). Annotation: The similarities and differences between autistic disorder and Asperger's disorder: A review of the empirical evidence. *Journal of Child Psychology and Psychiatry, 45*(3), 421–434.

Mahoney, W. (2002). Dual diagnosis in children. In D. Griffiths, C. Stavrakaki, & J. Summers (Eds.) Dual diagnosis: An introduction to the mental health needs of persons with developmental disabilities (pp. 483–507). Sudbury, ON: Habilitative Mental Health Resource Network.

Manett, J. (2007, December). Transitioning to the post-secondary environment: Factors for students with autism spectrum disorders. Paper presented at Erinoak Conference, Mississauga, ON.

Manjiviona, J., & Prior, M. (1995). Comparison of Asperger syndrome and high-functioning autistic children on a test of motor impairment. *Journal of Autism and Developmental Disorders, 25*(1), 23–39.

Mansell, S., & Sobsey, D. (2001). The Aurora project: Counseling people with developmental disabilities who have been sexually abused. Kingston, NY: NADD Press.

Marriage, K. J., Gordon, V., & Brand, L. (1995). A social skills group for boys with Asperger's syndrome. *Australian and New Zealand Journal of Psychiatry, 29*(1), 58–62.

Marriage, K. J., Miles, T., Stokes, D., & Davey, M. (1993). Clinical and research implications of the co-occurrence of Asperger's and Tourette syndromes. *Australian and New Zealand Journal of Psychiatry, 27*(4), 666–672.

Marriage, S., Wolverton, A., & Marriage, K. (2009). Autism spectrum disorder grown up: A chart review of adult functioning. *Journal of the Canadian Academy of Child and Adolescent Psychiatry, 18*(4), 322–327.

Marrs, R. W. (1995). A meta-analysis of bibliotherapy studies. *American Journal of Community Psychology, 23*(6), 843.

Matson, J. L. & Boisjoli, J. A. (2008). Autism spectrum disorders in adults with intellectual disability and comorbid psychopathology: Scale development and reliability of the ASD-CA. *Research in Autism Spectrum Disorders, 2*(2), 276–287.

Mawhood, L., & Howlin, P. (1999). The outcome of a supported employment scheme for high-functioning adults with autism or Asperger syndrome. *Autism: International Journal of Research and Practice, 3*(3), 229–254.

Mawson, D., Grounds, A., & Tantam, D. (1985). Violence and Asperger's syndrome: A case study. *British Journal of Psychiatry, 147*, 566–569.

Mayes, S. D., Calhoun, S. L., & Crites, D. L. (2001). Does DSM–IV Asperger's disorder exist? *Journal of Abnormal Child Psychology, 29*(3), 263–271.

McAlonan, G. M., Daly, E., Kumari, V., Critchley, H. D., van Amelsvoort, T., Suckling, J., et al. (2002). Brain anatomy and sensorimotor gating in Asperger's syndrome. *Brain, 125*(7), 1594–1606.

McBrides, J. A., & Panksepp, J. (1995). An examination of the phenomenology and the reliability of ratings of compulsive behavior in autism. *Journal of Autism and Developmental Disorders, 25*(4), 381–396.

McClure, I., & LeCouteur, A. (2007). Evidence-based approaches to autism spectrum disorders. *Child Care Health and Development, 33*(5), 509–512.

McDonald, S., Flanagan, S., Rollins, J., & Kinch, J. (2003). TASIT: A new clinical tool for assessing social perception after traumatic brain injury. *Journal of Head Trauma Rehabilitation, 18*(3), 219–238.

McDougle, C. J., Holmes, J. P., Carlson, D. C., Pelton, G. H., Cohen, D. J., & Price, L. H. (1998). A double-blind, placebo-controlled study of risperidone in adults with autistic disorder and other pervasive developmental disorders. *Archives of General Psychiatry, 55*(7), 633–641.

McDougle, C. J., Kem, D. L., & Posey, D. J. (2002). Case series: Use of ziprasidone for maladaptive symptoms in youths with autism. *Journal of the American Academy of Child and Adolescent Psychiatry, 41*(8), 921–927.

McDougle, C. J., Kresch, L. E., Goodman, W. K., Naylor, S. T., Volkmar, F. R., Cohen, D. J., et al. (1995). A case-controlled study of repetitive thoughts and behavior in adults with autistic disorder and obsessive–compulsive disorder. *American Journal of Psychiatry, 152*(5), 772–777.

McDougle, C. J., Naylor, S. T., Cohen, D. J., Volkmar, F. R., Heninger, G. R., & Price, L. H. (1996). A double-blind placebo–controlled study of Fluvoxamine in adults with autistic disorder. *Archives of General Psychiatry, 53*, 1001–1008.

McDougle, C. J., Scahill, L., Aman, M. G., McCracken, J. T., Tierney, E., Davies, M., et al. (2005). Risperidone for the core symptom domains of autism: Results from the study by the autism network of the research units on pediatric psychopharmacology. *American Journal of Psychiatry, 162*(6), 1142–1148.

McLaughlin-Cheng, E. (1998). Asperger syndrome and autism: A literature review and meta-analysis. *Focus on Autism and Other Developmental Disorders, 13*(4), 234–245.

Medical Research Council. (2001). MRC review of autism research: Epidemiology and causes. London: Author.

Meins, W. (1996). A new depression scale designed for use with adults with mental retardation. *Journal of Intellectual Disability Research, 40*(3), 222–226.

Mesibov, G. B. (1992). Treatment issues with high-functioning adolescents and adults with autism. In E. Schopler & G. B. Mesibov (Eds.), High-functioning individuals with autism (pp. 143–155). New York: Plenum Press.

Miles, J. H., Takahashi, T. N., Haber, A., & Hadden, L. (2003). Autism families with a high incidence of alcoholism. *Journal of Autism and Developmental Disorders, 33*(4), 403–415.

Miller, J. N., & Ozonoff, S. (2000). The external validity of Asperger disorder: Lack of evidence from the domain of neuropsychology. *Journal of Abnormal Psychology, 109*(2), 227–238.

Mishna, F., & Muskat, B. (1998). Group therapy for boys with features of Asperger syndrome and concurrent learning disabilities: Finding a peer group. *Journal of Child and Adolescent Group Therapy, 8*(3), 97–114.

Mnukhin, S. S., Isaev, D. N., & O'Tuama, L. (1975). On the organic nature of some forms of schizoid or autistic psychopathy. *Journal of Autism and Childhood Schizophrenia, 5*(2), 99–108.

Mohr, C., Curran, J., Coutts, A., & Dennis, S. (2002). Collaboration—together we can find the way in dual diagnosis. *Issues in Mental Health Nursing, 23*(2), 171–180.

Moldin, S. O., Rubenstein, J. L. R., & Hyman, S. E. (2006). Can autism speak to neuroscience? *Journal of Neuroscience, 26*(26), 6893–6896.

Moore, A. (2008, April 6). Love and Asperger's syndrome. Available at www.telegraph.co.uk.

Mortimer, A. M. (2007). Symptom rating scales and outcome in schizophrenia. *British Journal of Psychiatry, 191,* S7–S14.

Mouridsen, S. E., & Sorensen, S. A. (1995). Psychological aspects of von Recklinghausen neurofibromatosis (NF1). *Journal of Medical Genetics, 32*(12), 921–924.

Mousseau, C., Ludkin, R., Szatmari, P., & Bryson, S.E. (2006). Current issues for more able adults with autism spectrum disorder: An examination of quality of life, mental health, and physical well being. Hamilton ON: Woodview Manor.

Munro, J. D. (2010). An integrated model of psychotherapy for teens and adults with Asperger syndrome. *Journal of Systemic Therapies, 29*(3), 82–96.

Munro, J. D. & Burke, L. (2006). Clinical services for adults with Asperger syndrome. *The Autism Newslink, 3*(2), 11.

Murray, J. A. (1999). The widening spectrum of celiac disease. *American Journal of Clinical Nutrition, 69*(3), 354–365.

Murray, H. A., & Bellack, L. (1973). Thematic Apperception Test. San Antonio, TX: Psychological Corporation.

Murrie, D. C., Warren, J. I., Kristiansson, M., & Dietz, P. E. (2002). Asperger's syndrome in forensic settings. *International Journal of Forensic Mental Health, 1*(1), 59–70.

Muskat, B. (2005). Enhancing academic, social, emotional, and behavioural functioning in children with Asperger syndrome and nonverbal learning disability. In K. P. Stoddart (Ed.), Children, youth and adults with Asperger syndrome: Integrating multiple perspectives (pp. 60–71). London: Jessica Kingsley.

Myers, S. M., & Johnson, C. P. (2007). Management of children with autism spectrum disorders. *Pediatrics, 120*(5), 1162–1182.

Myhill, G., & Jekel, D. (2008). Asperger marriage: Viewing partnerships through a different lens. Focus CE Course, 1–11. Retrieved January 23, 2011 from http://www.naswma.org/

Myles, B. S., Bock, S.J., & Simpson, R. L. (2001). Asperger Syndrome Diagnostic Scale examiner's manual. Austin, TX: PRO-ED.

Nagy, J., & Szatmari, P. (1986). A chart review of schizotypal personality disorders in children. *Journal of Autism and Developmental Disorders, 16*(3), 351–367.

National Institute of Child Health and Human Development. (2003). Families and fragile X syndrome. NIH Publication. Retrieved from http://www.nichd.nih.gov/publications/

Nazeer, K. (2006). Send in the idiots: Stories from the other side of autism. New York: Bloomsburg.

Neihart, M. (2000). Gifted children with Asperger's Syndrome. *National Association for Gifted Children, 44*(4), 222–230.

Nettle, D. (2007). Empathizing and systemizing: What are they, and what do they contribute to our understanding of psychological sex differences? *British Journal of Psychology, 98*, 237–255.

Newman, S. S., & Ghaziuddin, M. (2008). Violent crime in Asperger syndrome: The role of psychiatric comorbidity. *Journal of Autism and Developmental Disorders, 38*(10), 1848–1852.

Newport, J., & Newport, M. (2002). Autism–Asperger's and sexuality: Puberty and beyond. Arlington, TX: Future Horizons.

Nicholson, R. P., & Szatmari, P. (2003). Genetic and neurodevelopmental influences in autistic disorder. *Canadian Journal of Psychiatry, 48*(8), 27–38.

Nikolov, R. N., Bearss, K. E., Lettinga, J., Erickson, C., Rodowski, M., Aman, M. G., et al. (2009). Gastrointestinal symptoms in a sample of children with pervasive developmental disorders. *Journal of Autism and Developmental Disorders, 39*(3), 405–413.

Nylander, L., & Gillberg, C. (2001). Screening for autism spectrum disorders in adult psychiatric out-patients: A preliminary report. *Acta Psychiatrica Scandinavica, 103*(6), 428–434.

Nylander, L., Lugnegard, T., & Hallerback, M. U. (2008). Autism spectrum disorders and schizophrenia spectrum disorders in adults—is there a connection? A literature review and some suggestions for future clinical research. *Clinical Neuropsychiatry, 5*(1), 43–54.

O'Neill, J. L. (1999). Through the eyes of aliens: A book about autistic people. London: Jessica Kingsley.

Ontario Partnership for Adults with Aspergers and Autism. (2008). Forgotten: Ontario adults with autism and adults with Aspergers. Toronto, ON: Autism Ontario and Ontario Partnership for Adults with Aspergers and Autism.

Ontario Partnership for Adults with Aspergers and Autism. (2009). Comments to the Minister of Municipal Affairs and Housing: Ontario's long-term affordable housing strategy. Toronto, ON: Autism Ontario and Ontario Partnership for Adults with Aspergers and Autism.

Opar, A. (2008). Search for potential autism treatments turns to 'trust hormone'. *Nature Medicine, 14*(4), 353–353.

Organization for Autism Research. (2006). Life journey through autism: A guide for transition to adulthood. Arlington, VA: Organization for Autism Research.

Organization for Autism Research. (2009a). Guidelines for college success. Retreived August 15, 2009 from http://www.researchautism.org.

Organization for Autism Research. (2009b). Understanding Asperger syndrome: A professor's guide. Retreived August 15, 2009 from http://www.researchautism.org.

Ornitz, E. M. (1985). Neurophysiology of infantile autism. *Journal of the American Academy of Child Psychiatry, 24*(3), 251–262.

Ozonoff, S. (1998). Assessment and remediation of executive dysfunction in autism and Asperger syndrome. In E. Schopler, G. B. Mesibov, & L. J. Kunce (Eds.), Asperger syndrome or high-functioning autism? (pp. 263–289). New York: Plenum Press.

Ozonoff, S., & Griffith, E. M. (2000). Neuropsychological function and the external validity of Asperger syndrome. In A. Klin, F. R. Volkmar, & S. S. Sparrow (Eds.), Asperger syndrome (pp. 72–96). New York: Guilford Press.

Ozonoff, S., Rogers, S. J. & Pennington, B. F. (1991). Asperger's syndrome: Evidence of an empirical distinction from high-functioning autism. *Journal of Child Psychology and Psychiatry, 32*(7), 1107–1122.

Ozonoff, S., South, M., & Miller, J. N. (2000). DSM-IV-defined Asperger syndrome: Cognitive, behavioural, and early history differentiation from high-functioning autism. *Autism: International Journal of Research and Practice, 4*(1) 29–46.

Panksepp, J. (2005). Melatonin–the sleep master. An emerging role for the over-the-counter supplement in the treatment of autism. Retrieved from http://legacy.autism.com/

Paradiz, V. (2002). Elijah's cup: A family's journey into the community and culture of high-functioning autism and Asperger's syndrome. New York: Free Press.

Pardhe, S., & Nandy, R. (2006). Asperger's syndrome: Management of anxiety and panic attacks. *Indian Journal of Occupational Therapy, 38*(2), 43–45.

Parloff, M. B., Kelman, H. C., & Frank, J. D. (1954). Comfort, effectiveness, and self-awareness as criteria of improvement in psychotherapy. *American Journal of Psychiatry, 111*(5), 343–352.

Pelletier, P. M., Ahmed, S. A., & Rourke, B. P. (2001). Classification rules for basic phonological processing disabilities and nonverbal learning disabilities: Formulation and external validity. *Child Neuropsychology, 7*(2), 84–98.

Percy, M., & Propst, E. (2008). Celiac disease: Its many faces and relevance to developmental disability. *Journal on Developmental Disabilities, 14*(2), 105–110.

Perlman, L. (2000). Adults with Asperger disorder misdiagnosed as schizophrenic. *Professional Psychology: Research and Practice, 31*(2), 221–225.

Perner, L. (2003). Selecting a college for a student on the autism spectrum. *Autism Asperger's Digest, November/December*(36), 28–31.

Perry, A., & Condillac, R. (2003). Evidence-based practices for children and adolescents with autism spectrum disorders: Review of the literature and practice guide. Toronto, ON: Children's Mental Health Ontario (CMHO).

Peters, E. R., Joseph, S. A., & Garetty, P. A. (1999). Measurement of delusional ideation in the normal population: Introducing the PDS (Peters et al Delusions Inventory). *Schizophrenia Bulletin, 25*(3), 553–576.

Pfadt, A., Korosh, W., & Sloane Wolfson, M. (2003). Charting bipolar disorder in people with developmental disabilities: An informant-based tracking instrument. *Mental Health Aspects of Developmental Disabilities, 6*(1), 1–10.

Phelps-Terasaki, D., & Phelps-Gunn, T. (2007). Test of Pragmatic Language—Second Edition. Austin, TX: PRO-ED.

Pierre, J. (2008). Deconstructing schizophrenia for DSM-V: Challenges for clinical and research agendas. *Clinical Schizophrenia and Related Psychoses, 2*(2), 166–174.

Pinsof, W. M., & Wynne, L. C. (1995). The efficacy of marital and family therapy: An empirical overview, conclusions, and recommendations. *Journal of Marital and Family Therapy, 21*(4), 585–613.

Pinto, D., Pagnamenta, A. T., Klei, L., Anney, R., Merico, D., Regan, R., et al. (2010). Functional impact of global rare copy number variation in autism spectrum disorders. *Nature, 466*(7304), 368–372.

Piven, J., Palmer, P., Jacobi, D., Childress, D., & Arndt, S. (1997). Broader autism phenotype: Evidence from a family history study of multiple-incidence autism families. *American Journal of Psychiatry, 154*(2), 185–190.

Plimley, L. A. (2007). A review of quality of life issues and people with autism spectrum disorders. *British Journal of Learning Disabilities, 35*(4), 205–213.

Polimeni, M. A., Richdale, A. L., & Francis, A. J. P. (2005). A survey of sleep problems in autism, Asperger's disorder, and typically developing children. *Journal of Intellectual Disability Research, 9*(4), 260–268.

Poindexter, A., Cain, N., Clarke, D. J., Cook, E. H. & Levitas, A. (1998). Mood Stabilizers. In S. Reiss & M. G. Aman (Eds.). Psychotropic Medications and Developmental Disabilities: The International Handbook. (pp. 215–246). Columbus, OH: The Ohio State University Nisonger Center.

Posey, D. J., & McDougle, C. J. (2000). The pharmacotherapy of target symptoms associated with autistic disorder and other pervasive developmental disorders. *Harvard Review of Psychiatry, 8*(2), 45–63.

Posey, D. J., Puntney, J. I., Sasher, T. M., Kem, D. L., & McDougle, C. J. (2004). Guanfacine treatment of hyperactivity and inattention in pervasive developmental disorders: A retrospective analysis of 80 cases. *Journal of Child and Adolescent Psychopharmacology, 14*(2), 233–241.

Posey, D. J., Aman, M. G., McCracken, J. T., Scahill, L., Tierney, E., Arnold, L. E., et al. (2007). Positive effects of methylphenidate on inattention and hyperactivity in Pervasive Developmental Disorders: An analysis of secondary measures. *Biological Psychiatry, 61*(4), 538–544.

Posserud, M. B., Lundervold, A. J., & Gillberg, C. (2006). Autistic features in a total population of 7–9-year-old children assessed by the ASSQ (Autism Spectrum Screening Questionnaire). *Journal of Child Psychology and Psychiatry, 47*(2), 167–175.

Potenza, M. N., Holmes, J. P., Kanes, S. J., & McDougle, C. J. (1999). Olanzapine treatment of children, adolescents, and adults with pervasive developmental disorders: An open-label pilot study. *Journal of Clinical Psychopharmacology, 19*(1), 37–44.

Powell, A. (2002). Taking responsibility: Good practice guidelines for services—adults with Asperger syndrome. London: National Autistic Society.

Powell, S. B., Bodfish, J. W., Parker, D., Crawford, T. W., & Lewis, M. H. (1996). Self-restraint and self-injury: Occurrence and motivational significance. *American Journal on Mental Retardation, 101*(1), 41–48.

Poysky, J. (2007). Behavior patterns in Duchenne muscular dystrophy: Report on the Parent Project Muscular Dystrophy behavior workshop 8–9 December 2006, Philadelphia, PA. *Neuromuscular Disorders, 17*(11–12), 986–994.

Prior, M. (2003). Is there an increase in the prevalence of autism spectrum disorders? *Journal of Paediatric Child Health, 39*(2), 81–82.

Prout, H. T., & Strohmer, D. C. (1991). Emotional Problems Scales: Professional manual for the Behavior Rating Scales and the Self-Report Inventory. Lutz, FL: Psychological Assessment Resources.

Psychological Corporation (2009). Advanced Clinical Solutions for WAIS-IV and WMS-IV Administration and Scoring Manual. San Antonio, TX: Psychological Corporation.

Quinn, C., Swaggart, B. L., & Myles, B. S. (1994). Implementing cognitive behavior management programs for persons with autism: Guidlines for practitioners. *Focus on Autism and Other Developmental Disabilities, 9*(4), 1–3.

Quinn, P. O. (1997). Attention deficit disorder: Diagnosis and treatment from infancy to adulthood. New York: Brunner/Mazel Publishers.

Quint, F. L. (2005). From despair to hope: A mother's Asperger story. In K. P. Stoddart (Ed.), Children, youth and adults with Asperger syndrome: Integrating multiple perspectives (pp. 323–333). London: Jessica Kingsley.

Raheja, S., Libretto, S. E., & Singh, I. (2002). Successful use of risperidone in an adult with the pervasive developmental disorder, Asperger's syndrome: A case report. *British Journal of Developmental Disabilities, 48*(94), 61–66.

Raja, M., & Azzoni, A. (2001). Asperger's disorder in the emergency psychiatric setting. *General Hospital Psychiatry, 23*(5), 285–293.

Raja, M., & Azzoni, A. (2008). Comorbidity of Asperger's syndrome and bipolar disorder. *Clinical Practice and Epidemiology in Mental Health, 4*(26). Retrieved from www.cpementalhealth.com/

Ramsay, J. R., Brodkin, E. S., Cohen, M. R., Listerud, J., Rostain, A. L., & Ekman, E. (2005). "Better strangers": Using the relationship in psychotherapy for adult patients with Asperger syndrome. *Psychotherapy, 42*(4), 483–493.

Rank, B. (1949). Adaptation of the psychoanalytic technique for the treatment of young children with atypical development. *American Journal of Orthopsychiatry, 19*(1), 130–139.

Reaven, J., & Hepburn, S. (2003). Cognitive–behavioral treatment of obsessive–compulsive disorder in a child with Asperger syndrome: A case report. *Autism: International Journal of Research and Practice, 7*(2), 145–164.

Regehr, C., Stern, S., & Shlonsky, A. (2007). Operationalizing evidence-based practice: The development of an institute for evidence-based social work. *Research on Social Work Practice, 17*(3), 408–416.

Reiss, R., & Aman, M. G. (Eds.). (1998). Psychotropic medication and developmental disabilities: The international consensus handbook. Columbus, OH: Ohio State University, Nisonger Center.

Reiss, S., Levitan, G., & Szyszko, J. (1982). Emotional disturbance and mental retardation: Diagnostic overshadowing. *American Journal of Mental Deficiency, 86*(6), 567–574.

Reiss, S., & Rojahn, J. (1993). Joint occurrence of depression and aggression in children and adults with mental retardation. *Journal of Intellectual Disability Research, 37*(3), 287–294.

Renty, J., & Roeyers, H. (2007). Individual and marital adaptation in men with autism spectrum disorder and their spouses: The role of social support and coping strategies. *Journal of Autism and Developmental Disorders, 37*(7), 1247–1255.

Reynold, S., & Lane, S. J. (2008). Diagnostic validity of sensory over-responsivity: A review of the literature and case reports. *Journal of Autism and Developmental Disorders, 38*(3), 516–529.

Reynolds, W. M. (1999). Multidimensional Anxiety Questionnaire (MAQ): Professional manual. Odessa, FL: Psychological Assessment Resources.

Reynolds, W. M., & Koback, K. A. (1995). Hamilton Depression Inventory (HDI): Professional Manual. Odessa, FL: Psychological Assessment Resources.

Rhoades, R. A., Scarpa, A., & Salley, B. (2007). The importance of physician knowledge of autism spectrum disorder: Results of a parent survey. *BMC Pediatrics, 7*, 37.

Rhode, M., & Klauber, T. (Eds.). (2004). The many faces of Asperger's syndrome. London: Karnac Books.

Rice, C., Nicholas, J., Baio, J., Pettygrove, S., Lee, L.-C., Van Naarden Braun, K., et al. (2010). Changes in autism spectrum disorder prevalence in 4 areas of the United States. *Disability and Health Journal, 3*(3), 186–201.

Ringman, J. M., & Jankovic, J. (2000). Occurrence of tics in Asperger's syndrome and autistic disorder. *Journal of Child Neurology, 15*(6), 394–400.

Ritvo, E. R., Freeman, B. J., Pingree, C., Mason-Brothers, A., Jorde, L., Jenson, W. R., et al. (1989). The UCLA–University of Utah epidemiologic survey of autism: Prevalence. *American Journal of Psychiatry, 146*(2), 194–199.

Ritvo, E. R., Ritvo, R., Freeman, B. J., & Mason-Brothers, A. (1994). Clinical characteristics of mild autism in adults. *Comprehensive Psychiatry, 35*(2), 149–156.

Ritvo, R. A., Ritvo, E. R., Guthrie, D., Yuwiler, A., Ritvo, M. J., & Weisbender, L. (2008). A scale to assist the diagnosis of autism and Asperger's disorder in adults (RAADS): A pilot study. *Journal of Autism and Developmental Disorders, 38*(2), 213–223.

Roberts, J. E., King-Thomas, L., & Boccia, M. L. (2007). Behavioral indices of the efficacy of sensory integration therapy. *American Journal of Occupational Therapy, 61*(1), 555–562.

Roberts, S. W., & Kagan-Kushnir, T. (2005). Integrating paediatrics and child development: Asperger syndrome and the role of the developmental paediatrician. In K. P. Stoddart (Ed.), Children, youth and adults with Asperger syndrome: Integrating multiple perspectives (pp. 140–154). London: Jessica Kingsley.

Robertson, M. A., Sigalet, D. L., Holst, J. J., Meddings, J. B., Wood, J., & Sharkey, K. A. (2008). Intestinal permeability and glucagon-like preptide-2 in children with autism: A controlled pilot study. *Journal of Autism and Developmental Disorders, 38*(6), 1066–1071.

Rodier, P. M. (2000, February). The early origins of autism. *Scientific American, 28*(2), 56–63.

Rogers, C. R. (1951). Client-centered therapy: Its current practice, implications, and theory. Oxford, UK: Houghton Mifflin.

Rosenblatt, M. (2008). I exist: A message from adults with autism in England. London: National Autistic Society.

Roth, R. M., Isquith, P.K., & Gioia, G.A. (2005). Behavior Rating Inventory of Executive Function—Adult Version: Professionals Manual. Lutz, FL: Psychological Assessment Resources.

Rourke, B. P. (Ed.). (1995). Syndrome of nonverbal learning disabilities: Neurodevelopmental manifestations. New York: Guilford Press.

Rourke, B. P., Ahmad, S. A., Collins, D. W., Hayman-Abello, B. A., Hayman-Abello, S. E., & Warriner, E. M. (2002). Child clinical/pediatric neuropsychology: Some recent advances. *Annual Review of Psychology, 53*, 309–339.

Roy, M., Dillo, W., Bessling, S., Emrich, H. M., & Ohlmeier, M. D. (2009). Effective methylphenidate treatment of an adult aspergers syndrome and a comorbid ADHD: A clinical investigation with fMRI. *Journal of Attention Disorders, 12*(4), 381–385.

Ruedrich, S. L., Grush, L., & Wilson, J. (1990). Beta adrenergic blocking medications for aggressive or self–injurious mentally retarded persons. *American Journal on Mental Retardation, 95*(1), 110–119.

RUPP Network. (2002). Risperidone in children with autism and serious behavioral problems. *New England Journal of Medicine, 347*(5), 314–321.

RUPP Network. (2005). Randomized, controlled, crossover trial of methylphenidate in pervasive developmental disorders with hyperactivity. *Archives of General Psychiatry, 62*, 1266–1274.

Rush, A. J., & Frances, A. (2000). Guideline 2: Informed consent. Expert consensus guideline series: Treatment of psychiatric and behavioral problems in mental retardation. *American Journal on Mental Retardation, 105*(3), 169.

Rush, A. J., & Frances, A. (2002). Expert consensus guidelines series: Treatment of psychiatric and behavioral problems in mental retardation. *American Journal on Mental Retardation, 105*(3), 159–228.

Russell, A. J., Mataix-Cols, D., Anson, M. A. W., & Murphy, D. G. M. (2009). Psychological treatment for obsessive–compulsive disorder in people with autism spectrum disorders: A pilot study. *Psychotherapy and Psychosomatics, 78*(1), 59–61.

Russell, E., & Sofronoff, K. (2005). Anxiety and social worries in children with Asperger syndrome. *Australian and New Zealand Journal of Psychiatry, 39*(7), 633–638.

Ryan, R. M. (1992). Treatment-resistant chronic mental illness: Is it Asperger's syndrome? *Hospital and Community Psychiatry, 43*(8), 807–811.

Ryden, E., & Bejerot, S. (2008). Autism spectrum disorders in an adult psychiatric population. A naturalistic cross-sectional controlled study. *Clinical Neuropsychiatry, 5*(1), 13–21.

Ryden, G., Ryden, E., & Hetta, J. (2008). Borderline personality disorder and autism spectrum disorder in females: A cross-sectional study. *Clinical Neuropsychiatry, 5*(1), 22–30.

Sackett, D. L., Rosenberg, W. M. C., Gray, J. A. M., Haynes, R. B., & Richardson, W. S. (1996). Evidence based medicine: What it is and what it isn't. *British Medical Journal, 312*(7023), 71–72.

Sacks, O. (2001). Henry Cavendish: An early case of Asperger's syndrome? *Neurology, 57*(7), 1347.

Sajatovic, M., Ramirez, L. F., Kenny, J. T., & Meltzer, H. Y. (1994). The use of clozapine in borderline-intellectual-functioning and mentally retarded schizophrenic patients. *Comprehensive Psychiatry, 35*(1), 29–33.

Santosh, P. J., & Mijovic, A. (2006). Does pervasive developmental disorder protect children and adolescents against drug and alcohol use? *European Child and Adolescent Psychiatry, 15*(4), 183–188.

Scahill, L. (2005). Diagnosis and evaluation of pervasive developmental disorders. *Journal of Clinical Psychiatry, 66*(10), 19–25.

Schain R. J. and Freedman D. X. (1961). Studies on 5-hydroxyindole metabolism in autistic and other mentally retarded children. *Journal of Pediatrics, 58*, 315–320.

Schneider, E. (1999). Discovering my autism: Apologia pro vita sua (with apologies to Cardinal Newman). London: Jessica Kingsley.

Schneider, K. (1923). Psychopathic personalities. Vienna: Deuticke.

Schnurr, R. G. (2005). Clinical assessment of children and adolescents with Asperger syndrome. In K. P. Stoddart (Ed.), Children, youth and adults with Asperger syndrome: Integrating multiple perspectives (pp. 33–46). London: Jessica Kingsley.

Schopler, E. (1985). Convergence of learning disability, higher level autism and Asperger's syndrome. *Journal of Autism and Developmental Disorders, 15*(4), 359–360.

Schwartz-Watts, D. M. (2005). Asperger's disorder and murder. *Journal of the American Academy of Psychiatry and the Law, 33*(3), 390–393.

Searcy, E., Burd, L., Kerbeshian, J., Stenehjem, A., & Franceschini, L. A. (2000). Asperger's syndrome, X-linked mental retardation (MRX23), and chronic vocal tic disorder. *Journal of Child Neurology, 15*(10), 699–702.

Seltzer, M. M., Shattuck, P., Abbeduto, L., & Greenberg, J. S. (2004). Trajectory of development in adolescents and adults with autism.

Mental Retardation and Developmental Disabilities Research Reviews, 10(4), 234–247.

Seltzer, M. M., & Wyngaarden Kraus, M. (n.d.). Report #7: Health-related needs for adolescents and adults with autism and their parents. Retrieved January 24, 2011 from www.waisman.wisc.edu.

Sensory Processing Disorder Resource Center. Adolescent Adult Sensory Processing Disorder Checklist. Retrieved March 21, 2009 from www.sensory-processing-disorder.com.

Shadish, W. R., Ragsdale, K., Glaser, R. R., & Montgomery, L. M. (1995). The efficacy and effectiveness of marital and family therapy: A perspective from meta-analysis. *Journal of Marital and Family Therapy, 21*(4), 345–360.

Shalock, R. L. (Ed.). (1996). Reconsidering the conceptualization and measurement of QoL. Washington, DC: American Association on Mental Retardation.

Shastri, M., Alla, L., & Sabaratnam, M. (2006). Aripiprazole use in individuals with intellectual disability and psychotic or behavioural disorders: A case series. *Journal of Psychopharmacology, 20*(6), 863–867.

Shattock, P., & Whiteley, P. (2002). Biochemical aspects in autism spectrum disorders: Updating the opioid-excess theory and presenting new opportunities for biomedical intervention. *Expert Opinion on Therapeutic Targets, 6*(2), 175–183.

Sherman, S. (2002). Epidemiology. In R. J. Hagerman & P. J. Hagerman (Eds.), Fragile X syndrome: Diagnosis, treatment and research (3rd Ed.) Baltimore, MD: Johns Hopkins University Press.

Shields, J. (1991). Semantic–pragmatic disorder: A right hemisphere syndrome? *British Journal of Disorders of Communication, 26*(3), 383–392.

Shinoda Bolen, J. (1989). Gods in everyman. New York: Harper & Row.

Shore, S. (2001). Beyond the wall: Personal experinces with autism and Asperger syndrome. Shawnee Mission, KS: Autism Asperger Publishing.

Shtayermman, O. (2007). Peer victimization in adolescents and young adults diagnosed with Asperger's syndrome: A link to depressive symptomatology, anxiety symptomatology, and suicidal ideation. *Issues in Comprehensive Pediatric Nursing, 30*(3), 87–107.

Sicile-Kira, C. (2004). Autism spectrum disorders: The complete guide to understanding autism, Asperger's syndrome, pervasive developmental disorder, and other ASDs. New York: Perigee.

Siegel, L. (2003). IQ-discrepancy definitions and the diagnosis of LD: Introduction to the special issue. *Journal of Learning Disabilities, 36*(1), 2–3.

Silva, J. A., & Haskins, B. G. (2006). Asperger's disorder and murder. *Journal of the American Academy of Psychiatry and the Law, 34*(1), 133–134.

Silva, J. A., Ferrari, M. M., & Leong, G. B. (2002). The case of Jeffrey Dahmer: Sexual serial homicide from a neuropsychiatric developmental perspective. *Journal of Forensic Science, 47*(6), 1347–1359.

Silva, J. A., Leong, G. B., & Ferrari, M. M. (2004). A neuropsychiatric developmental model of serial homicidal behavior. *Behavioral Sciences and the Law, 22*(6), 787–799.

Simblett, G. J., & Wilson, D. N. (1993). Asperger's syndrome: Three cases and a discussion. *Journal of Intellectual Disability Research, 37*(1), 85–94.

Sinclair, J. (1993). Don't Mourn for Us. Paper presented at Autism: A World of Options, Geneva Centre for Autism International Conference. Toronto, ON.

Singer, G. S., Ethridge, B. L., & Aldana, S. I. (2007). Primary and secondary effects of parenting and stress management interventions for parents of children with developmental disabilities: A meta analysis. *Mental Retardation and Developmental Disabilities Research Review, 13*(4), 357–369.

Slater-Walker, G., & Slater-Walker, C. (2002). An Asperger marriage. London: Jessica Kingsley.

Sloman, L. (2005). Medication use in children with high–functioning pervasive developmental disorder and Asperger syndrome. In K. P. Stoddart (Ed.), Children, youth and adults with asperger syndrome: Integrating multiple perspectives (pp. 168–183). London: Jessica Kingsley.

Sloman, L., Schiller, E., & Stoddart, K. P. (2008). The CAMH social interaction and education model: A manualized group intervention for children with Asperger syndrome and their parents. Unpublished manuscript, Toronto, ON.

Smalley, S. L., Asarnow, R. F., & Spence, M. A. (1988). Autism and genetics: A decade of research. *Archives of General Psychiatry, 45*(10), 953–961.

Smith, C. P. (2007). Support services for students with Asperger's syndrome in higher education. *College Student Journal, 41*(3), 515–531.

Smith, I. M. (2000). Motor functioning in Asperger syndrome. In A. Klin, F. R. Volkmar, & S. S. Sparrow (Eds.), Asperger syndrome (pp. 97–124). New York: Guilford Press.

Smith, K. A., & Gouze, K. R. (2004). The sensory-sensitive child. New York: HarperCollins.

Smith Myles, B., & Southwick, J. (1999). Asperger syndrome and difficult moments: Practical solutions for tantrums, rage, and meltdowns. Shawnee Mission, KS: Autism Asperger Publishing.

Sobsey, D., & Mansell, S. (2001). The Aurora Project. Counselling people with developmental disabilities who have been sexually abused. Kingston, NY: NADD Press.

Social Anxiety Institute. (2007). How is social anxiety different than Asperger's disorder? Retreived from www.socialanxietyinstitute.org/asperger.html.

Sofronoff, K., Attwood, T., & Hinton, S. (2005). A randomised controlled trial of a CBT intervention for anxiety in children with Asperger syndrome. *Journal of Child Psychology and Psychiatry, 46*(11), 1152–1160.

Sofronoff, K., Attwood, T., Hinton, S., & Levin, I. (2007). A randomized controlled trial of a cognitive behavioral intervention for anger management in children diagnosed with Asperger syndrome. *Journal of Autism and Developmental Disorders, 37*(7), 1203–1214.

Sofronoff, K., & Farbotko, M. (2002). The effectiveness of parent management training to increase self-efficacy in parents of children with Asperger syndrome. *Autism: International Journal of Research and Practice, 6*(3), 271–286.

Sofronoff, K., Leslie, A., & Brown, W. (2004). Parent management training and Asperger syndrome: A randomized controlled trial to evaluate a parent based intervention. *Autism: International Journal of Research and Practice, 8*(3), 301–317.

Southgate, V., & Hamilton, A. F. (2008). *Trends in Cognitive Science, 12,* 225–229.

Sovner, R., & DesNoyers Hurley, A. (1990). Assessment tools which facilitate psychiatric evaluations and treatment. *Habilitative Mental Healthcare Newsletter, 9*(11), 91–98.

Sparrow, S. S., Balla, D. A., & Cicchetti, D. V. (1984). Vineland Adaptive Behavior Scales—Survey Form Manual. Circle Pines, MN: American Guidance Service.

Sparrow, S. S., Cicchetti, D. V., & Balla, D. A. (2005). Vineland Adaptive Behavior Scales—Second Edition. Circle Pines, MN: American Guidance Services.

Speer, L. L., Cook, A. E., McMahon, W. M., & Clark, E. (2007). Face processing in children with autism. *Autism: International Journal of Research and Practice, 11*(3), 265–277.

Spicer, D. (2004). Parents on the autism spectrum. Autism–Asperger's Digest (January/February), 46–47.

Ssucherewa, G. E. (1926). Die schizoiden Psychopathien im Kindesalter [The schizoid psychopathy in childhood]. *Monatsschrift für Psychiatric und Neurologie, 60,* 235–261.

Stachnik, J. M., & Nunn-Thompson, C. (2007). Use of atypical antipsychotics in the treatment of autistic disorder. *Annals of Pharmacotherapy, 41,* 626–634.

Stahmer, A. C., & Aarons, G. A. (2009). Attitudes toward adoption of evidence-based practices: A comparison of autism early intervention providers and children's mental health providers. *Psychological Services, 6*(3), 223–234.

Stavrakaki, C., Antochi, R., & Emery, P. C. (2004). Olanzapine in the treatment of pervasive developmental disorder: A case series. *Journal of Psychiatry and Neuroscience, 29*(1), 57–60.

Steingard, R., & Biederman, J. (1987). Lithium responsive manic-like symptoms in two individuals with autism and mental retardation. *Journal of the American Academy of Child and Adolescent Psychiatry, 26*(6), 932–935.

Stewart, M. E., Barnard, L., Pearson, J., Hasan, R., & O'Brien, G. (2006). Presentation of depression in autism and Asperger syndrome: A review. *Autism: International Journal of Research and Practice, 10*(1), 103–116.

Stigler, K. A., Posey, D. J., & McDougle, C. J. (2004). Aripiprazole for maladaptive behavior in pervasive developmental disorders. *Journal of Child and Adolescent Psychopharmacology, 14*(3), 455–463.

Stigler, K. A., Desmond, L. A., Posey, D. J., Wiegand, R. E., & McDougle, C. J. (2004). A naturalistic retrospective analysis of psychostimulants in pervasive developmental disorders. *Journal of Child and Adolescent Psychopharmacology, 14*(1), 49-56.

Stoddart, K. P. (1998). The treatment of high-functioning pervasive developmental disorder and Asperger's disorder: Defining the social work role. *Focus on Autism and Other Developmental Disabilities, 13*(1), 45–52.

Stoddart, K. P. (1999). Adolescents with Asperger syndrome: Three case studies of individual and family therapy. *Autism: International Journal of Research and Practice, 3*(3), 255–271.

Stoddart, K. P. & Ratti, R. (1999) Poster Presentation: A therapeutic support group for developmentally delayed men. International Conference on Developmental Disabilities, sponsored by Reena, Toronto, ON.

Stoddart, K. P. (2003). Reported stress, personality, and mental health in parents of children with pervasive developmental disorders. Doctoral dissertation, University of Toronto.

Stoddart, K. P. (2005a). Depression and anxiety in parents of children and adolescents with Asperger syndrome. In K. P. Stoddart (Ed.), Children, youth and adults with Asperger syndrome: Integrating multiple perspectives (pp. 296–310). London: Jessica Kingsley.

Stoddart, K. P. (2005b). Introduction to Asperger syndrome: A developmental lifespan perspective. In K. P. Stoddart (Ed.), Children, youth and adults with Asperger syndrome: Integrating multiple perspectives (pp. 13–30). London: Jessica Kingsley.

Stoddart, K. P. (2005c). Young adults with Asperger syndrome: Psychosocial issues and interventions. In K. P. Stoddart (Ed.), Children, youth and adults with Asperger syndrome: Integrating multiple perspectives (pp. 84–97). London: Jessica Kingsley.

Stoddart, K. P. (2006a). Psychosocial issues in "more able" adolescents and adults with ASD. In Autism Society Ontario (Ed.), Living with ASD: Adolescence and beyond (pp. 45–59). Toronto, ON: Autism Society Ontario.

Stoddart, K. P. (2006b, April). Aging and autism spectrum disorders. The 15th roundtable on aging and intellectual disabilities, sponsored by International Association for the Scientific Study of Intellectual Disabilities, Toronto, ON.

Stoddart, K. P. (2007a, October). Asperger syndrome: Growing awareness, growing responsibility. Opening keynote presented at the Asperger Manitoba's First Annual Conference: Breaking Through, Winnepeg, MB.

Stoddart, K. P. (2007b, October). Youth and young adults with Asperger syndrome: Psychosocial issues and interventions. Paper presented at Asperger Manitoba's First Annual Conference: Breaking Through, Winnipeg, MB.

Stoddart, K. P. (2007c, November). Interventions for Asperger Syndrome: Current Research and Future Directions. National Autism Research Symposium sponsored by Canadian Institutes of Health Research, Toronto, ON.

Stoddart, K. P. (2009, February). Canadian youth and adults with autism spectrum disorders: Towards an inclusive approach to service. Opening keynote presented at the Second National Policy Forum on Autism: Autism across the Lifespan, sponsored by Centres of Excellence for Children's Well-being, Montreal, QC.

Stoddart, K. P. (2010). Redpath Social Anxiety Checklist. Unpublished.

Stoddart, K. P., & Burke, L. (2011). The Asperger Screening Questionnaire for Adults (ASQ-A): The development of a self-report screening tool for adults suspected of having Asperger syndrome. Manuscript in preparation.

Stoddart, K. P., Burke, L., & Temple, V. (2002a, April). The clinical needs and characteristics of adults with autistic spectrum disorders: A review of 100 cases. Paper presented at the State of the HART: Habilitative Achievements in Research and Treatment for Mental Health in Developmental Disabilities. University of British Columbia, Vancouver, BC.

Stoddart, K. P., Burke, L., & Temple, V. (2002b). Outcome evaluation of bereavement groups for adults with intellectual disabilities. Journal of Applied Research in Intellectual Disabilities, 15(1), 28–35.

Stoddart, K. P., & Duhaime, S. (2011). A cognitive–behaviour group for anxiety and depression in adults with Asperger syndrome. Manuscript in preparation.

Stoddart, K. P., & McDonnell, J. (1999). Addressing grief and loss in adults with developmental disabilities. *Journal on Developmental Disabilities, 6*(2), 51–56.

Stoddart, K. P., McDonnell, J., Temple, V., & Mustata, A. (2001). Is brief better? A modified brief solution-focused therapy approach for adults with developmental delays. *Journal of Systemic Therapies, 20*(2), 24–40.

Stoddart, K. P., Muskat, B., & Mishna, F. (2005). Children and adolescents with Asperger syndrome: Social work assessment and intervention. In K. P. Stoddart (Ed.), *Children, youth and adults with Asperger syndrome: Integrating multiple perspectives* (pp. 155–167). London: Jessica Kingsley.

Stokes, M., Newton, N., & Kaur, A. (2007). Stalking, and social and romantic functioning among adolescents and adults with autism spectrum disorder. *Journal of Autism and Developmental Disorders, 37*(10), 1969–1986.

Stonehouse, M. (2004). Stilted rainbow: The story of my life on the autistic spectrum and a gender identity conflict. In Autism Ontario (ed.). *In our own words: First hand accounts by adults on the autism spectrum.* (pp. 43–52) Toronto, ON: Autism Ontario.

Stores, G., & Wiggs, L. (1998). Abnormal sleep patterns associated with autism: A brief review of research findings, assessment methods, and treatment strategies. *Autism: International Journal of Research and Practice, 2*(2), 157–169.

Sturmey, P. (2005). Against psychotherapy with people who have mental retardation. *Mental Retardation, 43*(1), 55–57.

Sullivan, P., & Knutson, J. (1994). The relationship between child abuse and neglect and disabilities: Implications for research and practice. Omaha, NB: Boys Town National Research Hospital.

Sullivan, W. F., Heng, J., Cameron, D., Lunsky, Y., Cheetham, T., Hennen, B., et al. (2006). Consensus guidelines for primary health care of adults with developmental disabilities. *Canadian Family Physician, 52*(11), 1410–1418.

Suppes, T., Swann, A., Dennehy, E. B., Habermacher, E. D., Mason, M., Crismon, M. L., et al. (2001). Texas medication algorithm project: Development and feasibility testing of a treatment algorithm for patients with bipolar disorder. *Journal of Clinical Psychiatry, 62*(6), 439–447.

Sverd, J. (1991). Tourette syndrome and autistic disorder: A significant relationship. *American Journal of Medical Genetics, 39*(2), 173–179.

Sverd, J., Sheth, R., Fuss, J., & Levine, J. (1995). Prevalence of pervasive developmental disorder in a sample of psychiatrically hospitalized children and adolescents. *Child Psychiatry and Human Development, 25*(4), 221–240.

Szatmari, P. (1998). Differential diagnosis of Asperger disorder. In E. Schopler, G. B. Mesibov, & L. J. Kunce (Eds.), Asperger syndrome or high-functioning autism? (pp. 61–76). New York: Plenum Press.

Szatmari, P. (2003). The causes of autism spectrum disorders. BMJ, 326 (January 25), 173–174.

Szatmari, P. (2005). Developing a research agenda in Asperger syndrome. In K. P. Stoddart (Ed.), Children, youth and adults with Asperger syndrome: Integrating multiple perspectives (pp. 229–241). London: Jessica Kingsley.

Szatmari, P. (2007, November). What happens when he grows up, Doctor? Paper presented at the National Autism Research Symposium, Toronto, ON.

Szatmari, P., Bartolucci, G., & Bremner, R. (1989). Asperger's syndrome and autism: Comparison of early history and outcome. *Developmental Medicine and Child Neurology, 31*(6), 709–720.

Szatmari, P., Bartolucci, G., Bremner, R., Bond, S., & Rich, S. (1989). A follow-up study of high-functioning autistic children. *Journal of Autism and Developmental Disorders, 19*(2), 213–225.

Szatmari, P., Bartolucci, G., Finlayson, A., & Krames, L. (1986). A vote for Asperger's syndrome. *Journal of Autism and Developmental Disorders, 16*(4), 515–518.

Szatmari, P., Bremner, R., & Nagy, J. (1989). Asperger's syndrome: A review of clinical features. *Canadian Journal of Psychiatry, 34*(6), 554–560.

Szatmari, P., Bryson, S. E., Boyle, M. H., Streiner, D. L., & Duku, E. (2003). Predictors of outcome among high functioning children with autism and Asperger syndrome. *Journal of Child Psychology and Psychiatry, 44*(4), 520–528.

Szatmari, P., Bryson, S. E., Streiner, D. L., Wilson, F., Archer, L. & Ryerse, C. (2000). Two-year outcome of preschool children with autism or Asperger's syndrome. *American Journal of Psychiatry, 157*(12), 1980–1987.

Szatmari, P., Georgiades, S., Duku, E., Goldberg, J., & Bennett, T. (2008). Alexithymia in parents of children with autism spectrum disorder. *Journal of Autism and Developmental Disorders, 38*(10), 1859–1865.

Szatmari, P., Tuff, L., Finlayson, A., & Bartolucci, G. (1990). Asperger's syndrome and autism: Neurocognitive aspects. *Journal of the American Academy of Child and Adolescent Psychiatry, 29*(1), 130–136.

Sze, K. M., & Wood, J. J. (2008). Enhancing CBT for the treatment of autism spectrum disorders and concurrent anxiety. *Behavioural and Cognitive Psychotherapy, 36*(Special Issue 04), 403–409.

Tager-Flusberg, H., & Joseph, R. M. (2003). Identifying neurocognitive phenotypes in autism. Philosophical Transactions of the Royal Society of London Series B—*Biological Sciences, 358*(1430), 303–314.

Tammet, D. (2006). Born on a blue day: Inside the extraordinary mind of an autistic savant. New York: Free Press.

Tandon, R., Harrigan, E., & Zorn, S. H. (1997). Ziprasidone: A novel antipsychotic with unique pharmacology and therapeutic potential. *Journal of Serotonin Research, 4,* 159–177.

Tani, P., Lindberg, N., Nieminen-von Wendt, T., von Wendt, L., Alanko, L., Appelberg, B., et al. (2003). Insomnia is a frequent finding in adults with Asperger syndrome. *BMC Psychiatry, 3,* 12.

Tantum, D. (1988). Annotation Asperger syndrome. *Journal of Child Psychology and Psychiatry, 29*(3), 245–255.

Tantum, D. (2000). Psychological disorder in adolescents and adults with Asperger syndrome. *Autism: International Journal of Research and Practice, 4*(1), 47–62.

Tantum, D. (2003). The challenge of adolescents and adults with Asperger syndrome. *Child and Adolescent Psychiatric Clinics of North America, 12*(1), 143–163.

Tateno, M., Tateno, Y., & Saito, T. (2008). Letter to the editor: Comorbid childhood gender identity disorder in a boy with Asperger syndrome. *Psychiatry and Clinical Neurosciences, 62,* 238.

Taylor, B., Miller, E., Farrington, C. P., Petropoulos, M. C., Favot-Mayaud, I., Li, J., et al. (1999). Autism and measles, mumps, and rubella vaccine: No epidemiological evidence for a causal association. *Lancet, 353*(9169), 2026–2029.

Taylor, D. C., Neville, B. G. R., & Cross, J. H. (1999). Autistic spectrum disorders in childhood epilepsy surgery candidates. *European Child and Adolescent Psychiatry, 8*(3), 189–192.

Taylor, J. L. (2005). In support of psychotherapy for people who have mental retardation. *Mental Retardation, 43*(6), 450–453.

Thalayasingam, S., Alexander, R. T., & Singh, I. (2004). The use of clozapine in adults with intellectual disability. *Journal of Intellectual Disability Research, 48*(6), 572–579.

Thede, L. L., & Coolidge, F. L. (2006). Psychological and neurobehavioral comparisons of children with Asperger's disorder versus high-functioning autism. *Journal of Autism and Developmental Disorders, 37*(5), 847–854.

Thompson, B. (2008). Counselling for Asperger couples. London: Jessica Kingsley.

Tidmarsh, L., & Volkmar, F. R. (2003). Diagnosis and epidemiology of autism spectrum disorders. *Canadian Journal of Psychiatry, 48*(8), 517–525.

Tietz, J. (2002). The boy who loved transit: How the system failed an obsession. *Atlantic Monthly, 304,* 43–51.

Tinsley, M., & Hendrickx, S. (2008). Asperger syndrome and alcohol: Drinking to cope? London: Jessica Kingsley.

Tivey, B. (1989, June). AIDS education and outreach in Toronto bath houses. Paper presented at the International Conference on AIDS, Montreal, PQ.

Tonge, B. J., Brereton, A. V., Gray, K. M., & Einfeld, S. L. (1999). Behavioural and emotional disturbance in high-functioning autism and Asperger syndrome. *Autism: International Journal of Research and Practice, 3*(2), 117–130.

Towbin, K. E. (2003). Strategies for pharmacologic treatment of high functioning autism and Asperger syndrome. *Child and Adolescent Psychiatric Clinics of North America, 12*(1), 23–45.

Townsend, E. A., & Polatajko, H. J. (2007). Enabling occupation II: Advancing an occupational therapy vision for health, well-being and justice through occupation. Ottawa, ON: Canadian Association of Occupational Therapists (CAOT).

Tsai, L. (2000). Children with autism spectrum disorder: Medicine today and in the new millennium. *Focus on Autism and Other Developmental Disabilities, 15*(3), 138–145.

Tyrer, P., Nur, U., Crawford, M., Karlsen, S., MacLean, C., Rao, B., et al. (2005). The Social Functioning Questionnaire: A rapid and robust measure of perceived functioning. *International Journal of Social Psychiatry, 51*(3), 265–275.

Underwood, L., McCarthy, J. & Tsakanikos, E. (2010). Mental health of adults with autism disorders and intellectual disability: Prevalence and patterns of psychopathology. *Current Opinion in Psychiatry, 23*(5), 421–426.

van den Eijnden, R. J. J. M., Spijkerman, R., Vermulst, A. A., van Rooij, T. J., & Engels, R. C. M. E. (2010). Compulsive internet use among adolescents: Bidirectional parent-child relationships. *Journal of Abnormal Child Psychology, 38*(1), 77–89.

van Engeland, H., & Buitelaar, J. K. (2008). Autism Spectrum Disorders. In M. Rutter, D. V. M. Bishop, D. S. Pine, S. Scott, J. Stevenson, E. Taylor, et al. (Eds.), Rutter's child and adolescent psychiatry (5th ed.). Malden, MA: Blackwell.

van Krevelen, D. A. (1971). Early infantile autism and autistic psycho-pathology. *Journal of Autism and Childhood Schizophrenia, 1*(1), 82–86.

Virani, A. S., Bezchlibnyk-Butler, K. Z. & Jeffries, J. J. (Eds.) (2009). Clinical handbook of psychotropic drugs (18th revised edition). Ashland, OH: Hogrefe and Huber Publishing.

Vismara, L. A., Young, G. S., Stahmer, A. C., Griffith, E. M., & Rogers, S. J. (2009). Dissemination of evidence-based practice: Can we train therapists from a distance? *Journal of Autism and Developmental Disorders, 39*(12), 1636–1651.

Volkmar, F. R., Klin, A., Schultz, R. T., Rubin, E. & Bronen, R. (2000). Asperger's Disorder. *American Journal of Psychiatry, 157*(2), 262–267.

Wallace, G., & Hammill, D. D. (2002). Comprehensive Receptive and Expressive Vocabulary Test—Second Edition: Examiner's Manual. Austin, TX: PRO-ED.

Wan, C. Y., Demaine, K., Zipse, L., Norton, A., & Schlaug, G. (2010). From music making to speaking: Engaging the mirror neuron system in autism. *Brain Research Bulletin, 82*(3–4), 161–168.

Warwick, T.C., Griffith, J., Reyes, B., Legesse, B., & Evans, M. (2007). Effects of vagus nerve stimulation in a patient with temporal lobe epilepsy and Asperger syndrome: Case report and review of the literature. *Epilepsy and Behavior, 10*(2), 344–347.

Watzlawick, P., Beavin, J., & Jackson, D. D. (1967). Pragmatics of human communication: A study of interactional patterns, pathologies, and paradoxes. New York: Norton.

Webb, E., Morey, J., Thompsen, W., Butler, C., Barber, M., & Fraser, W. I. (2003). Prevalence of autistic spectrum disorder in children attending mainstream schools in a Welsh education authority. *Developmental Medicine and Child Neurology, 45*(6), 377–384.

Wechsler, D. (1999). Wechsler Abbreviated Scale of Intelligence Manual. San Antonio, TX: Psychological Corporation.

Wechsler, D. (2008). Wechsler Adult Intelligence Scale—Fourth Edition (WAIS–IV). San Antonio, TX: Psychological Corporation.

Weisbrot, D. M., Gadow, K. D., DeVincent, C. J., & Pomeroy, J. (2005). The presentation of anxiety in children with pervasive developmental disorders. *Journal of Child and Adolescent Psychopharmacology, 15*(3), 477–496.

Weiss, J. A., & Lunsky, Y. (2010). Group cognitive behaviour therapy for adults with Asperger syndrome and anxiety or mood disorder: A case series. *Clinical Psychology & Psychotherapy, 17*(5), 438–446.

Weiss, L. (1992). Attention deficit disorder in adults: Practical help for sufferers and their spouses. Dallas, TX: Taylor Publishing.

Weller, E. B., Rowan, A., Elia, J., & Weller, R. A. (1999). Aggressive behavior in patients with attention-deficit/hyperactivity disorder, conduct disorder and pervasive developmental disorders. *Journal of Clinical Psychiatry, 60*(Suppl. 15), 5–11.

Wentz, E., Lacey, J. H., Waller, G., Rastem, M., Turk, J., & Gillberg, C. (2005). Childhood onset neuropsychiatric disorders in adult eating disorder patients: A pilot study. *European Child and Adolescent Psychiatry, 14*(8), 431–437.

Wermter, A.-K., Kamp-Becker, I., Hesse, P., Schulte-Korne, G., Strauch, J., & Helmut Remschmidt, H. (2010). Evidence for the involvement of genetic variation in the oxytocin receptor gene (OXTR) in the etiology of autistic disorders on high-functioning level. *American Journal of Medical Genetics* (Part B), 153B, 629–639.

West, O. L., Casarino, J. P., Dibella, G. P., & Gross, R. A. (1980). Partial hospitalization: Guidelines for standards. *Psychiatric Annals, 70*(8), 43–55.

Wheeler, M., & Kalina, N. (2000). The road to post-secondary education: Questions to consider. *The Reporter, 5*(2), 3.

White, S., Oswald, D., Ollendick, T., & Scahill, L. (2009). Anxiety in children and adolescents with autism spectrum disorders. *Clinical Psychology Review, 29*(3), 216–229.

Wilkinson, L.A., (2008). The gender gap in Asperger Syndrome: Where are the girls? *Teaching Exceptional Children Plus, 4*(4), Article 3. Retrieved from: http://escholarship.bc.edu/

Willemsen-Swinkels, S. H., & Buitelaar, J. K. (2002). The autistic spectrum: Subgroups, boundaries, and treatment. *Psychiatric Clinics of North America, 25*(4), 811–836.

Willey, L. H. (1999). Pretending to be normal: Living with Asperger's syndrome. London: Jessica Kingsley.

Williams, D. (1992). Nobody nowhere. Toronto, ON: Doubleday.

Williams, D. (1994). Somebody somewhere. Toronto, ON: Doubleday.

Williams, D. (2005). The website of Donna Williams. Autism and Medications. Downloaded from http://www.donnawilliams.net.

Williams, J. H., Waiter, G. D., Gilchrist, A., Perrett, D. I., Murray, A. D., & Whiten, A. (2006). Neural mechanisms of imitation and "mirror neuron" functioning in autistic spectrum disorder. *Neuropsychologia, 44*(4), 610–621.

Wilson, B. A., Alderman, N., Burgess, P. W., Emslie, H., & Evans, J. J. (1996). *Behavioural Assessment of the Dysexecutive Syndrome*. Bury St. Edmunds, UK: Thames Valley Test Company.

Wilson, W.J., Heine, C., & Harvey, L.A. (2004). Central auditory processing and central auditory processing disorder: Fundamental questions and considerations. *Australian and New Zealand Journal of Audiology, 26*(2), 80–93.

Wing, L. (1981). Asperger's syndrome: A clinical account. *Psychological Medicine, 11*(1), 115–129.

Wing, L. (1991). The relationship between Asperger's syndrome and Kanner's autism. In U. Frith (Ed.), Autism and Asperger syndrome (pp. 93–121): Cambridge, UK: Cambridge University Press.

Wing, L., & Potter, D. (2002). The epidemiology of autistic spectrum disorders: Is the prevalence rising? *Mental Retardation and Developmental Disability Research Reviews, 8*(3), 151–161.

Wing, L., & Shah, A. (2000). Catatonia in autistic spectrum disorders. *British Journal of Psychiatry, 176*, 357–362.

Wiznitzer, M. (2004). Autism and tuberous sclerosis. *Journal of Child Neurology, 29*(9), 675–679.

Wolff, S. (1996). The first account of the syndrome Asperger described?: Translation of a paper entitled "Die schizoiden Psychopathien im Kindesalter." *European Child and Adolescent Psychiatry, 5*(3), 119–132.

Wolff, S. (2000). Schizoid personality in childhood and Asperger syndrome. In A. Klin, F. R. Volkmar, & S. S. Sparrow (Eds.), Asperger syndrome (pp. 278–305). New York: Guilford Press.

Wolff, S., & Barlow, A. (1979). Schizoid personality in childhood: A comparitave study of schizoid, autistic, and normal children. *Journal of Child Psychology and Psychiatry, 20*(1), 29–46.

Wolff, S., & Chick, J. (1980). Schizoid personality in childhood: A controlled follow-up study. *Psychological Medicine, 10*(1), 85–100.

Wood, J. J., Drahota, A., Sze, K., Har, K., Chiu, A., & Langer, D. A. (2009). Cognitive behavioral therapy for anxiety in children with autism spectrum disorders: A randomized, controlled trial. *Journal of Child Psychology and Psychiatry, 50*(3), 224–234.

Woodbury-Smith, M. R., Robinson, J., Wheelwright, S., & Baron-Cohen, S. (2005). Screening adults for Asperger syndrome using the AQ: A preliminary study of its diagnostic validity in clinical practice. *Journal of Autism and Developmental Disorders, 35*(3), 331–335.

World Health Organization (2007). International Statistical Classification of Diseases and Related Health Problems 10th Revision. Retrieved from: http://apps.who.int.

Yardley, L., McDermott, L., Pisarski, S., Duchaine, B., & Nakayama, K. (2008). Psychosocial consequences of developmental prosopagnosia: A problem of recognition. *Journal of Psychosomatic Research, 65*(5), 445–451.

Yates, J. R. W. (2006). Tuberous sclerosis. *European Journal of Human Genetics, 14*, 1065–1073.

Yatham, L. N., Kennedy, S. H., O'Donovan, C., Parikh, S., & MacQueen, G. (2005). Canadian Network For Mood And Anxiety Treatments (CANMAT) guidelines for the management of patients with bipolar disorder: Consensus and controversies. *Bipolar Disorders, 7*, 5–69.

Yeargin-Allsopp, M., Rice, C., Karapurkar, T., Doernberg, N., Boyle, C., & Murphy, C. (2003). Prevalence of autism in a U.S. metropolitan area. *Journal of the American Medical Association, 289*(1), 49–55.

Yirmiya, N., & Shaked, M. (2005). Psychiatric disorders in parents of children with autism: A meta-analysis. *Journal of Child Psychology and Psychiatry, 46*(1), 69–83.

Youth in Transition Project. (2010). Adolescent Autonomy Checklists. Adolescent Health Transition Project: University of Washington Division of Adolescent Medicine. Retrieved September 4, 2010 from: http://depts.washington.edu/healthtr.

Yrigollen, C. M., Han, S. S., Kochetkova, A., Babitz, T., Chang, J. T., Volkmar, F. R., et al. (2008). Genes controlling affiliative behavior as candidate genes for autism. *Biological Psychiatry, 63*(10), 911–916.

Zelenski, S. (2002). Evaluation for and use of psychopharmacologic treatment in crisis intervention for persons with mental retardation and mental illness. In R. H. Hanson, N. A. Wieseler, & K. C. Lakin (Eds.), Crisis: Prevention and response in the community (pp. 245–256). Washington, DC: American Association on Mental Retardation.

INDEX

In this index, *b* denotes box, *f* denotes figure, and *t* denotes table.

AA. *see* Alcoholics Anonymous (AA)
AAMFT. *see* American Association of Marriage and Family Therapy (AAMFT)
ABA. *see* applied behavior analysis (ABA)
ABAS-II. *see* Adaptive Behavior Assessment System-2nd edition (ABAS-II)
ABC. *see* Aberrant Behavior Checklist (ABC)
Abell, F., 113
Aberrant Behavior Checklist (ABC), 230, 270
abstract thinking, in gifted students, 131
abuse. *see* anger and anger management; posttraumatic stress disorder (PTSD); sexual abuse, vulnerability to
Abuse and Disability Project, 96, 100
academic advising, 258, 263–64, 265*f*–66*f*
accommodations
  for employment, 183, 197
  for environments, 255
  for eye contact, 44
  for post-secondary education, 185–86, 197, 263–64, 265*f*–66*f*
  for sensory functioning, 255
  for special interests, 210
  see also disclosure, of diagnosis

ACS. *see* Advanced Clinical Solutions (ACS)
ACT. *see* assertive community treatment (ACT)
activities of daily living. *see* adaptive behavior; housing and life skills
activity-based groups, 261–62
adaptive behavior
  in adults with ASDs, 28–29
  anger management, 168–69
  as an assessment theme, 55, 64–65
  catatonia and, 112
  cognitive-behavior modification to improve, 256–57
  as diagnostic criteria, 13
  interests and repetitive behaviors as, 89
  life skills coaching to improve, 256
  self-medication in lieu of, 167
  serial murders and, 167, 168
  see also housing and life skills
Adaptive Behavior Assessment System-2nd edition (ABAS-II), 65, 161
adaptive behavior scales, 64–65
addictions
  ADHD and, 134
  families as enablers in, 217, 249
  Internet and video games as, 211
  as an issue in intimate relationships, 175
  lack of support systems and, 161

ASD-CA. *see* Autism Spectrum
Disorder-Comorbidity for
Adults (ASD-CA)
ASDI. *see* Asperger Syndrome
Diagnostic Interview (ASDI)
ASDs. *see* autism spectrum disorders
(ASDs)
asexuality, 178
ASHA. *see* American Speech-
Language-Hearing Association
(ASHA)
ASO. *see* Asperger Society of Ontario
(ASO)
Asperger, H.
on attention difficulties, 134
on depression, 103
gender differences, 19
observations of, 1, 8, 9–10
prognosis in adults, 26, 33
on sensory difficulties, 135
Asperger Integrated Psychotherapy
(AIP), 200
Asperger Society of Ontario (ASO),
160, 163, 262
Asperger Syndrome (AS)
ASDs and, 1–2, 7–8, 22–23, 44, 56,
137
cross-generational effects in, 15, 17
developmental lifespan perspective
and, 1
diagnosis confusion and controversy
about, 21–23, 111–12
diagnostic criteria, 3*f*–4*f*, 22, 23, 60,
63, 64, 130
discovery of, 8–13
HFA versus, 22–23
historical figures with, 32
NLDs and, 129–30
spectrum within a spectrum, 30–33
variability of adult presentation of,
25–29
Asperger Syndrome Diagnostic
Interview (ASDI), 52
ASRS-v1.1. *see* Adult ADHD Self-
Report Scale (ASRS-v1.1)
assaults, 164, 169
see also sexual abuse, vulnerability
to; victimization, sexual
assertive community treatment (ACT),
270
assessment process
for challenging behaviors and mental
health, 117–23, 169
comorbidity issues in, 194–95
environments and, 197
informants in the interview, 45–47

multidisciplinary input in, 41–42
outcome of, 75–77
reevaluations in, 245
refusal of, 249
sample protocol for, 73*b*
themes within, 55–56, 57–72, 57*b*
see also clinical observations;
measurement tools
Aston, M., 172, 174, 181, 250
attachment, oxytocin and, 17
attention-deficit/hyperactivity
disorder (ADHD)
bipolar disorder versus, 105
CAPD and, 136
differential diagnosis and, 74
dual diagnosis and, 83, 84
Duchene's muscular dystrophy
(DMD) and, 146
eating disorders and, 153
executive functions (EFs)
and, 67
FraX disorder and, 145
measurement tools for, 67
as misdiagnosis, 194
overview of, 134
see also stimulants and other
options
attention to detail. *see* central
coherence
Attwood, T.
on ADHD, 134
on ASD characteristics in women,
115
Australian Scale for on Asperger's
Syndrome (ASAS), 54
on delusions versus superhero
identity, 63
on intimate relationships, 174
on introduction to AS, 245
on paranoia, 113
on stalking behavior, 165
atypical antipsychotics. *see*
antipsychotics
audiologists, 41, 137
auditory hallucinations, 110
auditory sensitivities, 136
Australian Scale for Asperger's
Syndrome (ASAS), 53–54
Autism Clinical Trials Network
(ACTN), 225
Autism Diagnostic Interview-Revised
(ADI-R), 51, 52
Autism Diagnostic Observation
Schedule-Generic (ADOS-G),
51, 52–53
autism quotient (AQ), 219